THE HIPPOCRATIC PREDICAMENT

THE
HIPPOCRATIC
PREDICAMENT

Affordability, Access, and Accountability in American Medicine

ROBERT M. KAPLAN

Division of Health Care Sciences
Department of Family and Preventive Medicine
University of California, San Diego
La Jolla, California

ACADEMIC PRESS, INC.

Harcourt Brace Jovanovich, Publishers

San Diego   New York   Boston
London   Sydney   Tokyo   Toronto

This book is printed on acid-free paper.

Academic Press, Inc.
1250 Sixth Avenue, San Diego, California 92101-4311

United Kingdom Edition published by
Academic Press Limited
24–28 Oval Road, London NW1 7DX

Library of Congress Cataloging-in-Publication Data

Kaplan, Robert M.
    The Hippocratic predicament : affordability, access, and
accountability in American medicine / Robert M. Kaplan.
        p.   cm.
    Includes bibliographical references and index.
    ISBN 0-12-397370-8
    1. Medical care–United States.   2. Medical care, Cost of–United
States.   3. Medical policy–United States.   I. Title.
    [DNLM: 1. Cost Control.   2. Health Policy–United States.
3. Health Priorities–economics–United States.   4. Health Services
Accessibility–economics–United States.   W 84 AA1 K17]
RA395.S3K35   1992
362.1'0973–dc20
DNLM/DLC
for Library of Congress   92-11085
                                                                    CIP

PRINTED IN THE UNITED STATES OF AMERICA
92 93 94 95 96 97   BC   9 8 7 6 5 4 3 2 1

Contents

CHAPTER SIX

The Oregon Experiment / 129

CHAPTER SEVEN

Problems and Concerns / 157

CHAPTER EIGHT

Summary and Conclusions / 181

APPENDIX

Preface

Two trends are apparent in contemporary health services research. The first trend is the growing recognition that the American health care system is in serious financial trouble. Scores of analysts, politicians, and citizens are calling for reform in the financing and delivering of health services. The second trend is the emergence of outcomes research and a series of new methodologies for evaluating the effectiveness of medical care. These methods involve assessment of the costs, risks, and benefits of various treatments and interventions. This book summarizes progress resulting from the interface between these two trends. Specifically, we recommend that information on health outcomes be used to direct health care resource allocations. The purpose of this exercise is to suggest health policies that control cost, improve access, and maximize health benefits for the population.

In theory, application of outcomes research for policy analysis seems relatively simple. In practice, however, important methodological, practical, and ethical concerns become apparent. Oregon was the first American state to enact legislation that considered these ideas. The bold move by the Oregon State Legislature stimulated discussion and provoked heated debate about the feasibility of formal resource allocation. Because of the importance of the Oregon exercise, several chapters are devoted to a review of these policies and responses to them.

This book deals with controversial issues and it is certain that the message will not be well received by all readers. As author, I must bear responsibility for the text. Yet I gratefully acknowledge the many individuals who contributed to the development of the theory that underlies the presentation. Many of the ideas reflected in this manuscript result from collaborative work with colleagues at the University of California, San Diego. My interest in this topic was originally stimulated by the late J. W. Bush and has been developed through ongoing collaborations with close colleagues John Anderson, Charles Berry, Larry Schneiderman, and Richard Kronick. Important colleagues at other institutions who have contributed to these ideas include Pennifer Erickson from the National Center for Health Statistics and Donald Patrick from the University of Washington.

The manuscript also benefited from critical review. Graduate students Elizabeth Eakin, Matthew Mintz, and Maria de Nuncio Zuniga read the entire manuscript as did medical students Ram Duriseti and Nelson Soohoo. In addition, Dr. Oscar Kaplan reviewed the entire manuscript and gave critical feedback with tact only a father can provide. Critical review and technical support for putting the manuscript together were provided by Robin Nordmeyer, Rachel Ingrahm, and Beverly Jones.

Finally, I would like to express my sincere appreciation to the sponsors for this project. The bulk of the work was completed under a grant from the California Policy Seminar. In addition, some subsections of the manuscripts were developed as part of the University of California Health Net Award lecture and as a special lecture to the Royal Society of Medicine in London. My participation in several activities provided special access to much of the material used for this manuscript. I am indebted to the Oregon Health Services Commission for providing regular and detailed information about its work. Further, participation in the advisory panel for the U.S. Congress Office of Technology Assessment Panel reviewing the Oregon Medicaid waiver provided access to material and discussions that helped shape the content of the manuscript.

Overview and
Executive Summary

In 1987 a young boy in Oregon developed acute leukemia and his physicians decided that he needed a bone marrow transplant. In addition to his serious illness, the boy became the victim of a new change in the Oregon Medicaid program. With the state unable to afford many basic health services, there was some concern about whether the underfunded public program should be paying for very expensive organ transplantation procedures. The state legislature recognized that 34 transplants to Medicaid patients during the period 1987 to 1989 used the same financial resources as prenatal care and delivery for 1500 pregnant women. The legislature decided that it should use its limited resources to provide a small benefit to a large number of pregnant women instead of providing a larger benefit to a small number of people needing organ transplantation. The family of the young leukemia sufferer protested this policy, but the boy died while the case was under appeal. After the case attracted substantial media attention, the Oregon legislature began to grapple with some very serious questions.

The ethical issue in Oregon is essentially similar to those in all other states. The costs of health care are expanding much more rapidly than are the budgets for Medicaid. The state could not afford all the services it wanted to provide. There was not enough money for both organ transplantation and prenatal care and there was a need to either choose between them or find some other place to cut the budget. If the state was unwilling to drop some services, the only other alternative was to strip some individuals from the Medicaid rolls. Indeed, most states took the easy way out and revised the Medicaid eligibility criteria to exclude people. Oregon also recognized that health care was not a two-tiered system, but rather a three-tiered system. The three-tiered system included people who had regular insurance and could pay for their care; people enrolled in Medicaid; and a growing third tier of people who had no health insurance at all. In 1991, this third tier

1

represented about one-fifth the population of the state, or about 450,000 Oregon citizens. In addition, another 230,000 were underinsured. The trend indicated the number of uninsured and underinsured was steadily increasing. Collectively, Oregon citizens spent approximately $6 billion on health care in 1989, which is about three times what they spend in state income taxes.

Rarely is there consensus that social reform is necessary. However, there is near consensus that the American health care system needs reconstruction. Only one quarter of the American public believes that the current system is working (Jajich-Toth & Roper, 1990), and this dissatisfaction has stimulated calls for reform from Republicans and Democrats, conservatives and liberals, management and labor. Health care was placed under the spotlight by the 1990 Conference of Governors, and legislatures throughout the United States are searching for innovative solutions to the problem. Suddenly, and unexpectedly, health care reform became a major issue in the 1992 presidential election. In November of 1991, congressional Democrats toured the county collecting horror stories about average citizens who had been ruined by lack of health insurance or poor access to health care. This book examines the problems and offers a new method to guide long-range thinking about the problems. A preliminary tryout of the model in the state of Oregon is described and evaluated.

PROPOSED SOLUTIONS

There are plenty of proposed solutions to the troubling problems of American health care. However, the proposals are often overly simplistic. The problem cannot be resolved by limiting lawsuits, controlling physician groups, or doing away with health care administrators. When analyzed, each of these solutions is unlikely to produce lasting benefits because none addresses all three problems (the three A's). Policy changes such as prospective payment or reimbursing physicians based on the resources required to produce a service may have an impact upon health care costs. However, they do not necessarily resolve the access problem and may do very little to improve health outcome. The last two sessions of Congress saw at least a dozen proposals on health care reform. The proposals came from all aspects of the political spectrum. They included those from the far left and those from the far right, as well as a substantial number of proposals from the middle. The backing for these bills ranged from groups such as the American Medical Association and the American Hospital Association, to specific politicians, to political advocate groups such as the American Heritage Foundation. Several of the proposals enhance access. However, only a few of the proposals take on the issue of affordability and none of the proposals specifically attempts to produce more health care for the invested dollar. We believe that a successful proposal must attack all three problems. In order to accomplish this, we have proposed a General Health Policy Model.

A GENERAL HEALTH POLICY MODEL

Mathematical models of decision making can be useful aids for making resource allocation decisions. These models have been suggested for use in European, Australian, and American health care systems. Despite variability in the approaches taken by different countries, virtually all western countries have come to recognize that health care resources are very limited. The United Kingdom National Health Service, for example, has recognized the need to prioritize because there are many more demands for service than there are resources to provide them (Williams, 1988). As a result of these discussions, health care has become one of the most important political issues in Great Britain.

Prioritization schemes make little sense without some consideration of outcome. The most important challenge in developing a formal model for resource allocation is in defining a common unit of health benefit. Typically, the value of each specific intervention in health care is determined by considering a measure specific to the intervention or the disease process. Treatments for hypertension, for example, are evaluated in terms of blood pressure while those for diabetes are evaluated by blood glucose. Yet it is difficult to compare the relative value of investing in blood glucose versus blood pressure reduction. Traditional public health measures, such as life expectancy, are usually too crude to allow appropriate prioritization.

In order to understand health outcomes, it is necessary to build a comprehensive theoretical model of health status. This model includes several components. The major aspects of the model include mortality (death) and morbidity (health-related quality of life). Diseases and disabilities are important for two reasons. First, illness may cause the life expectancy to be shortened. Second, illness may make life less desirable at times prior to death (health-related quality of life) (Kaplan & Anderson, 1988a, 1990).

Our approach to these problems is reflected in a General Health Policy Model (Kaplan & Anderson, 1988a). The purpose of the system is to express benefits and side-effects of any health care program in terms of equivalents of completely well years of life. The years-of-life figure is adjusted for diminished quality of life produced by disease or disability. The health outcomes are measured using a method known as the Quality of Well-Being Scale Scores. This measure classifies people according to their observed levels of mobility, physical activity, and social activity. Scales to assess these attributes are derived from common national health surveys, such as the National Health Interview Survey. In addition, symptoms and other self-reported health problems are taken into consideration.

Many approaches to measuring health outcomes consider only whether a person is dead or alive. The General Health Policy Model attempts to use the information about functioning and symptoms to evaluate quantitatively all of the levels of health between death and wellness. In order to accomplish this, each of the observable levels of functioning and symptoms is given a weight derived from community surveys to reflect social preference or utility for the state on a scale ranging from 0 (dead) to 1.0 (for optimum functioning). A score of .64, for example, suggests that an individual was in an observable state for which the societal preference was 64% of the distance between optimum functioning and death. The person remaining in this state for 1 year would have lost .36 (or 1.0 – .64) well-years. Prognoses in the model are defined by transitions among observable states over time. These are represented in all calculations of well-years. Using this system, it is possible to estimate the number of well-year equivalents a program produces. Dividing the cost of the program by the well-year production results in an estimate of the cost/utility of the program. The cost/utility ratio can be used to compare the relative value of different programs, thereby providing a common metric for comparison of programs with different specific objectives.

The general nature of the Health Policy Model leads to some different conclusions than more traditional medical approaches. For example, the traditional medical model focuses on specific diseases and on pathophysiology. Characteristics of illness are quantified according to blood chemistry or in relation to problems in a specific organ system. Often, focusing on disease-specific outcome measures leads to different conclusions than those evaluated using a more general outcome measure. Many treatments produce benefits for a specific outcome but induce side effects that are often neglected in the analysis. Estimates of the benefits of surgery must take into consideration the fact that surgery causes dysfunction through wounds that must heal prior to any realization of the treatment benefits. Further, surgeries often create complications. The general approach to health status assessment attempts to gain a global picture of the net treatment benefits, taking into consideration treatment benefits, side effects, and estimates of their relative importance.

THE OREGON EXPERIMENT

Led by John Kitzhaber, the Physician President of the state Senate, the Oregon legislature recognized that the state was rationing health care. The problem was that rationing was implicit and not open to public scrutiny. Medicaid has a finite budget and the costs of the program have grown much faster than have available resources. Over the past few years, the costs of the Oregon Medicaid program have been growing at a rate of 25% per year. In response to financial pressures, the eligibility criteria have needed to be revised. In other words, people were being rationed rather than services. Many individuals in need of care received none because they were in the wrong category. A young woman employed as an hourly worker, for example, may be ineligible for health care while an unemployed twin sister would become eligible for Medicaid if she became pregnant. Thus, the system creates incentives to become pregnant in order to have a regular source of health care. The system allowed health care under Medicaid for poor families with young children but disallowed coverage for poor families with older children. Oregon, like many other states, defined Medicaid eligibility for the Aid to Families with Dependent Children (AFDC) as 50% of the poverty line. That policy set the criterion income at about $5700 per year for a family of three. A hard-working independent carpenter earning $11,000 a year might be completely excluded by the system even though he was at high risk for injury.

In response to this problem, Oregon passed three pieces of legislation, including the controversial Senate Bill 27, which mandated that health services be prioritized using a process similar to the General Health Policy Model. The justification for the prioritization was to eliminate services that did not provide benefit. The process of creating the prioritized list was an extremely difficult one. The Commission began by creating a prioritized list of all health services. However, it soon became apparent that this was a nearly impossible task. Thus, the Commissioners began searching for combinations of conditions and treatments that could be lumped together. For example, the problem of rectal prolapse was paired with the treatment partial colectomy, while osteoporosis was paired with medical treatment. A Health Services Commission was created in order to create the prioritized list.

The Health Services Commission obtained several sources of information. First, they held public hearings to learn about preferences for medical care in the Oregon communities. These meetings helped clarify how citizens viewed medical services. Various approaches to care were rated and discussed. On the basis of 48 town meetings attended by more than 1000 people, thirteen community values emerged. These values included prevention, cost/effectiveness, quality of life, ability to function, length of life, and so on. The major lesson from the community meetings was that citizens wanted preventive services. Further, the people consistently stated that the state should forego expensive heroic treatments for individuals or small groups in order to offer preventive services for everyone. On the basis of this information, the commission decided to make prevention a high priority. The U.S. Preventive Services Task Force had carefully reviewed over 100 interventions for 60 different illnesses and conditions. In each case, data on clinical outcomes were carefully considered. The Commission agreed to follow the recommendations in the published "Guide to Clinical Preventive Services" (See U.S. Preventive Services Task Force, 1989).

In order to pay for preventive services, it was necessary to reduce spending elsewhere. A major portion of the Commissioners' activity was to evaluate services using the Quality of Well-Being (QWB) Scale from the General Health Policy Model. The Commissioners could not have possibly conducted clinical trials for each of the many condition–treatment pairs. Further, estimation of treatment benefit using the QWB cannot be left to laymen. So, the Commission formed a medical committee which had expertise in essentially all specialty areas and had the participation of nearly all of the major provider groups in the state.

Working together, the Committee estimated the expected benefit from 709 condition–treatment pairs.

The QWB which was used to estimate the effect of services requires weights. These weights are not medical expert judgments, but should be obtained from community peers. The Oregon citizens were particularly concerned about using weights from California in order to assign priorities in their state. Thus, 1001 Oregon citizens participated in a separate weighting experiment. The weights were obtained in a telephone survey that was conducted by Oregon State University. In 1990, the Commission published its first prioritized list. Unfortunately, many of the rankings seemed counterintuitive and the approach drew serious criticism in the popular press. As a result, the system was reorganized according to three basic categories of care: essential, very important, and valuable to certain individuals. Within these major groupings there were 17 subcategories. The Commissioner decided to place greatest emphasis on problems that were acute and fatal. In these cases treatment prevents death and there is full recovery. Examples include appendectomy for appendicitis, nonsurgical treatment for whooping cough, and so on. Other categories classified as essential included maternity care, treatment for conditions that prevent death but do not allow full recovery, preventive care for children, and so on. There were nine categories classified as essential. Listed as very important were treatments for nonfatal conditions that would return the individual to a previous state of health. Also included in this category were acute nonfatal one-time treatments that might improve quality of life. These might be hip replacements, cornea transplants, and so on. At the bottom of the list were treatments for fatal or nonfatal conditions that did not improve quality of life or extend life. These might be progressive treatments for the end stages of diseases such as cancer and AIDs or care for conditions in which the treatments were known not to be effective. In the revised approach, the Commission decided to ignore cost information and to allow their subjective judgments to influence the rankings on the list. Unfortunately, the final exercise in Oregon resulted in many deviations from the General Health Policy Model. However, the exercise demonstrates an attempt to resolve the health care crisis on the basis of health outcome. In the next section we will consider several of the ethical issues raised by the Oregon experiment.

ETHICAL ISSUES RAISED BY THE OREGON EXPERIMENT

The Oregon experiment has been a target for many legal, social, and ethical critics. A few of these concerns are briefly reviewed. They include:

> Community preferences cannot be used to make decisions about individual cases. Further, the process was unfair because preferences of non-Medicaid recipients were used to prioritize services for the poor.

One of the most robust findings relevant to the General Health Policy Model is that preferences do not differ greatly across social or demographic groups. Data from Oregon and other sources were used to evaluate this concern. Comparisons were made between women and men, between Medicaid recipients and non-recipients, and between patients and nonpatients. In each of the comparisons, there was remarkable similarity between the preferences. Even using completely different methodologies, preferences obtained from citizens in Oregon are remarkably similar to those obtained from residents of California. These findings have been replicated in several other studies.

The Rule of Rescue

Hadorn (1991a) expressed serious concerns about the original Oregon priority list. As an emergency room physician, Hadorn was also troubled because many technologies may relieve pain and reduce disability but do not rescue people from imminent death. The rule of rescue argues that there is a moral obligation to invest in rescue whenever saving a life is a possibility. Specifically, life-saving procedures should always rank above those that can be delayed. In other words, we should not spend money on prevention if it detracts from the opportunity for rescue, even if the rescue effort is highly likely to fail.

According to Hadorn, the ranking provided by the Commission did not make intuitive sense. However, careful analysis of Hadorn's statement suggests that there were problems with his analysis. For example, Hadorn reviewed the original version of the list and pointed out that tooth capping produced the same expected benefit as surgery for ectopic pregnancy. However surgery for ectopic pregnancy saves lives in almost all cases. The reason that these two were similar was that tooth capping provides a small benefit at a small cost, while ectopic pregnancy provides a big benefit at a big cost. The cost/utility ratio appears to be the same. However, a review of Hadorn's analysis identified several problems. For example, it appears that Hadorn underestimated the cost of tooth capping. In fact, the cost he used ($38.00) was less than one-tenth of prevailing charges. Further, Hadorn apparently overestimated the effect of treatment for tooth capping. Hadorn correctly identified that there were a substantial number of errors in the early construction of the list. However, the list that Hadorn referred to was quickly abandoned by the Commissioners. Further, the Oregon law allows continual revisions of the list when new data become available. Through successive review and critiques, the list will be improved.

The program discriminates against children

The Children's Defense Fund (CDF) attacked the Oregon program because they thought it discriminated against children. In Oregon, poor women and children make up about 75% of Medicaid recipients. Further, the blind and the disabled were excluded from the initial version of the proposal. Critics charge that the proposal was a way of denying health care to those who needed it most. Although these arguments are compelling, it is also important to consider the benefits the program provides for poor women and children. Currently, thousands of women and children have no health care coverage at all. The Oregon proposal will make funding available to an estimated 60,000 children and women who now receive no care. The General Health Policy Model in no way discriminates against children. Usually services for children are well evaluated because they have the potential to produce many well-years of benefit. In fact, many criticisms of the model have suggested that the model is biased in favor of children. For example, prevention of a birth defect may produce large numbers of well-years over the course of a life span. Lasting treatment effects accumulate years of benefit as the person ages.

Legal Challenges

The Children's Defense Fund vowed to launch several legal challenges against the Oregon proposal. The rationale for some of these challenges is unclear. However, the term children's *defense* is informative. The group advocates programs for children through legal and political action. The major advocates are attorneys who have expressed deep concerns about one essential component of the proposal. In order to have a prioritized list, it is necessary to offer malpractice immunity for physicians who deny some services to patients. The CDF felt this was not acceptable. In order to stop the experiment, the CDF argued that the Oregon plan creates a form of social experimentation in which women and children are forced to participate without consent. Further, they suggested that the program was unconstitutional because it discriminated on the basis of race and sex. The Office of Technology Assessment retained legal counsel to evaluate these challenges. Although it is always difficult to predict with certainty how the court will receive particular challenges, the independent counsel suggested that the program did not violate the equal protection clauses nor did it require the approval of a human subjects committee.

Perhaps the most peculiar aspect of the CDF argument is the assertion that the program would be bad for the socially disadvantaged. The Oregon Medicaid program now denies access to substantial numbers of women and children. These people are unable to get any medical services except in emergency rooms. Apparently this situation is acceptable to CDF. In order to protect the current system, they vowed to submit petitions that will interfere with any attempt to broaden coverage so that 60,000 currently uninsured women and children can receive needed medical care. The aspect of the Oregon plan that apparently was missed by the CDF is that there is little evidence that the implementation of the plan will damage people. Indeed the funds to expand coverage and increase benefit would be captured by the elimination of services that provide little or no benefit.

In August of 1992, the Department of Health and Human Services denied Oregon's application to proceed with their experiment. The rationale for this decision was that the Oregon proposal violated the Americans with Disabilities Act.

Specifically, the Department expressed concern that persons with disabilities received lower scores on the Quality of Well-Being scale than persons without disabilities. They regarded this as discriminatory and in violation of the Americans with Disabilities Act which was implemented in July of 1992. Unfortunately, detailed analysis failed to support the justification for this decision. For example, the statement that people without disabilities undervalue health status of people with disabilities is simply not supported by the majority of studies. Further, if any bias exists it is *in favor* of people with disabilities because lower initial scores leave more room for improvement. Systematic analyses suggest that if there is a bias, it is relatively small. Unfortunately, the August 1992 decision makes it unlikely that the Federal Government will allow experimentation in which health outcomes are considered part of the evaluation process.

WHERE DO WE GO FROM HERE?

We need a new paradigm for thinking about alternatives in health care. The proposed model is consistent with the thinking of several groups, including scholars in the United States (Weinstein & Stason, 1976, 1977; Office of Technology Assessment, 1979; Russell, 1986, 1987), the United Kingdom (Williams, 1988; Drummond et al., 1987; Maynard, 1991), Canada (Torrance, 1986, 1987), and Australia (Richardson, 1991). Although the exact methodologies proposed by these different research groups vary slightly, the theory is nearly identical. Recently, Patrick & Erickson (1992) offered a detailed account of the methodological steps required to implement the system. Methods are now available to begin guiding policy decisions. However, our information base for the implementation of the model is still incomplete.

Three Needs for the Future: Data, Data, and More Data

In addition to the financial problems in American health care, there is a second crisis—the crisis of ignorance. Our understanding of the effects of contemporary health care upon health outcomes is shameful. When new treatments are introduced, we typically know something about the biologic theory, the mechanism of action, and the effect of treatment upon some specific biologic outcome. However, the effects of treatment upon everyday functioning and quality of life are rarely evaluated. When the Oregon Health Services Commission began to prioritize health services, they recognized that there was no good information to help them appraise the value of many current services. The U.S. Congress, in recognition of our ignorance about outcomes, recently created the Agency for Health Care Policy and Research (AHCPR) to focus on medical outcome studies. A recent emphasis on outcomes by the Food and Drug Administration (FDA) has stimulated the measurement of health outcomes in the evaluation of pharmaceutical products. Further, the National Heart Lung and Blood Institutes (NHLBI) now requires quality-of-life assessment in its clinical trials. Other NIH institutes have also encouraged the measurement of health-related quality of life. New data are becoming available. Yet, it may be several decades before we have enough information to apply the model with great confidence. Nevertheless, many steps toward the implementation of the model can be taken even while we await new information.

In the future, we will need at least three types of new data: information on the general population, outcome data, and cost data.

Health of the Population

With the failure of the current health care system, it is often argued that greater expenditures on health care in the United States have no effect upon common public health indicators. The indicator most commonly cited is infant mortality. Despite our higher expenditures on health care, it is not possible to demonstrate that the United States has a lower infant mortality rate than other westernized countries. The great majority of services in health care have no effect on infant mortality because services for individuals older than 1 year of age (except pregnant women) are neglected by this indicator. Further, a substantial number of services have no effect on life expectancy. In effect, the value of investments in health care is being evaluated against very crude measures.

When the U.S. Department of Health and Human Services released the *Health Promotion, Disease Prevention Objectives for the Nation, Year 2000,* it emphasized that the number one overall goal for the nation for the year 2000 was to increase the years of healthy life—a concept identical to well-years or quality-adjusted life years. The life expectancy in the United States was 73.7 years in 1980. It is estimated that about 11.7 years were lost to diseases and disabilities. Fries and colleagues (1989) argued that we may be reaching the point at which it is unlikely that we will be able to extend the life expectancy. Once a human being reaches a certain age, he or she experiences multiple biological failures that are beyond remedy. However, Fries and colleagues have suggested that we may be able to make life better during these later years of life. Better quality of life can be reflected in well-years of life but would not be captured with measures of life expectancy.

Because of the new interest in health-related quality of life, the National Center for Health Statistics has proposed using the Quality of Well-Being Scale as part of the National Health Interview Survey. New data on well-years of life will greatly advance our understanding of the wellness of the population.

Outcome Data

As mentioned above, we know too little about the effects of medical care. Outcome data must be obtained from several sources. Ideally, the data will come from randomized clinical trials. However, in the interim, we must depend on judgments from expert peer panels. In addition to outcome data, we need further information about preferences for various conditions and for health outcomes. Many of the analyses that are currently in the literature are based on preferences from very small samples of subjects. For instance, a study of 867 individuals in San Diego, California, has been used in a variety of different analyses for people in different locations and from different social circumstances.

Cost Data

Finally, we need considerably more information on costs. Not only do we need to understand the variations in the costs of procedures, but much more information is needed on the resources required to produce health outcomes. Currently, the resource base for most medical charges is poorly understood. The recent trend toward cost shifting in hospital charges makes cost accounting even more difficult.

CONCLUSIONS

A General Health Policy Model can contribute to the resolution of the current health care crisis. When properly applied, the model uses the best scientific information on the costs, risks, and benefits of treatment. The model is directed toward using available resources to produce the greatest benefit for the largest number of people. Most ethical challenges to the model are important, but can be addressed. The greatest problem facing implementation of the model is lack of scientific data. We need considerably more research on the efficacy of clinical interventions. Until this information becomes available, we must recognize that the application of the model is an iterative process in which the best data available should be used. However, it is also important to recognize that we have limitations in our current understanding. Thus, evaluations must be continually modified as we learn more. Ultimately, policy science can contribute to the health and well-being of the population.

CHAPTER ONE

Three Problems Contributing to the Crisis in American Health Care

The strong, masculine, Minnesota auto sales manager was nearly in tears when he addressed Senator Kennedy's Senate Labor Subcommittee investigating access to health care in a June 1991 hearing. The Minnesota resident had always been employed but was in the process of changing jobs when his young son was diagnosed with lymphocytic leukemia. Physicians told the man that the chances of saving his son were excellent. However, the treatments would be very costly. The sales manager had already signed up for health insurance coverage with his new employer, but the start date was nullified by his son's preexisting condition. Neither the insurance from the new or the old employer would cover the medical expenses. For starters, these costs would exceed $300,000.

The man took a brief time off work to care for his son and investigate the problem. Even without insurance, the family could go into debt and pay the bills through wages. Yet when he returned to work the man discovered that the company had hired someone else to take over his new responsibilities. Like many other companies, the auto dealership was self-insured and could not take the risk of employing someone with a catastrophic illness in the family. To do so would affect their entire rate structure and would force the company either to lower wages or to significantly reduce profits. This situation, the man explained to Senator Kennedy's committee, made him essentially unemployable in a field where he had been a highly respected employee.

The family sought the best advice from lawyers and social workers. What they learned made a bad situation even worse. Their only alternative was to spend down the family assets so that they would sink significantly below the poverty line, to declare bankruptcy, and to file for public assistance. This would allow them to get medical help for their son under Minnesota's Medicaid program. The proud father and his wife had always regarded themselves as hard working middle-class Americans. Yet a nearly random situation, one that could happen to any American, had created a situation where it was inadvisable to seek employment even though they were able, willing, and anxious to do so. Under the federal bankruptcy, law they were able to keep their home. However, they realized that only one additional unexpected financial crisis stood between them and living on the street.

Senator Kennedy's committee responded with sympathy. Each Senator commented on the tragedy and assured the family they would do something about the insane health care system that they held responsible for these problems. Yet this case was not unique or unusual. Indeed, the senators had spent the entire afternoon hearing testimony on very similar cases. Further, these themes had been presented to the committee repeatedly. Those with frighteningly personal cases came from nearly all states and nearly all income and education levels. Not only were senators familiar with these types of cases, they were also familiar with proposals for a solution. Senator Kennedy had been introducing legislation on national health insurance for nearly 20 years. The committee had entertained many national health insurance proposals and had heard testimony that each would fail. Recognizing the potential of health care reform as a political weapon, congressional Democrats conducted a tour to collect similar horror stories during the fall of 1991. Sad stories were not hard to find. However, concrete suggestions for a solution to the problem were few.

In this book we examine the problem of health care financing and consider different approaches to the resolution of this important problem. This chapter attempts to summarize the problem. For most readers, this will only provide a restatement of information that is well known and widely disseminated.

The second chapter will evaluate some of the simple solutions that are commonly offered in the popular press. For example, we will introduce and dismiss such beliefs as the problem can be resolved by making a one-time cut in administrative costs, by funding all medical services for all people, or by shifting our emphasis from allopathic medicine to prevention.

Chapter Two also will examine some of the successes and failures of the administrative remedies that have been attempted. These include reimbursement by diagnostic-related groups (DRGs), reimbursement by resource-based relative value scales (RBRVS), and the introduction of managed care to health maintenance organizations (HMOs) and preferred provider organizations (PPOs). There have been dozens of proposals to address the crisis in health care. A sampling of these proposals is critically analyzed in Chapter Three.

The fourth chapter introduces a General Health Policy Model as a new way of thinking about problems of health care. The basic components of the model are used to estimate the expected benefits of various health care services. A unique aspect of the model is that it uses a general measurement unit to characterize the outcomes of any service, be it medicine, surgery, prevention, or policy change. A second component of the model is cost. Ultimately, a ratio was formed to evaluate the costs, risks, and benefits of various programs or treatments. The emphasis is to provide the greatest health benefit, given limited resources.

The fifth chapter offers several examples of the application of the model. These include analyses of common clinical treatments for diseases such as diabetes, heart disease, high blood pressure, and Acquired Immune Deficiency Syndrome (AIDS). The chapter also reviews applications for some public health controversies, such as the decision to have male children circumcised, the use of public funds to screen for breast cancer using mammography, and the use of excise taxes to reduce cigarette smoking.

Chapter Six explores applications of the model. We will touch upon applications in clinical medicine but the major emphasis will be on public policy and resource allocation considerations. Particular attention will be given to the proposed application of the model for resource allocation in Oregon.

The seventh chapter reviews the ethical and methodological difficulties with this approach. The final chapter (Chapter Eight) summarizes the problem and identifies research needs for the implementation of the General Health Policy Model, as well as other approaches.

COMMON MISCONCEPTIONS TO BE CHALLENGED

This book will challenge several widely held beliefs about health care in the United States.

Common Myths about Health Care

There are several common misconceptions about health care in the United States. Dispelling these common myths will provide an important framework for analyzing the health care system.

Myth 1: The United States is second to none in health care. The United States is second to none in its expenditures on health care. However, we have little evidence that these expenditures pay off in terms of health benefits. The United States is seventeenth in the world in infant mortality and leads the westernized world in the proportion of its population that has no way of paying for medical care.

Myth 2: Cost-cutting efforts have been a "death sentence" for some people. There have been several major efforts in the United States to cut health care costs (see Chapter Two). For example, policies have been enacted to shorten the length of hospital stays and to change the rate at which physicians are reimbursed for various services. Each time one of these policies has been enacted, it has met with editorials arguing that cost cutting will cost lives. However, changes in reimbursement patterns have not resulted in measurable changes in health status. Many countries with much less expensive health care systems have better scores on common health indicators.

Myth 3: The free-market system will resolve our problems. Medical care is a peculiar market. Consumption choices are different because of the nature of the service. Given full freedom of choice, it is unlikely that someone will select a surgeon for a life-threatening procedure because he or she offers the lowest cost. Further, consumers are often unaware of the pricing structure and cannot make informed choices. Another problem is that the nature of the doctor–patient relationship places the consumer in a compromised position. When they are sick, patients are anxious and vulnerable. Under these circumstances, a provider can easily sell services. This is often justified by identifying very rare, but serious consequences if action is not taken. In addition, there is the problem of the third-party payer. Many consumers are unconcerned about their choices because the bill goes to an insurance company or to the federal government. As a result of these problems, market forces cannot be expected to adequately regulate the consumption of health care.

Myth 4: Interfering with the doctor–patient relationship will have disastrous consequences. Medical groups have long argued that decisions should be left to the doctor–patient dyad. However, considerable evidence presented in Chapter Two suggests that physicians sometimes recommend procedures that are not useful. When these physicians are simply given feedback that they are doing too many procedures, expenditures are reduced and there is no harm to patients. The uninterrupted doctor–patient decision process, with a third party paying the bill, makes an expensive process more expensive. Simply adding a neutral referee could reduce expenses.

Myth 5: The American public will never allow health care to be rationed. Although concerned about their own health care system, many Americans are grateful that they do not face the distasteful prospects of England and other countries that "ration" health care. Such moral bankruptcy will never be allowed here. Or will it? There is considerable evidence that the American system does, indeed, ration. There are differences. In England some services are not available to people covered by the publicly funded National Health Service. Renal dialysis, for example, is not given to all people with end-stage kidney disease. Services are allocated based on need and chances of benefit. In the United States, rationing is different because people are rationed. Some whole classes of people cannot get care because they are uninsured and have no resources to pay for expensive services. The only refuge is the hospital emergency rooms. However, these services are so overburdened that they cannot handle the masses of people in need. Jerry Buckingham, executive director of the Los Angeles County–USC Medical Center acknowledged that his system was like many other inner-city hospitals that keep emergency room patients waiting as long as 24 hours. "The much-dreaded era of 'rationing' is upon us" Buckingham (1991) recently proclaimed.

WHAT IS WRONG WITH THE HEALTH CARE SYSTEM?

There are few items in contemporary America upon which there is consensus. One of the exceptions is the current concern about the health care system. Public opinion polls consistently show that only about 25% of Americans have faith in the current health care system (Jajich-Toth & Roper, 1990). Those calling for reform in the health care system include peculiar bedfellows. They are Republicans and Democrats, conservatives and liberals, management and labor. In June of 1991, hundreds of labor organizations joined forces to participate in "Health Care for All Week." Pickets were joined by the American Association of Retired Persons (AARP). That same week a coalition of more than 150 interest groups launched a massive rally to demand guaranteed medical care for all California citizens. The groups involved included the Catholic charities, the Congress of California Seniors, and a coalition of health care reform groups. Traditionally, these groups would have faced opposition from the establishment. Yet at roughly the same time, delegates of the American Medical Association were meeting in Chicago and calling for similar reforms. As we will see, the solutions suggested by these groups are not the same. Yet the conclusion that something is seriously wrong is hard to avoid.

Relman (1989) suggested that there are three basic deficiencies in our health care system. First, health care costs too much. Those who pay for health care, primarily large employers and governments, can no longer afford to offer high levels of services. A second problem is that our system is inequitable. Despite the fact that we spend more on health care as a proportion of the Gross National Product (GNP) than any other country, we still have between 22 and 39 million persons who have no insurance or inadequate resources to cover their medical care. The third, and perhaps most challenging, problem is that we have failed to be good consumers of health care. Theoretically, we purchase health care in order to obtain health. We know very little about the relationship between care and health outcomes. Many of the services we purchase may either be unnecessary or ineffective (Brook & Lohr, 1986). A simple mnemonic for these three problems is "The Three A's: Affordability, Access, and Accountability." We will briefly address each of these issues in the following sections.

Cost: The Problem of Affordability

No one denies that health care is expensive and many feel that it is appropriate that we spend much of our resources on health care. However, the proportion of all expenditures devoted to health care is troubling. Figure 1.1 shows expenditures on health care estimated at the beginning of each decade between 1940 and 1990. In the 1940–1949 period, approximately 4 billion dollars were spent on health care each year in the United States. That amount had tripled by the 1950–1959 period. As Fig. 1.1 illustrates, the rate of increase has been staggering—the 1990 expenditure of 666.2 billion was 166 times greater than the 1940 expenditure. Today,

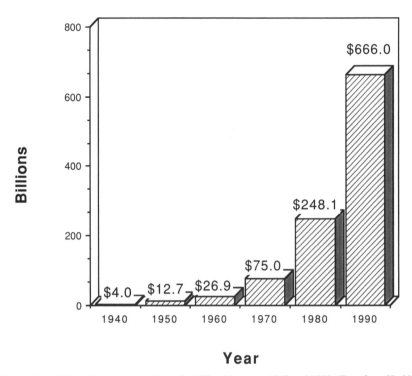

Figure 1.1 U.S. health care expenditures (in billions) between 1940 and 1990. (Data from Health Care Financing Administration, 1990).

we spend the same amount every other day that was spent in the entire year of 1940. On the average, 1 billion dollars are spent on health care each half day. These increases far exceed what would be expected on the basis of inflation. In 1990 medical care costs increased 10.5% while the GNP expanded by 5.1%. Perhaps most informative is the proportion of the GNP that is devoted to health care. Figure 1.2 shows the proportion of the GNP that is devoted to health care for the United States and for the average nations reporting to the Organization of Economic Cooperation and Development (OECD) (Health Care Financing Administration, 1988). As the figure suggests, health care costs have risen more rapidly in the United States than in the other countries reporting to OECD. In 1960 medical services accounted for only about 5% of the U.S. GNP. By 1990 medical services had increased to 12.2% of the GNP (*The Nation's Health,* 1991). Some estimates suggest that health care spending could reach three-fourths of a trillion dollars by the end of 1992. The 1990 expenditures are expected to double by 1995 and triple by the turn of the century. If these forecasts are correct, the United States

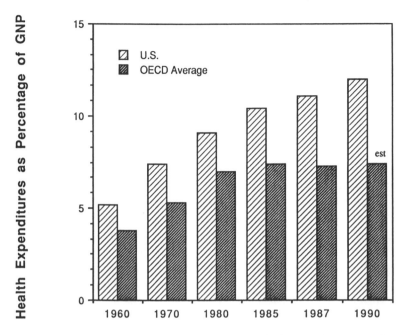

Figure 1.2 Comparison of United States and average from OECD countries on expenditures in health care between 1960 and 1990. (Data from Health Care Financing Administration, 1990.)

will spend more than 15% of its GNP on health care by the year 2000 even under conservative estimates of economic growth (Relman, 1989).

The consequences of devoting a high percentage of the GNP to health care have been debated. High expenditures on health care have raised serious concerns about the likelihood that American products can successfully compete with those offered by foreign competitors. For example, it has been estimated that the Chrysler Corporation spends about $700 per automobile on health care while the comparable figure for Japanese auto makers is less than $300. Discrepancies in health insurance account for a major proportion of the cost differences required to produce products in different countries. In 1986, Great Britain spent only about 6% of its GNP on health care, Japan spent less than 7%, while West Germany spent only about 8%. If these discrepancies continue, it is likely that American products will fail in international competition and that the balance of trade will be even more severely distorted. Some economists suggest that a full 20% of the GNP could be devoted to health care early in the twenty-first century. Reinhardt (1990) believes that there is little danger that health care expenditures, by themselves, will cause the economic ruin of American society. The real issue, according to Reinhardt, is in the distribution of care. Denying access to the poor may have more serious effects on society than cost. This is an issue that we will explore in the next section. However, another difficult problem is in the costs of health care for individual employers. Consider, as an example case, health care costs within the University of California.

THE MEDICAL CARE CRISIS AT THE UNIVERSITY OF CALIFORNIA: A CASE STUDY

The University of California is one of the largest employers in the state of California. With 93,000 employees, 19,000 retirees, and more than 100,000 family members, the system is one of the largest systems of public education and research in the United States. In 1990 the University spent $365 million on health benefits for its employees. In 1970 the University made a monthly contribution of $8 for each employee while the employee contributed 73% of the costs of the insurance plan. However, the total cost per employee for health insurance was less than $30 per month. By 1989 the University was paying $276 for each employee with the employee paying only about 3% of the total plan premium. Between 1970 and 1990 the University's total cost for health and welfare insurance for its employees had increased over 3000%. Yet it is interesting to consider the employees' contribution. Adjusted for inflation, the 1970 and 1990 employee contributions out of their paychecks were comparable (between $8 and $30 per month). What had really happened was that health insurance costs had gone completely out of control.

Many of the increased costs are accounted for by new medical technologies. However, the higher use of services was also a significant factor. For example, claims by University employees increased 12.5% between 1988 and 1989 and cost/employee claims jumped 73% between 1983 and 1989. The cost of prescription drugs used by employees increased 36% between 1987 and 1989. Further, there was a large increase in the number of psychiatric and substance abuse claims.

By 1990, the University needed to explore options for providing benefits to its employees. Although the University always prided itself on its employee benefits program, it became apparent that the University could no longer afford its own programs. To make things worse, the University itself owns and operates five of its own major medical centers and numerous clinics in association with its five medical schools. In fact, the University is one of the major health care providers in the state of California. The system is both part of the cause and a victim of the consequence of the problem. By 1990, the University needed to inform its employees that big changes were ahead. Although most employers will continue to provide health insurance coverage, the era of unrestricted use of resources has come to an abrupt end. In the 1990s, experimentation with alternative ways for financing employee benefits had become the rule rather than the exception.

GUIDELINES AND MODELS

Practice guidelines require formal decision-making models. Mathematical models for decision making are now being proposed in a variety of health care systems. For example, these models have been suggested for use in European, Australian, and American health care systems. More experts are proclaiming that health care resources are very limited. Many services routinely performed by physicians may be unassociated with benefit. In fact, some analyses indicate that at least 30% of current medical services are unnecessary (Brook & Lohr, 1986). Hadorn & Brook (1991) suggested the development of basic benefit insurance packages that use practice guidelines to guide physician decision making. These guidelines would direct providers away from excessively costly and unnecessary procedures. The assumption is that enough money would be saved by elimination of unnecessary services to create access to basic services for all people. However, the identification of effective and efficacious services might not solve the problem. Future iterations of the proposal will need to consider comparisons across diagnoses and they may need to recognize the possibility of prioritized funding. For example, we may need to invest in some services, but not others. In the United Kingdom, the National Health Service has acknowledged the need to prioritize competing demands on its very limited budgets (Rosser, 1992). Oregon has also proposed prioritized funding. Yet prioritization schemes make little sense without some consideration of outcome.

The most important challenge in developing a formal model for net benefit and a model of resource allocation is in defining a common unit of health benefit. Typically, the value of each specific intervention in health care is determined by considering a measure specific to the intervention or the disease process. For example, treatments for hypertension are evaluated in terms of blood pressure while those for diabetes are evaluated by blood glucose. Yet it is difficult to compare the relative value of investing in blood glucose versus blood pressure reduction. Traditional public health measures, such as life expectancy, are usually too crude to allow appropriate prioritization. However, we believe a general model of health outcome is both feasible and practical. Although the guidelines often mention net benefit, they do little to operationalize this construct. We believe the definition of outcome is central to the process. Our approach to this problem will be described in Chapter 4.

Pointed Fingers

By 1990, everyone recognized that there was a problem. Yet no one group was willing to take responsibility. Hospitals blamed the high cost of technology and the extravagant practices of some physicians. Doctors blamed lawyers for pursuing poorly justified malpractice claims. Lawyers blamed doctors. Insurance companies blamed everyone, including overutilizing patients, hospitals that extended lengths of stay, and physicians who overdiagnosed and overtreated. In exchange, everyone blamed insurance companies for permitting administrative costs to become excessive (Woolhandler & Himmelstein, 1991). Further, the culpable role of the federal government was often cited. The vilification of a single responsible group has led to many proposals for simple solutions. These naive proposals will be discussed in Chapter Two. Some groups offered specific evidence that they had not contributed to the cost problem. The left-hand portion of Fig. 1.3 is based on an ad sponsored by the Pharmaceutical Manufacturers Association that appeared in several newspapers. The ad replicated the proportion of the GNP devoted to health care (open hatched bars) and also showed that there has been no change in

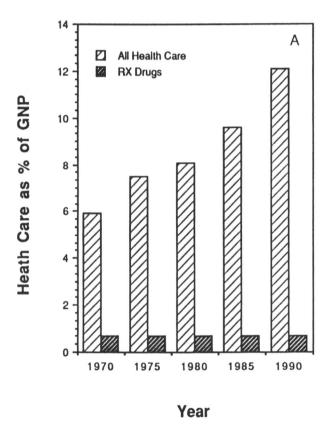

Year

Figure 1.3 (A) Comparison of growth in all health care and growth in pharmaceuticals as proportion of the GNP. (Data from *Washington Post*, 1991.) (B) Percentage change from previous year for physician charges, hospital charges, and pharmaceutical/sundries charges between 1978 and 1990. (Data from Statistical Bulletin, January-March, 1991.) *(Figure continues)*

the percentage of the GNP that is devoted to prescription medications. As the figure shows, prescription medications have remained less than 1% of the GNP between 1970 and 1990. The ad included a quote from Gerald J. Mossinghoff, President of the Pharmaceuticals Manufacturers Association, stating, "If every element of the health care system were as constant a percentage of GNP as pharmaceuticals, the health care share would not be ramping up" (Washington Post, 1991).

But must we accept this statement as true? The right-hand portion of Fig. 1.3 shows year-to-year changes in the cost of physician services, hospital care, and drugs and sundries from 1979 through 1989. There have been consistent year-to-year increases. Although there was a substantial increase in physician and hospital charges in 1980 and 1981, the yearly increases in pharmaceuticals were comparable to hospital and physician charges in the other years. The left-hand portion of Fig. 1.4 summarizes the increase in hospital care, physician services, drugs and sundries, and nursing home care between 1979 and 1989. The graphs suggest that

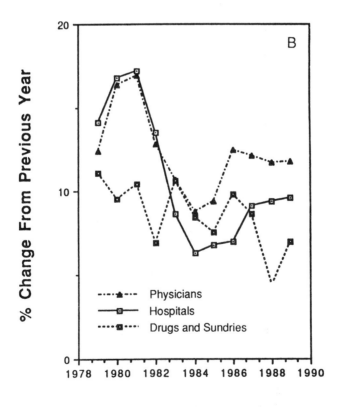

Year

Figure 1.3 *(continued)*

the greatest increase has been for hospital care followed by physician services. However, these graphs can be deceptive. The right-hand portion of Fig. 1.4 presents data from the same Health Care Financing Administration (HCFA) table. The bars in the figure are the ratios of 1989 to 1979 costs. During this decade most of the increases were comparable. Physician costs increased 3.2 times while nursing home costs increased 3.28 times. Hospital costs, which appeared to increase most in the left-hand section of the figure, were actually ranked third (2.64 times increased). Although pharmaceutical costs showed the lowest rate of in-

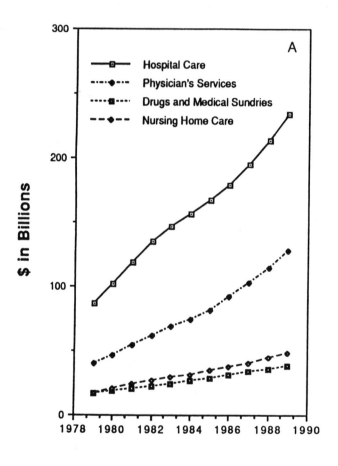

Year

Figure 1.4 (A) Cost (in billions) of hospital care, physician services, drugs and sundries, and nursing home care between 1978 and 1989. (B) Ratio of 1989/1979 costs for hospitals, physicians, pharmaceuticals, and nursing homes. (Data from Health Care Financing Administration, 1990.) *(Figure continues)*

crease (2.23 times), they were actually quite comparable to the increase in costs of other services.

The Pharmaceutical Manufacturers Association graph and the left-hand portion of Fig. 1.4 make increases in pharmaceutical costs look small because they are a small proportion of total health care expenditures. For example, the choice of method for graphing the data can be deceptive. Overall, rapid rates of cost increase were apparent for most sectors of the health care industry (Iglehart, 1992). No longer were professional organizations discussing the issues in a reasonable and responsible way. Instead, the era of the defensive public relations campaign had begun.

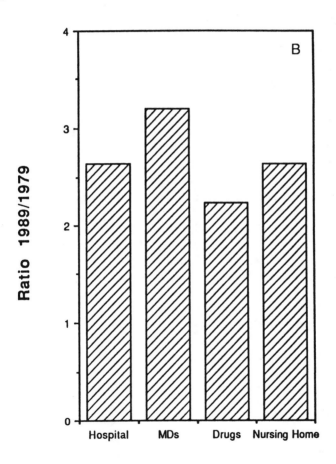

Figure 1.4 *(continued)*

The Access Problem

Despite the amount we spend on American health care being remarkably high, a substantial proportion of the American population is completely locked out of the system. Over the last decade congressional committees have repeatedly listened to stories about seriously ill people who could have been helped but were denied access to hospitals because of their inability to pay the bills. John Bunker, an anesthesiologist and former chair of several different departments at the Stanford Medical School, emphasized the inequities of the system. He stated:

> The American public has been warned that medical care may soon have to be rationed. . . . The truth is that medical care is already rationed and it always has been. One of the disgraces of national policy is that the poor and unemployed who cannot afford to pay for medical care or have no medical insurance must often accept inferior treatment, if they can get treatment at all. [Lee & Estes (1990), p. 293]

Although the exact numbers are uncertain, nearly all observers agree that substantial numbers of Americans are uninsured. The number 37 million is cited most frequently, while other estimates range between 32 and 38 million. The 1987 National Medical Expenditure Survey (NMES) found that 47.8 million Americans did not have health insurance during some part of the calendar year 1987. On any particular day during that year, between 34 and 36 million people were uninsured, while 24.5 million were uninsured throughout the entire year (Short et al., 1989; Short, 1990).

Similar reports have emerged from the Bureau of the Census. The Bureau reported that from the first quarter of 1986 through the last quarter of 1988, 63.6 million people had no regular health insurance for at least 1 month. During the final quarter of 1988, 31.5 million were uninsured (Nelson & Short, 1990). Another study by a completely independent group, The Employee Benefit Research Institute, suggested that 33 million Americans lacked health insurance and were ineligible for it in 1988 (Chollet et al., 1990). Although these estimates do vary, it is probably safe to assume that well over 30 million Americans have no regular source of health care at any one time. Further, these figures substantially increase if the window of inquiry is expanded to 1 or 2 years.

Those who are uninsured are not a random sample from the general population. The only group that is really immune is the elderly since virtually all Americans older than 65 years are covered under Medicare. Although those in the age range of 19–25 years are most likely to be uninsured (23.3% in the 1987 NMES survey), the second most likely group to be excluded is children and adolescents under 18 years of age. In 1988, 17% of children and adolescents had no health insurance from either public or private sources (Bloom, 1990).

Members of different racial and ethnic groups have very different rates of health care coverage. The NMES suggested that 18.6% of non-Hispanic whites were uninsured for all or part of 1987. This stands in contrast to 29.8% of black respondents and 41.4% of Hispanic residents. The Hispanic group, which is least likely to be insured, also represents the most rapidly growing demographic group in the United States.

The uninsured are not necessarily the unemployed. In fact, the majority of the uninsured are working but are not employed in professions that provide adequate health insurance coverage. One might think that those closest to the health care system would be most likely to be well insured. However, an analysis of health insurance among health and insurance workers suggested some surprising conclusions. The March 1991 Current Population Survey evaluated health insurance among 6182 civilian health personnel and 1498 insurance workers under the age of 65 years. About 9% of civilian health workers had no health insurance; 5.1% of insurance workers were themselves uninsured, while 6% of those working in physician offices had no health insurance. Remarkably, 52.2% of health and insurance workers received no employer contribution toward their health care. About 20% of nursing home employees had no health insurance. Projecting these results to the nation, it was estimated that nearly 1 million health and insurance workers themselves had no coverage for their health care expenses (Himmelstein & Woolhandler, 1991a).

In California, the 1990 Census revealed that more Californians were uninsured than had been anticipated. An estimated 6 million Californians were uninsured according to the census, and 90% of these individuals either worked or were from a family with a working adult. This means that about 22.5% of Californians under age 65 were uninsured in comparison to the 16.5% national average. When insurance coverage was broken down by industry, it was of interest that public administrators, those in the best position to influence public policy, are almost universally insured through their employers. Conversely, agricultural and construction workers are rarely insured by their employers and are very likely to have no insurance at all. Yet it is precisely these workers that have the highest probability of job-related injuries and toxic exposures (*Los Angeles Times,* 1991).

Very low-income individuals may qualify for a Medicaid program. Originally, Medicaid was designed to help low income women and children and those with certain defined disabilities. However, Medicaid covers families with dependent children and thus may also include coverage for some men. In contrast to Medicare, which is a federal program, Medicaid is administered by the states. This allows each state to define its own threshold for eligibility. The national average for Medicaid eligibility is set at less than 50% of the federal poverty level. With the current federal poverty level at about $12,000 per year, this means that a family of three with a yearly income of $6,000 is too rich to be considered eligible for Medicaid support. As a result, the great majority of low-income people are simply out of luck. In a 1987 survey, 47.5% of individuals or families with incomes below the poverty level were uninsured. The situation does not get much better for people between the poverty line and 125% of poverty (between about $11,000 and $13,750 in 1990 dollars). Among this group about 45% have no source of health insurance.

Medicaid recognizes certain peculiar categories. For example, Congressional action in the 1980s required Medicaid coverage for pregnant women. Governors of 49 states have asked Congress to cease requesting special coverages as states simply do not have the money to expand services. Yet current policies lead to nonsensible actions. For example, most states provide Medicaid coverage for pregnant women. For many low-income women the only way to obtain health insurance is to become pregnant. Further, most states allow low-income families support for dependent children. Yet the age criteria for coverage vary. A family may get coverage for young children but may get left out in the cold if the children are adolescents.

Medicaid also has become highly political. Governors or legislators attempting to win votes have sometimes committed large sums of money that have taken large pieces of the expenditure pie. These decisions typically make access worse. For example, the state of Illinois passed a 1985 bill that guaranteed reimbursement of up to $200,000 for any citizen who needed an organ transplant. At the same time, more than 60% of black children in Chicago's inner cities did not receive routine medical care and were not even immunized against common diseases such as polio. In 1990, Florida's Governor Martinez committed $100,000 to a heroic attempt to save the life of a single child who had nearly drowned in a swimming pool accident. All experts agreed that the case was futile. While the governor received great acclaim for his compassion, thousands of Florida children were denied basic services through Florida's underfunded Medicaid program (Kitzhabar, 1990).

COST SHIFTING

Hospitals are required to provide emergency services or face litigation. As a result, hospitals do provide services for the medically uninsured. But what happens to the charges for the services? Essentially, hospital costs are deferred. In other words, bills to patients who have insurance or who are capable of paying are inflated in order to cover the losses for treating the uninsured. This process is known as cost shifting.

As a result of cost shifting, facilities that care for the uninsured need to charge insured patients higher rates to offset their losses. Recent studies have suggested that cities with more uninsured patients have higher average health insurance costs. For example, Fig. 1.5 summarizes average monthly costs for insurance premiums for employees in small firms in selected U.S. cities. Los Angeles has the highest rate in the nation ($631 per month). In other words, the average small business in Los Angeles needs to pay twice as much for health insurance as the average small business in Seattle ($310 per month). Although cost shifting does not account for all of these differences, a substantial proportion is related to the high rate of medically uninsured in Los Angeles.

The consequences of cost shifting can be serious. By moving from Los

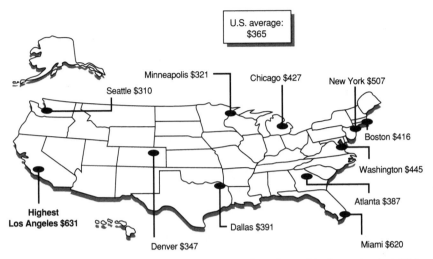

Figure 1.5 Average monthly insurance premiums per employee for small businesses in selected U.S. cities. (From *Los Angeles Times,* September 1991.)

Angeles to Seattle, a business can reduce its health insurance cost by nearly half and still provide the same level of benefits to its employees. Certainly, this makes Los Angeles, Miami, and New York unattractive homes for small businesses. The alternative is for businesses to decline health insurance for their employees. When this happens the cost to businesses offering insurance goes even higher and the vicious spiral becomes more severe.

In summary, the current system has failed miserably in providing adequate access to health care. It is a widely held assumption that health care is a basic right rather than a luxury. Despite our willingness to spend more on health care than any other country in the world, we still have substantial proportions of our population who have no health insurance at all. The poor and members of certain ethnic and minority groups are disproportionately stuck with no insurance and no regular source of care. Although proposed solutions differ, few groups are willing to defend the current system.

Outcome: The Problem of Accountability

Health care may be the only major American industry that is not held accountable for what it produces. Until recently the health care system seemed disinterested in studying whether it made patients better or worse. A recent growth of interest in "outcomes research" grew out of observations of small-area variation. Small-area variation refers to differential rates of service use across demographically homogeneous communities.

It has always been assumed that medical need is the primary reason for receiving medical care. Doctors perform procedures when people are sick. Yet we know that in demographically homogeneous communities the need for these services should be about the same. The number of children who need a tonsillectomy in Dayton should be about the same as the percentage who need the procedure in Toledo. However, observational studies suggest that there is substantial variability from community to community in how often procedures are performed. For example, in the early 1970s only 10% of the children in Middlebury, Vermont, had their tonsils out before age 15. In contrast, more than 60% of the 15-year-olds in Morrisville, Vermont (equivalent community) have had their tonsils removed. When physicians in Morrisville learned about this discovery, the rate of tonsillectomy dropped precipitously and the low rate has persisted. Differences in the rate at which procedures are used in similar communities are known as small-area variation. Small-area analysis has had a profound effect upon our understanding of the use of medical services.

Examples of small-area variation abound. For example, the per capita costs of hospitalization in New Haven, Connecticut, have been about half of what they are in Boston, Massachusetts. Small-area variation can be quantified in a variety of different ways. One of the simplest ways is to look at the ratio of the number of procedures of the highest-use community divided by that of the lowest-use community. For some procedures there is very little variation. For example, cholectomy has a highest-to-lowest ratio of 1.47. On the other hand, total knee replacement has a variation ratio of 7.42, while carotid endarterectomy (a procedure that reams out obstructed arteries that carry blood to the brain) has a variation ratio of 19.39. This means that nearly 19 people in some communities get carotid endarterectomy for every 1 person that gets it in a very similar environment. This variation applies to hospitalizations for illnesses as well as for medical procedures. Illnesses such as upper respiratory tract infections have variation ratios of nearly 16. We also know that medicine is practiced differently in different communities. For example, prior to the implementation of the prospective payment system, there was remarkable variation from community to community in how long patients stayed in the hospital. This is still true if comparisons are made between systems. Cardiac surgery, for example, may have a much longer length of stay in a VA hospital than in a private for-profit setting (Wennberg, 1990). International comparisons are also of great interest. For example, about 8 out of every 10 well-insured patients receive angiography following a myocardial infarction (MI) (heart attack) in a certain private hospital in San Diego, California. In the same city, about 40% of VA patients receive the procedure following a heart attack. In Vancouver, only about 20% of post-MI patients get angiography. Only about 10% receive the procedure in Sweden (Nicod et al., 1991). Clearly there is small-area variation for many procedures. Many would argue that small-area variation represents differences in the quality of medical care. If this is true, areas where procedures are used more aggressively should be the ones where people live longer or have higher qualities of life. Yet, we have no evidence whatsoever that aggressive medical care results in better patient outcomes. The probability of surviving myocardial infarction, accounting for the seriousness of the heart attack, is the same in San Diego, Vancouver, and Sweden. Children in Middlebury, Vermont do not live longer than children in Morrisville, and there is little evidence that they suffer more illnesses. Life expectancy in New Haven is about the same as life expectancy in Boston. All other indicators suggest that the quality of health in these same communities, controlling for some demographic variables, is quite comparable. Small-area variation has helped us understand that there is variation in costs and effort devoted to medical care, but there is not necessarily variation in health outcome.

International comparisons help emphasize this point. Figure 1.6 summarizes the increases in health care spending as a proportion of the Gross Domestic Product (GDP) for six OECD countries between 1970 and 1989. The countries are

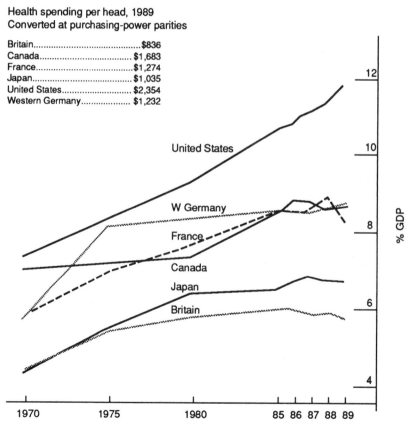

Figure 1.6 Changes in health care expenditure between 1970 and 1990 for Britain, Canada, France, Japan, the United States, and West Germany. (Data adapted from OECD.)

the United States, West Germany, France, Canada, Japan, and Great Britain. As the figure shows, the increase in spending as a proportion of the GDP increased in all countries except Canada between 1970 and 1975. However, these increases leveled off in West Germany, Japan, and Britain. Although there have been some increases in France and Canada, the rate of increase in the United States is much more rapid than in any other country. We would expect that different levels of expenditure would be associated with better outcomes. The various portions of Fig. 1.7 consider this issue using data from seven OECD countries. Figure 1,7A considers the relationship between the percentage of GDP devoted to health care and the infant mortality rate. The result goes in the wrong direction. It appears that the more countries spend on health care the higher is the infant mortality rate. Indeed, the relationship appears to be linear with the exception of Great Britain, which has a low expenditure on health care and relatively high infant mortality rate. Figure 1.7B shows the relationship between the number of doctors per 10,000 persons in the population and the percentage of the GNP devoted to health care. This relationship is statistically significant. Countries with high GNPs have greater numbers of physicians. However, as shown in the lower portion of the figure, GNP

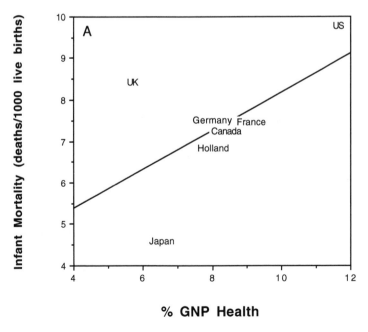

% GNP Health

Figure 1.7 Relationship of the Gross National Product expenditures on health care to infant mortality, physicians/10,000 in the population, and life expectancy. (From *The Economist*, July 1991.) *(Figure continues)*

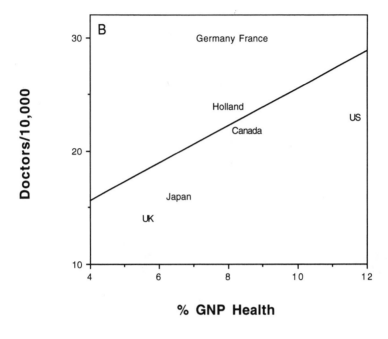

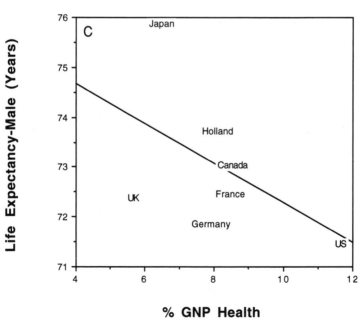

Figure 1.7 *(continued)*

and number of physicians are unrelated to life expectancy. In fact, the relationship is significant in the opposite direction. Those countries that devote a greater proportion of their GNP to health care have shorter life expectancies, at least for males (Fig. 1.7C).

Many social critics believe that the solution to problems of public health is to spend more money. In fact, there is a significant relationship between health expenditures and wealth as demonstrated in Fig. 1.8. At least among nations reporting to OECD, countries with higher GDP per person were also those who spent the greatest amount of their resources on health care. Yet, these analyses can be deceptive because of the way funds are distributed. For example, Japan, which spends less than 7% of its GNP on health care, has well more than twice as many medical beds per 10,000 persons in the population than do Canada, Britain, or the United States. In fact, the United States has fewer medical beds per 10,000 persons than Britain, Canada, Italy, France, West Germany, Holland, and Japan. Similarly, we would expect high expenditures to be related to long hospital stays. Yet the average length of stay for an American patient is less than one-fifth of that for patients in Japan. Among these eight countries, the United States has the shortest length of stay while Japan has the longest.

The outcomes movement, which will be the focus of Chapter Four, questions the relationship between expenditures and health benefits. Careful analyses have challenged the frequent use of many procedures. Brook and colleagues (1990) at

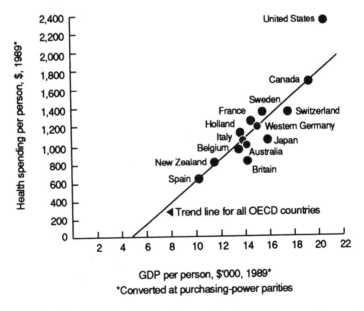

Figure 1.8 The relationship between per capita expenditures on health care and gross domestic product. (From *The Economist,* July 1991.)

the RAND Corporation, for example, have studied carotid endarterectomies. These are operations that are used to open arteries in the neck in order to reduce the chances of strokes. When carefully reviewed, the RAND researchers found that between 25 and 33% of the surgeries probably should not have been done. For many patients, these surgeries were unlikely to lead to better health outcomes and may have created new risks. After reviewing the latest clinical trial, an editorialist for the *Journal of the American Medical Association* concluded, "Endarterectory adds a little—but not a lot. It is useful to a small proportion of patients but can subject persons who are not eligible for endarterectomy to the risks of angiography" (Levy, 1991, p. 3333). Like many medical and surgical procedures, it does some good for some people. Too often it is used when the chances of benefit are slim.

Careful reviews of a wide variety of other procedures have suggested that the use of medical procedures in the United States is out of control. In many cases, the procedures have no likelihood of improving patients' health and, in many cases, medical procedures place patients at risk. For the most part, however, the effect of most medical treatments upon patient outcomes is unknown. This has caused such a concern that the U.S. Congress created the Agency for Health Care Policy and Research (AHCPR) in 1989 and gave it special responsibilities for evaluating medical effectiveness. The agency created Patient Outcomes Research Teams (PORTS) in an effort to determine how medical procedures and investments in medical care have an impact upon patient outcomes (Salive, Mayfield, & Weissman, 1990). As obviously beneficial as these efforts would seem, they have been largely neglected throughout the history of medical care.

WHO IS CONCERNED ABOUT THE PROBLEM?

Clearly the health care system has problems. But who is complaining about it? As we shall see in the next sections, the problem has stirred reaction from many different sectors, including consumers, politicians, business, and labor.

Consumers

A common belief about the marketplace is that there is a relationship between satisfaction and willingness to pay. We might expect that those countries with higher expenditures on health care would be more satisfied with their systems. Indeed, this is generally true as suggested in Fig. 1.9. For the United Kingdom, Japan, West Germany, and Canada greater expenditures are associated with greater satisfaction. However, there is an unusual point on the figure. In the United States, where expenditures on health care are the highest, satisfaction is the lowest. Several lines of evidence suggest that American consumers are unhappy with their health care. Most of them would prefer some national health insurance program. A 1990 Gallup Poll in California demonstrated that 83% endorsed the item, "Do you think the United States Government should develop some form of national

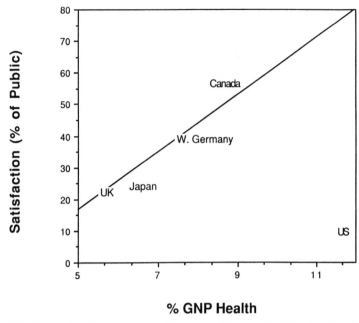

% GNP Health

Figure 1.9 The relationship between expenditures on health care and public satisfaction with health services. (Adapted from Blue Cross of California, 1990, p. 17).

health insurance program for everyone?" The same poll demonstrated that the most important concern for consumers was the cost of care. Seventy-three percent of California residents and 77% in a U.S. national sample indicated a willingness to pay more taxes in order to support indigent care. However, a resounding 78% stated that they would be unwilling to accept a lower quality of care if it costs less. Health care has the potential to become a political issue since more than half of the voters disapprove of the California legislature's performance on health care issues (Christiansen & Nielsen, 1990).

Despite beliefs that the government is doing a poor job in health care, citizens seem to distrust greater government involvement. This is illustrated in Fig. 1.10, which shows whether citizens favor or oppose various solutions to health care financing. In a poll conducted by the Health and Insurance Association of America, private insurance was favored most commonly, while expansion of Medicare programs to the nonelderly was opposed most often. These findings might appear to be in contrast with preferences for type of system. Although public opinion polls indicate that consumers would oppose the expansion of the Medicare system, it is remarkable that they are attracted to the Canadian system which has many similarities. Figure 1.11 summarizes results from two public opinion polls, one con-

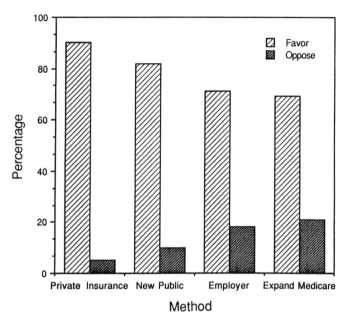

Figure 1.10 Preference for centralized health care system by type of insurance. (From Jajich-Toth & Roper, 1990.)

ducted by Harris and Blendon and another conducted by the Roper Organization. The figure summarizes the percentage of the population that would prefer a Canadian-like system or prefer their own system. In both polls, American citizens expressed preference for the Canadian system, and in the Harris/Blendon study the preference for the Canadian system was sizable (Jajich-Toth & Roper, 1990). Starfield (1991) reported on a "satisfaction–expense" ratio. The numerator of the ratio was the percentage of people who felt their health care system needed only minor changes divided by the percentage expressing the need for complete overhaul. The denominator for the ratio was per capita cost of health care expressed in thousands of dollars. Comparing 10 westernized countries on this index, Starfield found the United States to be at the bottom with a score of 2. The Netherlands obtained the highest score, 9.0, while Canada also obtained a high rating of 7.6. The poor placement of the United States reflects the combination of high expense and low satisfaction. Other countries with low satisfaction, such as the United Kingdom, had low expenses as opposed to the high U.S. costs. Thus their overall rating was not as low as that of the United States (the rating was 2.1 for the United Kingdom).

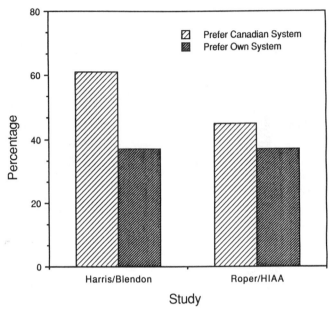

Figure 1.11 Preference for Canadian or American health care systems in two public opinion polls. (From Jajich-Toth & Burns, 1990.)

Business

Business has traditionally opposed any centralized approach to a social problem. However, recent evidence suggests that the tides have turned. Lee Iacocca, CEO of the Chrysler Corporation, was among the first to publicly argue that irresponsible health care policy was damaging business opportunities. A 1991 poll of business executives showed that 90% believe that the health care system needs to be completely rebuilt or to undergo radical alteration. Business executives liked the idea of selective contracting for Medicaid and Medicare services and tax incentives for small businesses to provide health care for their employees. Further, more than half of the business executives wanted government intervention to control costs (Cantor et al., 1991).

The reason that business supports fundamental change in the health care system is that high health insurance costs are bad for the bottom line. Since 1982, more than 50% of pre-tax corporate profits have been spent on health insurance. Employee benefits are the fastest-rising component of employee compensation packages and the 1989 increase in health insurance premiums averaged 20%. In 1989, employers spent more than $176.8 billion to provide insurance for their employees (Marwick, 1991).

Political Leaders

Another poll surveyed 201 physicians, 50 union leaders, 1175 corporate executives, 251 hospital executives, 21 major health insurers, 260 members of Congress, 25 key committee staff, 50 state health commissioners, and 15 executives from the Department of Health and Human Services. This study was conducted by representatives of the insurance industry (Metropolitan Life Insurance). Despite the heterogeneity of the group, there was near consensus that the health care system is in serious condition. There was, however, disagreement on how the changes should be achieved. Seventy percent of the union leaders thought that the system needed to be totally rebuilt while only 4% of physicians favored a major overhaul. Nevertheless, requests for reform have been plentiful. In a June 1991 address to the American Medical Association, Department of Health and Human Services Secretary Louis Sullivan, himself a physician, requested reform. Unexpectedly, Sullivan's challenge to traditional organized medicine was well received by the delegates. Both the editors of the *New England Journal of Medicine* and the *Journal of the American Medical Association* dedicated many of their journal pages in 1990 and 1991 to proposed solutions for health care financing and health care access. Today, few physicians are unaware or unconcerned about the problem (Schramm, 1991).

THE HIPPOCRATIC PREDICAMENT

Physicians throughout the world celebrate the transition from being a student to being a physician by taking the Hippocratic Oath. The Hippocratic Oath, which dates back to ancient Greece, provides the guiding ethical code for the practice of medicine. The first part of the oath defines the duties of physicians and the obligation to transmit medical knowledge. The second part of the oath offers general guidelines for the treatment of disease. Although the oath was first developed in the fourth century B.C., it only gradually came to influence medical ethics. In 1948 a modern version of the oath was developed at a conference in Geneva. The oath was amended in 1968 and is now administered upon graduation from medical school to all new physicians in the United States and throughout the western world.

Portions of the oath emphasize that patients will always be given the first consideration. Further, the oath emphasizes strong loyalty to fellow physicians. For example, it includes the statement, "I will maintain by all the means in my power, the honor and the noble traditions of the medical profession" and it also states that, "my colleagues will be my brothers." The oath emphasizes social responsibility. It underscores that patients shall not be discriminated against on the basis of religion, race, nationality, party politics, or social standing. The oath also states "the health of my patient will be my first consideration."

Herein lies the Hippocratic predicament. On the one hand, physicians have taken a solemn oath to do everything in their power to help individual patients. Further, they have pledged not to consider social standing as a factor in treatment decisions. Yet the American system has evolved such that there is discrimination on the basis of income and social standing. Further, resources are limited to the extent that we are unable to provide basic services for all people. The pledge that physicians honor the traditions of the medical profession contradicts the movement toward professional management of health care. Along several dimensions, the Hippocratic Oath is at odds with the directions of contemporary health care.

Contemporary physicians truly face a Hippocratic predicament. However, the problem may have a solution. Physicians throughout the western world take the Hippocratic Oath. Yet the problems in health care delivery are much more severe in the United States than in other countries. One of the goals of this book is to explore ways to work with the profession, respect the teachers of medicine, and keep the health of the patient as the most important consideration.

SUMMARY

The conclusions of this chapter are not surprising. Our health care system is in trouble. The problem with health care in America has at least three components. First, health care is *unaffordable*—we are devoting too much of our GNP to health care. The second problem is *access* to health care, despite our high expenditures. Between 32 and 38 million Americans are uninsured or underinsured. The third problem is *accountability*. Despite our high expenditures on health care, we have little evidence that the system is making people healthier or that Americans are more satisfied with the care they receive.

There is broad consensus that something needs to be done about these problems. Many different solutions have been proposed and we will consider some of them in the next chapters. However, it is important to emphasize that a good solution must address all three aspects of the problem. It must reduce costs or at least control them. Further, it must expand access. Finally, and perhaps most importantly, we must address the outcomes problem. Expenditures on health care must be directed toward achieving better health. In the following chapters we will consider various solutions to these problems in relation to the major issues of affordability, access, and accountability.

CHAPTER TWO

A Look at Solutions

Analogies between medicine and the health care system are common. Many medical patients present themselves with signs and symptoms of illness. Few physicians would deny that there is a problem when a patient is observed with high fever, elevated white blood cell counts, nausea, and vomiting. Yet physicians may take different approaches to the diagnostic work-up and may differ in the level of therapeutic aggressiveness they pursue.

Problems in the American health care system may be analogous to the doctor–patient relationship. The signs and symptoms of sickness of the system are apparent to all. However, onlookers have proposed radically different diagnoses and treatment plans. In this chapter, we will consider several proposed remedies for this problem. The various remedies will be evaluated against the three A's: affordability, access, and accountability. We will begin by reviewing "naive" solutions to the problem and then proceed to provide an overview of some of the approaches that have been tried. In the next chapter we will review current proposals.

Before reviewing any specific proposal it may be valuable to trace the history of government intervention in health care. Perhaps the first recorded instance of government intervention was in 2200 B.C. At this time, Hammurabi, the King of Babylon, enacted laws that limited physician fees. This policy was directed toward affordability. Further, laws in ancient Babylon were directed toward outcome and accountability. Physicians could be punished by law for using treatments that injured their patients. Accountability was also apparent in ancient Chinese societies where physician payments were made contingent upon patient improvement. By the fourteenth century, most parts of the Holy Roman Empire had laws regulating medical education and physician fees (*The Economist*, 1991).

In contemporary America, government intervention is rarely seen as the ideal policy. Yet organized labor is now begging for universal, government-based health insurance (*AFL–CIO Health Security Action News*, 1989). Even the president of the Chrysler Corporation declared "business has lost the war on hospital costs" and suggested that the time for government intervention had come (Iacocca, 1989). In the last few years, the Congress has seen a growing tide of new bills designed to overhaul the health care system. Yet few of the bills have passed (Kinzer, 1990).

SIMPLE SOLUTIONS

Whatever the solution, it will not be simple. But many simple solutions never-theless have been proposed. In the next few pages we will briefly review some of these simplistic solutions. These include increasing spending, raising taxes, na-tionalizing hospitals, letting medical associations prevail, restricting lawyers, and eliminating administrators.

Increase Spending

Some people believe that we can resolve the problem through increased spending on health care (Weiner, 1991). After all, we can spend our money any way we would like. No one knows for certain that the economy will fall apart if health care costs rise beyond 12% of the GNP. What would happen if we devoted 20% of the GNP to health care? After all, we devote nearly a third of the federal budget to defense. Why not reallocate some of these military resources to health care? As the Physicians for Social Responsibility have so adeptly argued, each nuclear submarine translates into literally thousands of vaccinations or preventive care programs for children.

Despite the appeal of increased spending, this position has few serious advo-cates. Although we spend an enormous amount on defense, people often confuse percentage of federal budget spent on defense and percentage of GNP. Spending about one-third of the federal budget on defense represented only about 6.23% of the GNP in 1990. In fact, we spend nearly twice as much of the GNP on health care as we do on either defense or education (see Fig. 2.1). The fact that we spend for other purposes does not necessarily justify our spending more on health care.

One of the major problems is that spending, by itself, addresses none of the major issues. It makes health care less affordable and does not necessarily increase access. The great acceleration in health care spending in the United States was accompanied by decreased rather than increased access for low-income people. Of course, most proposals for increased spending are designed to improve access and it is likely that universal health insurance would provide at least some basic coverage for low-income individuals.

The major concern about increased spending is that it does nothing to ensure improved outcomes. Indeed, as argued in Chapter One, there appears to be no relationship between expenditure and health outcome in industrialized countries. Further, there is at least some evidence that there are negative consequences of overexpenditure because patients are overtreated and exposed to the occasional

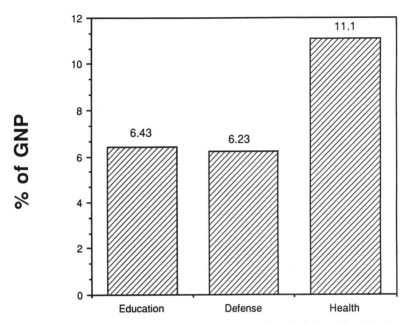

Figure 2.1 Percentage of GNP devoted to education, defense, and health. (Adapted from DOD data.)

toxic consequences of modern medicine. Many medications have side effects. When these drugs are taken unnecessarily, patients are exposed to the consequences without the expectation of benefit. Surgeries are similar. As noted in Chapter One, many complex surgical procedures such as carotid endarterectomy are performed on patients with little chance of being helped. These patients, however, are not excused from the risk of surgical complications (Levy, 1991).

The consequences of devoting growing percentages of the GNP to health are uncertain. However, there are important balance-of-trade issues. Auto makers now spend more for health care than they do for steel. Figure 2.2 shows the proportion of sticker price in Chryslers and Toyotas devoted to employee health care. As the figure shows, the cars manufactured in Japan have a significant competitive advantage due exclusively to health insurance costs. As differentials in health insurance costs among the United States, West Germany, and Japan increase, so might the differentials in automotive sales. The United States is already losing the balance-of-trade war. We import more than we export, while both Germany and Japan export more than they import. Figure 2.3 shows the merchandise balance of trade between 1960 and 1988. Between 1960 and 1975, the United States exported about as much merchandise as it imported. Recent years have witnessed a new strong trend in which imports significantly exceed exports. Cost differentials attributed to differences in health insurance rates are likely to make this problem worse.

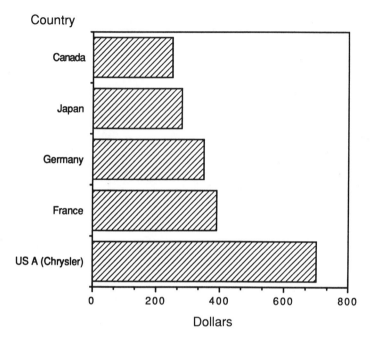

Figure 2.2 Proportion of sticker price devoted to health care costs for Chryslers in comparison to automobiles manufactured in Canada, Japan, France, and West Germany. (Adapted from Relman, 1989.)

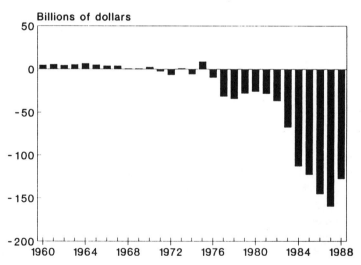

Figure 2.3 United States balance of trade for merchandise, 1960–1988. (Data from U.S. Department of Commerce, 1989.)

Economists suggest that rising health care costs cause "displaced consumption." As we spend more for health care we have less to spend on goods and other services. Studies have demonstrated that as health care costs have increased there has been a significant reduction in the consumption of personal goods and in savings. For example, the consumption of durable goods has declined from 49% in 1950 to 30% in 1990 (Thorpe & Spencer, 1991). For each dollar earned in the United States, only 88 cents are left after we pay for health care. This is in contrast to 93 cents in Japan and 94 cents in England. If the proportion of GNP devoted to health care continues to expand we will continue to take earning potential away from other sectors of the economy. Simply stated, uncontrolled spending will not resolve the problem.

Raise Taxes

A related solution would be to increase taxes. In comparison to other OECD countries, the United States has relatively low tax rates. Our taxes as a percentage of our gross domestic product are about 30%. This compares to 50% and higher in Scandinavian countries. Figure 2.4 summarizes the percentage of gross domestic product that is devoted to tax for 23 nations reporting to OECD. Among these countries, the United States has a surprisingly low tax rate.

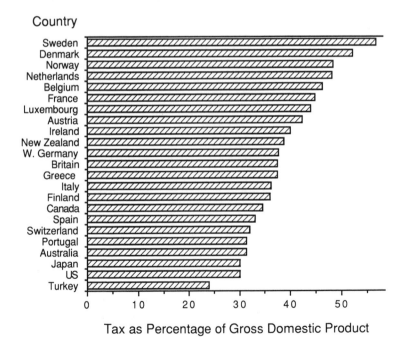

Figure 2.4 Tax as a percentage of gross domestic product in western countries. (Adapted from 1987 OECD data.)

Increased taxes would provide greater revenues that could be used to fund health care. Although new tax revenues could be used to pay for the medically uninsured, increasing taxes would be politically unpopular. With tax increases in other areas, few politicians are willing to run on a platform that includes increased taxpayer expenditures, although a 1989 Gallup Poll in California did suggest that 73% of Californians would be willing to pay more taxes to fund indigent health care as compared with 77% of a national sample. However, when asked about the most they would be willing to pay per month, the most common responses were in the lowest category of less than $25 per month. A 1990 poll showed that less than 9% would be willing to pay $100 or more per month (Christiansen & Nielsen, 1990).

Although tax increases may improve access by providing a funding source for the uninsured, they also contribute to the cost problem and there is no assurance that they improve accountability.

Nationalize Hospitals and Place All Doctors on a Government Salary

A second solution is to nationalize hospitals and place doctors and other health workers on salaries. A truly socialized system, it is argued, provides access to all at a reasonable cost. Further, centralization of the system can enhance quality. Or can it? Perhaps the best example of a completely centralized system is the National Health Service in Great Britain.

After facing continuous criticism for several decades, it is worth noting that the British system has actually fared well. It gains high marks for affordability since the United Kingdom has now maintained the lowest percentage of GDP devoted to health among the major industrialized countries. The system also gets reasonably good marks for access and accountability. The major public health indicators (infant mortality and life expectancy) for the United Kingdom are quite comparable with countries that spend nearly twice as much on health care. However, there are serious problems. First, satisfaction with health care is very low. The system is not "user friendly" and public opinion polls suggest that the British want alternatives to their current health care. By the early 1990s it became apparent that the British system needed revision and that market-based alternatives got the nod. New policies in the United Kingdom now allow general practitioners to purchase services from hospitals and specialists. The general practitioners control funds and they can allocate their own budget in order to maximize benefits for their patients. This new system stimulates competition between hospitals and between specialists (Vall-Spinosa, 1991).

The option of completely socializing medicine has few serious advocates. Where it has been tried, such as in the United Kingdom, it has not worked well. In fact, health care reform is now one of the major political issues in Britain. Thus, the British system should not be considered a truly viable alternative.

Medical Associations Know Most about Health Care— Get Government off Their Backs!

A third simplistic solution is to trust organized medicine. Advocates for this position suggest that doctors know most about medicine. They argue that, after all, doctors are honest, well educated, and intelligent. They have chosen the profession because they care about people.

Unfortunately, trusting medical associations helped create the current predicament. Medical trade associations have been extremely influential in shaping the system we now have. The increase in the percentage of GNP devoted to health care is no accident. Persuasive lobbies have supported legislation that allowed reimbursement for a wide variety of medical procedures. Although medical organizations have argued for increased access, they have consistently resisted attempts to control costs or to improve accountability.

The Whole Problem Is Caused by Lawyers—Indemnify Doctors against Malpractice!

A commonly held belief is that lawyers drive the escalation in health care costs. Physicians, fearing malpractice suits, order many unnecessary tests. Thus, it has been suggested that simply limiting malpractice claims would reduce unnecessary expenditures.

Public opinion polls show that lawyers are among the most disliked groups in contemporary society. Certainly, blaming the whole problem on them is appealing. Further, there is at least some reason to believe that fear of malpractice litigation does accelerate costs. On the other hand, attempts to demonstrate that malpractice claims are a major factor in health care costs have not been persuasive. The total cost of malpractice litigation is hard to estimate. Newer evidence suggests that the rapid increase in malpractice claims peaked in the 1970s and 1980s and has now leveled off. Malpractice premiums cannot be blamed as the major cause of health care cost inflation. Total costs for insurance premiums are estimated to be about $7 billion, which is only about 1% of American health care expenditures (Weiler & Brennan, 1990).

Insurance costs probably do not tell the entire story. It is commonly argued that excessive test ordering is "defensive medicine" stimulated by fear of litigation. However, research evidence challenges the notion that excessive test ordering is primarily driven by fear of being sued. Clearly there are other incentives for detailed work-ups. For example, studies have demonstrated that doctors order more tests when they have a financial interest in the laboratories that perform them (Hillman et al., 1989). Some studies have found that there is a financial incentive for those who overuse tests. When there is no longer a financial incentive to order tests or procedures, the use of services promptly declines (Hillman et al., 1989). These results do not support the position that the doctor–patient relationship should remain uninterrupted. In fact, factors other than the patient's best interest appear to determine the use of some services.

It is often assumed that patients and lawyers are "malpractice crazy." Poorly grounded lawsuits do get filed. However, analyses suggest that many legitimate claims are never pursued. One study matched medical records from a random sample of 31,429 patients who had been hospitalized in New York with data on medical malpractice claims. Using this technique, it was possible to identify patients who had made claims against physicians or hospitals. The medical record file allowed examination of the incidence of injuries to patients that may have been caused by medical mismanagement. With this system, the investigators were able to determine how many patients who had been mistreated actually filed malpractice litigation. The study identified 280 patients who had suffered adverse events as a result of medical negligence. Among these, only 8 filed malpractice claims. In other words, 1.53% of those who had legitimate complaints actually filed malpractice lawsuits. On the other hand, many malpractice suits do not arise from strict medical negligence. Overall, the authors of this study concluded that most patients who suffer as a result of medical malpractice are not compensated. Further, the malpractice system does a poor job of holding providers accountable for offering poor medical care (Localio et al., 1991).

It might also be argued that fear of litigation has a positive impact on accountability. Fear of malpractice litigation may also stimulate physicians to perform well. Although extremely crude, the tort system does force a certain level of responsibility.

There Is Too Much Management in Health Care—Cut Administrative Costs.

Steffie Woolhandler and David Himmelstein describe American medicine as a "spectator sport." Patients along with their doctors and other providers stand in the arena and are observed by an increasing number of cost-containment experts, health care managers, and public administrators. In 1983, administrators in American medicine used 60% more resources than their colleagues in Canada and 97% more than health care administrators in Great Britain. Figure 2.5 summarizes the growth in administrative costs between 1970 and 1987. The figure suggests that the percentage increase for administration is severely out of line with the percentage increase for physician services. In 1987, the per capita expenditure for insurance administration was $106 in the United States, while in Canada it was $17. One estimate of total health care cost devoted to health care administration in the United States was $497 million in comparison to $156 million in Canada (Woolhandler & Himmelstein, 1991). Much of the cost might be attributed to waste (or administrative inefficiency) in the insurance industry. For example, Blue Cross/Blue Shield of Massachusetts provides insurance for 2.7 million subscribers. In order to administer the program they employ 6682 workers. This is more than all of the employees of the Canadian Provisional Health Plans, which provide

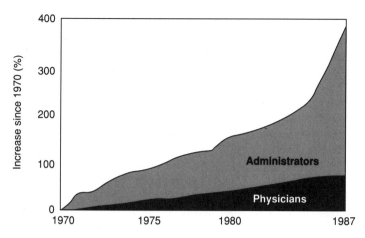

Figure 2.5 Growth in the number of physicians and health care administrators between 1970 and 1987. (From Woolhandler & Himmelstein, 1991.)

coverage to 25 million people. Comparable service to that provided to a larger number of Canadian residents in British Columbia is delivered by only 435 Prudential employees. According to this analysis, the solution to the problem is to get rid of insurance companies.

Clearly we cannot call this a "simplistic" solution. Administrative costs in American medicine are embarrassing and, as we will see in the next chapter, a move toward a universal payer system is very appealing. However, the belief that a move toward a Canadian system will resolve the major problems is not supported by all the evidence. For example, the problem of small-area variation in the use of services is more pronounced in some areas of Canada than it is in the United States (Fedson et al., 1992; Roos, 1989; Roos et al., 1990). The focus of attention on administrators does not do justice to the differential in physician pay. Doctors would like to blame administrators for all the problems while, in reality, it appears that the blame should be split between administrators and others. For example, a detailed analysis by Fuchs & Hahn (1990) found that the higher per capita spending on health care in the United States is largely attributed to physician fees. When carefully evaluated, it appeared that the quality of physician services per capita was actually better in Canada than in the United States, and fees for procedures were more than three times higher in the United States. Despite charging more money for individual services, however, net incomes for physicians were only about one-third higher in the United States than in Canada. This suggests that Canadian physicians respond to the lower fee structure by increasing their activity. This may be good because the universal access allows more patients to obtain more attention.

The major concerns about the Canadian system are that its costs are increasing. In fact, evaluation of Fig. 1.6 shows that Canada is among the countries experiencing rapid increases in the costs of health care. There are incentives for physicians to increase the use of procedures; placing controls on these will require more administrators. In 1987, the per capita health care costs in Canada were $1483, which was second among nations reporting to OECD (the United States was first at $2051). Like the United States, Canada has an expanding national debt and there will be increased pressures to reduce health care costs in order to address general fiscal problems. We will return to the issues involving the use of a central payer in the next chapter.

Table 2.1 summarizes some of the simple solutions as evaluated against the three principles of affordability, access, and accountability.

As Table 2.1 suggests, none of these solutions does well in jointly addressing the three concerns of affordability, access, and accountability. These solutions will not work because each addresses only one part of a three-component problem. In the next section we will look at several strategies that have been implemented to control costs. It is worth noting that problems in the health care system have stimulated experimentation in alternative solutions. This is one field in which ideas translate into practice quickly. As we will see, new ideas such as prospective payment through diagnostic-related groups (DRGs) and resource-based relative value scaling (RBRVS) often become national policy shortly after having been introduced.

THE ALPHABET SOUP OF POLICIES TO CONTROL COSTS

During the 1980s there was a variety of innovative experiments designed to control the rising costs of health care. These included the prospective payment

TABLE 2.1			
Summary of Simple Solutions as They Address Affordability, Access, and Accountability[a]			
Solution	Affordability	Access	Accountability
Increase spending	−	+	−/0
Increase taxes	−	+	−/0
Nationalize hospitals/doctors	+	0/+	−
Trust medical associations	−	−	−
Indemnify doctors	0/+	0	−
Eliminate administrators	0/+	0	−

[a]+, improves problems; 0, has no effect; −, may negatively impact problem.

system (PPS), which included reimbursement by DRGs. In addition, there was a growth of health maintenance organizations (HMOs) and preferred provider organizations (PPOs). More recently there have been proposals for changing the way physicians are reimbursed and basing these payments on RBRVS. The next sections, besides providing a guide to the acronyms, will review several of these experiments.

Prospective Payment System/Diagnosis-Related Groups

Prior to the enactment of Medicare in 1965, hospitals were reimbursed by Blue Cross on the basis of their cost. Essentially, hospital costs were passed through to third-party payers. The payers were either private insurance companies or the federal government. Until October of 1983, hospitals were allowed to bill for "reasonable costs." Many believe that this system provided hospitals with a license to steal. Whatever the motivation, the system permitted remarkable increases in hospital expenditures.

The Reagan administration, disturbed by the high costs of hospital care, adopted a new system of hospital reimbursement based largely on the ideas of Robert Fetter, a Yale professor (Fetter et al., 1980). This new Medicare payment approach, known as the prospective payment system (PPS), became effective on October 1, 1983. The system established rates of payment to hospitals based on medical diagnoses. Under this system, hospitals were paid a prospectively determined rate for each of 468 DRGs. The DRGs were based on estimates of the median length of hospital stay for each diagnosis. The rate for the DRG covers operating costs, exclusive of unusual outlier patients. The DRG covers capital-related costs, medical education costs, kidney acquisition costs, and bad debts. The major determiner of the reimbursement is the median length of stay for each condition. Under the previous system, hospitals were rewarded for keeping patients in house for a long time. The PPS created an incentive to discharge patients early since the hospital would be reimbursed the same amount for either a short or a long stay. The DRG payment system does allow for local adjustments. For example, the system takes into consideration the wages in a particular area, the number of resident physicians in training, and the hospital's location. The 468 DRGs were developed on the basis of detailed analysis of the cases treated, the patient's age, sex, and treatment procedure, and the usual length of stay. The PPS came with a variety of safeguards including peer review organizations (PROs) that review diagnoses, quality of care, appropriateness of admissions, and the handling of unusual cases. In addition, a prospective payment assessment committee (PROPAC) was created through the Congressional Office of Technology Assessment. PROPAC advises on the implementation of the system and recalibrates DRG payments based on new information.

The early analyses of the DRG system suggested that it was very effective. The early analysts, however, also expressed great fears that, although the system reduced cost, it consequently restricted access to care and resulted in poor health outcomes. The hospital industry made massive cuts in personnel and began aggressively bargaining with various suppliers and labor negotiators (Ries, 1990).

The cost savings realized through the PPS were met with significant complaints about effects upon patients. For example, one group of investigators suggested that patients with hip fractures received fewer inpatient services and eventually had poorer health outcomes. These patients were more likely to be sent to nursing homes and to stay there longer than patients with the same condition prior to the 1983 implementation of the PPS (Fitzgerald et al., 1988). While in the hospital, patients may receive fewer services than prior to the PPS. Although the intensity of care may be greater, this does not compensate for shorter length of stay (Palmer et al., 1989).

Although the initial promise for cutting health care costs with the PPS was great, newer analyses suggest that PPS will not resolve the major problems in the health care system. Figure 2.6 summarizes the number of inpatient days from 1982 through 1988. Schwartz & Mendelson (1991) analyzed data from the American Hospital Association and the Health Care Financing Administration to determine the rates of change in inpatient hospital use in this period. Between 1982 and 1988 there was a 28% decrease in the number of hospital inpatient days. This trend was sharpest in 1984 and 1985 after the implementation of the PPS. However, by 1988 there was virtually no further reduction in the total number of inpatient hospital days. The decreased number of inpatient hospital days was partially offset by increases in outpatient services. Overall, the underlying rate of increase in health care costs was not greatly affected by the implementation of the PPS.

The PPS was designed to restrict Medicare spending. This was necessary because Medicare spending was increasing by 9.2% per year between 1976 and 1982, while non-Medicare expenses were rising at about half that rate. The implementation of the PPS slowed the rate of spending on Medicare patients to

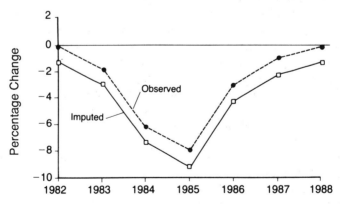

Figure 2.6 Observed and imputed reduction in the number of inpatient days per year, 1982–1988. (From Schwartz & Mendelson, 1991.)

.6% per year. However, as a consequence, non-Medicare spending rose by 9%. Shorter stays do reduce hospital costs. However, there are fixed costs of hospital admissions, including administrative time, insurance, and costs associated with the admission. At the margin, reducing hospital days does not linearly reduce costs. Schwartz and Mendelson estimate that the cost of days saved was only about 65% of the average patient day.

In summary, the PPS had some effect on cost. However, it may have had a negative impact on access, and effects on outcome have been largely unstudied. Many have argued that the PPS damaged patients. However, the few systematic studies that have examined the issue indicate that the system has not adversely affected patients (Rogers et al., 1990).

Managed Care in Health Maintenance Organizations

Health maintenance organizations provide all care for patients based on a flat fee. HMOs have been of great interest because the financial incentives are the reverse of those in traditional fee-for-service medicine. In HMOs there is an incentive to provide less care. The exception is when avoidance of care results in a preventable complication or a serious illness that is more expensive for the program.

Health maintenance organizations have been highly encouraged by the federal government. In 1973 the Health Maintenance Organization Act made formal grants available to HMOs. The compelling argument behind HMOs was that they would lower cost and increase efficiency. HMOs are appealing because they have the capability of lowering costs and improving accountability. During the Reagan administration there was continued acknowledgement of HMOs, but the grant and loan program was set aside and replaced with encouragement to increase private investment in these organizations (Luft, 1985).

Health maintenance organizations have been very successful, as evidenced by their remarkable growth. In California, HMO users grew from 8.3% of all hospital admissions in 1983 to nearly 17% in 1988 (Robinson, 1991). However, there have also been concerns. For example, some have suggested that HMOs "skim" by encouraging enrollment among healthier individuals and discouraging participation by those with serious diseases (Jackson-Beck & Kleinman, 1983). The success of HMOs may have also helped in other ways to control costs. Because they are important alternative selections among employees, HMOs have forced competition among other health plans and thus may have lowered costs (Enthoven, 1980, 1991).

Despite the attractiveness of HMOs, they may not provide the ultimate solution to the health care problem. In California for example, the large expansion in HMOs did increase competition in the mid-1980s. Nevertheless, analysis suggests that their effect has been modest, since hospital cost inflation rose by 74.5% during these years (Robinson, 1991). Several other problems suggest that HMOs will not provide the ultimate solution. First, HMOs are not attractive to everyone because they limit consumer choice. HMOs also differ considerably in the contractual agreements they offer to providers. The incentive structure in HMOs has recently become the focus of some very interesting investigations. For example, Hillman (1990) compared HMOs that offered different financial incentives for their providers. Physicians who are salaried and who do not receive extra income from hospitalizing their patients tend to send their patients to the hospital less often. There have also been studies of situations in which primary-care physicians have a fixed sum that can be used to pay for patient referrals and there is a financial disincentive for physicians to overexpend the money. Under these circumstances, fewer patients are referred to specialists or for special evaluative tests.

Many HMOs allow physicians to be partners in the business. However, there is growing evidence that financial conflicts of interest do not always benefit patients. One of the best illustrations of this was recently reported by Bruce Hillman and colleagues at the University of Arizona (Hillman et al., 1990). These investigators compared the use of radiographic imaging for patients with four conditions: acute upper respiratory symptoms (URI), pregnancy, low back pain, and male difficulty in urinating. Using private insurance claims data, the investigators compared costs based on physicians who owned their own imaging equipment (self-referring) and those who did not own equipment and who referred their patients to radiologists (radiologist-referring). Figure 2.7 summarizes the charges per episode of care for self-referring and radiologist-referring physicians. As the figure shows, there were substantial discrepancies. In fact, the charges were 7.5 times higher for obstetrical ultrasonography when the physician self-referred. Among the four procedures that were considered, the lowest ratio in cost differ-

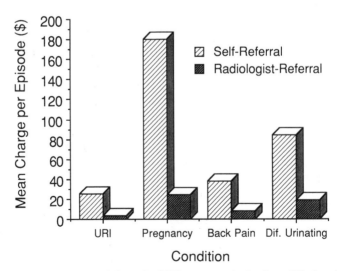

Figure 2.7 Charges per episode of diagnosis of URI, pregnancy, back pain, or difficulty urinating for self-referred and radiologist-referred patients. (Adapted from Hillman et al., 1990.)

ence was for evaluating men who had difficulty urinating. Here, charges for self-referring physicians were 4.4 times greater than for physicians that referred to radiologists. Costs for evaluating upper respiratory symptoms were 6.2 times higher, while those for low back pain were 4.8 times higher. These and similar studies in the literature raise important questions about the impact of financial incentives. One report developed for the Florida state legislature suggested that 40% of the doctors in Florida (an estimated 7600 physicians) have an interest in a free-standing facility to which they refer patients. Concerned about these apparent conflicts of interest, the AMA Council on Ethical and Judicial Affairs issued a statement in September of 1991 warning physicians about the potential problems associated with self-referral (Inglehart, 1991). Overall, the incentive structures in HMOs reduce the likelihood of abuse. The HMO solution does address costs but is neutral with regard to access. The effect of HMOs on outcomes has been addressed in relatively few studies.

Resource-Based Relative Value Scaling

The majority of cost-containment policies have been directed toward hospitals. In 1991 a new policy was introduced to directly affect physician payments. This strategy is known as resource-based relative value scaling (RBRVS). One of the difficulties in reimbursing physicians is that specialists with approximately the same years of training are paid differently depending on what they do. An ophthalmologist, for example, may get reimbursed $2500 to conduct a 15-minute cataract extraction with lens replacement. A medical school classmate who became a pediatrician may only get reimbursed $40 to devote the same amount of time to the physical examination of a sick child. The years and intensity of training for these physicians might be quite comparable.

A study suggested that five characteristics are closely related to the resource costs of patient visits. These are (1) the time the physician spends with patients; (2) the site of service; (3) whether the patient is referred from another physician; (4) whether the patient is established or is there for a first encounter; and (5) whether or not the care is continuing or physician initiated.

The RBRVS approach is to be taken very seriously. In 1989 as part of the Omnibus Budget Reconciliation Act, Congress appointed a Physician Payment Review Commission (PPRC) in order to overhaul the Medicare fee schedule. Under the current Medicare program, physicians are reimbursed according to current procedural terminology (CPT) codes for evaluation and management services. Some physician groups have been concerned because they are underpaid for their services relative to their colleagues in other specialties. Further, physicians in different locations use the CPT codes quite differently. This has led to inequitable payment and may be responsible for some cost escalation.

Because of these concerns, the PPRC decided to adopt a methodology originally proposed by William Hsaio, a health services researcher at Harvard University (Hsaio et al., 1990). The methodology uses physician judges to estimate the amount of work required to perform different medical services. Overall, the amount of work required is largely a function of the number of minutes a patient encounter lasts. Although various components of service do affect the predicted amount of work, the amount of time required is the major driving force in the total work estimated by these physician judges. Figure 2.8 shows a comparison between follow-up consultation, established patient office visit, and subsequent hospital visit ratings of estimated total work. Follow-up consultations are regarded as about 6 units of work greater than office visits for established patients in a 15-minute encounter and 15 units work greater for a 30-minute consultation.

The RBRVS system is an attempt to "level the playing field." It is estimated that the system will increase payments to general practitioners and family physicians by as much as 34%. Payments to thoracic surgeons are expected to decrease by about 26% (Eisenberg, 1991). As might be expected, the concept is warmly endorsed by primary care physicians and aggressively challenged by technical subspecialists.

One of the major concerns about RBRVS is that it may not result in significant cost reductions. Total costs are a product of unit cost (physician fee) and volume (number of patients or procedures). One possible reaction is that physicians will respond to reductions in unit cost by increasing volume. To counteract this force, Medicare has proposed volume performance standards and increases in volume will be carefully monitored.

RBRVS was not taken lightly by medical groups. Before implementing the

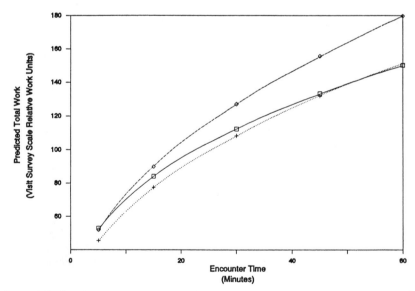

Figure 2.8 Relationship between encounter time and total work for follow-up consultations (◊), established patient office visits (□), and subsequent hospital visits (+). (From Lasker et al., 1991.)

system, the HCFA invited public comment. In response to this request, it received more than 95,000 responses. That exceeded its previous high of 60,000. Many physicians were irate, suggesting that the system was "inherently socialistic" because it reimbursed for time and effort rather than for value to the patient (*Medical World News,* September 2, 1991). There were also methodological complaints. For example, Maloney (1991) analyzed RBRVS codes and concluded that surgical services would be paid less per hour than would evaluation and management services. However, Maloney's conclusions have been seriously challenged. Apparently, Maloney used physician salary estimates based on university resident physicians and salaried physicians in academic settings. These work schedules are not at all representative of American physicians in general and, when used to estimate wage per hour, give incorrect results. Several published critiques of Maloney's work support the original RBRVS finding that procedure-oriented practices generate significantly more income than consultation services (Hsaio et al., 1992; Radecki et al., 1992). However, even some insiders were concerned about the final product. For example, Phillip Lee, who headed the PPRC ultimately challenged the final fee schedule (Lee & Ginsburg, 1991).

The RBRVS system was implemented on January 1, 1992. It is expected to reduce costs of physician services. The program will have no effect on access since it is directed exclusively toward Medicare. Further, the program is not designed to have an impact upon outcomes.

Utilization Review

Another approach is utilization review (UR). The purpose of UR is to reduce inappropriate hospital care through second opinions or through professional review of physician practices. It is suggested that at least 10–20% of hospital admissions are inappropriate. Utilization review might involve several different activities including preadmission certification, concurrent review, and or a retrospective review of admissions. Utilization review was first implemented in 1972 through Public Law 92-603. It created professional standards review organizations (PSROs) that monitored payments to hospitals under the Medicare and Medicaid programs. In recent years, UR has expanded and it is now commonly used in the private insurance sector. Most evidence suggests that UR has been at least partially successful in reducing hospital use. However, a detailed review of the literature by Wickizer (1990) noted that impact of UR upon costs has been less clear. Further, Wickizer was unable to conclude that UR enhanced patient outcome.

SUMMARY

In this chapter we have considered a variety of different approaches to the troubling problems in American health care. The solutions to the problems are sometimes overly simplistic. It is difficult to attribute the problems exclusively to lawyers, physician groups, or administrators. Major policy interventions have focused almost exclusively on the cost side. Policies such as PPS and RBRVS address cost regulation but do not specifically consider the issues of access or outcome. Furthermore, most of these programs are directed only at the Medicare program, for which access is not a major problem. In the next chapter we will consider some current proposals for resolving the American health care crisis.

CHAPTER THREE

Review of Current Proposals

It seems that everyone has a suggestion for how to resolve our health care crisis. The last chapter considered simple solutions and reviewed solutions that focus on cost. This chapter provides a brief overview of several of the national health insurance proposals that are currently under consideration. These proposals are considered as background for a general health policy model that will be introduced in Chapter Four.

A DOZEN SOLUTIONS

A single solution to the problem would be welcomed. However, at least a dozen different solutions have already been introduced to the Congress and it is likely that several other alternatives will be offered in the coming sessions. The proposers come from all angles of the political spectrum. They include those on the far left and those on the far right as well as a substantial number of proposals from the middle. The groups backing bills range from the American Medical Association and the American Hospital Association to specific politicians and political groups such as the American Heritage Foundation. In the following pages we will briefly consider some of the proposals. We start with the proposals further to the right and move through the political spectrum to those emphasizing more fundamental social reform.

The Heritage Foundation

Perhaps the most conservative approach has been recommended by the Heritage Foundation. This plan is based on an overhaul of the tax structure. The major premise behind this plan is that underinsurance in the United States results from the tax exclusion for company-provided health care plans. The Heritage Foundation plan calls for an elimination of the tax exclusion for health insurance. In its place, the Foundation would support refundable tax credits for those who purchase health insurance and pay their own medical expenses.

The vast majority of Americans receive health insurance through their employers (see Fig. 3.1). Employers provide health insurance as a pre-tax benefit. Resources that are used to attract employees are divided into wages and benefits so that the package looks attractive to employees. By shifting the proportion of wages that the employee would pay for health care to a benefit the employee receives health insurance without having to pay tax on this portion of his or her wage (Butler, 1991). Estimates suggest that the federal government loses considerable revenue by allowing pre-tax insurance benefits. If health insurance benefits were reported as income and taxed, the yield to the federal government could exceed $50 billion per year. This could almost cover federal contributions to Medicaid.

The American Heritage Foundation believes that the tax exclusion for company-based health insurance causes several problems. For example, they argue that the current system is inequitable. Highly paid employees receive substantial benefits while low-income employees, who do not earn enough to pay taxes, do not receive any benefits. A second problem is that the current system provides a disincentive to change jobs because some employees may have difficulties obtaining insurance, particularly those with preexisting medical conditions. A third concern is that, under the current system, employees have little incentive to be conscientious consumers of care. Since their employer is paying the bill, the system encourages waste and this ultimately results in health care cost inflation.

There are two basic principles of the Heritage Foundation proposal. The first is to replace the tax exclusion with a new system of refundable tax credits for health care. These tax credits would be adjustable and would accelerate as higher percentages of the family income are devoted to health care. The second provision of the proposal is to establish a health care social contract. Under this contract, the

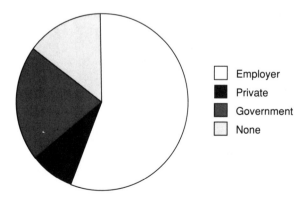

Figure 3.1 Health insurance payment sources. (Adapted from Enthoven & Kronick, 1989.)

head of household would be required to provide health insurance for all family members. The health insurance would include the minimum basic benefits package. Catastrophic insurance for all who accept the contract would prevent extreme losses in the event of serious illness. The social contract would consider differences in income. Low-income families would be eligible for more government assistance. Framers of the plan believe that it would reduce health care costs. The plan would create greater competition and the consumer decision making might drastically reduce the administrative costs because inefficient insurers would not be selected. The plan also provides greater autonomy to consumers. There would be an incentive for many different insurers to join the competition and the ordinary consumer would have many options.

There are also some serious concerns about the Heritage Foundation proposal. For example, the proposed system would make the access problem worse. Despite credits for low-income individuals, it is highly likely that there will be great disparities in access. High-income individuals may be more likely to use their resources to purchase good quality health care even though they get a lesser tax credit. Low-income and less engaged individuals may not recognize that insurance is a wise investment and may not participate.

One of the major concerns with the Heritage Foundation proposal is that it will cause adverse selection. Well individuals or those without chronic illnesses will be able to purchase lower-cost insurance than those who have the misfortune of a chronic disease. The Heritage Foundation argues that there could be a cross-subsidy that allows those with high health care expenses to obtain a greater tax write-off. Yet the proposal provides little assurance to those unfortunate enough to be limited in income because of their illnesses. Another major problem is that the proposal does not provide for long-term care. Purchase of long-term care insurance is left to the discretion of the consumer. Those with fewer resources would be less likely to obtain this type of coverage. Overall, the Heritage Foundation proposal may reduce costs. It claims to increase access or at least be neutral with regard to access. However, the effect on *equal* access should be reviewed. Our most important concern is that the proposal does not address outcome and is likely to have either adverse effects or no impact upon health status.

U.S. Chamber of Commerce

The U.S. Chamber of Commerce has opposed employer-mandated health insurance programs. Their argument is that these programs would cripple business. The Chamber estimates that employer-mandated programs would put 3.3 million people out of work. Employers are simply unable to afford premiums and remain competitive. The Chamber of Commerce also opposes the notion of "pay or play." The pay-or-play provision is common in several of the proposals discussed below. Under these rules, a small company must provide coverage for its employees (play) or pay into a pool that would be used to cover the uninsured.

The Chamber of Commerce does not have a specific proposal to remedy any of the major problems. They favor an "incentive/competition approach." However, this remedy is not clearly defined and, whatever form it takes, would be phased in over the course of time.

The American Medical Association

The American Medical Association has now proposed its own solution. The proposal is complex, with 6 fundamental principles and 16 key points. The 6 principles of the AMA proposal are summarized in Table 3.1.

The proposal retains private insurance companies. However, the key provision of the proposal is that it creates state risk pools to cover those who are difficult to insure. The proposal would expand Medicaid coverage to all people below the poverty line. Currently, the poverty line is about $12,700 for a family of four. Nationwide, only about 40% of those below the poverty line are now covered by Medicaid programs.

The AMA proposal maintains employers as the basic sponsor of health insurance. It emphasizes that 26 million of the approximately 33 million individuals who currently do not have health insurance are working or are from families with a working head of household. In order to confront this problem, the proposal creates risk pools so that small businesses and new businesses can afford the cost of coverage. Risk pools are necessary because the cost of a single high-risk employee (i.e., someone with diabetes or heart disease) can make insurance costs to a small business unaffordable. Pooling costs across businesses spreads the risk and reduces cost. There would be a 100% tax credit for people who obtain their health insurance through the risk pool.

TABLE 3.1

Six Principles of the AMA Proposal[a]

1. Improvements to the American health care system should preserve the strengths of our current system.
2. Affordable coverage for appropriate health care should be available to all Americans regardless of income.
3. Particular efforts are needed to assure continued access by the elderly to affordable health care services.
4. Health care services should be designed with high quality at appropriate costs.
5. Patients should be free to determine from whom and the manner in which health care benefits are delivered.
6. All physicians should be committed to the highest ethical standards in the delivery of care to the patients.

[a]Adapted from Todd et al. (1991).

There are many attractive features to the AMA proposal. For example, it provides universal access and it represents a concern for quality health care. However, this is clearly a medicine-sponsored proposal. For example, it provides many provisions that reinforce the current system. The AMA emphasizes that it is "better to build on a system that is currently serving effectively the vast majority of the nation's population" (Todd et al., 1991).

One of the key issues in the AMA proposal is the requirement for federal reform of medical malpractice awards. On the assumption that medical malpractice has a detrimental effect on health care costs, the AMA proposal would cap malpractice awards to patients. The AMA proposal downplays the role of physicians and hospitals in the accelerating costs of health care. Instead, the proposal is designed to alter the practices of patients, attorneys, and insurance companies. The only modification of physician practice that the proposal recognizes is development of practice parameters or guidelines. However, the AMA describes these only as nonbinding recommendations for physician practice and underscores the physician's right to use a range of procedures in a given case.

The AMA proposal would probably have little effect upon health care costs. They report preliminary actuarial studies showing that the cost to the federal government would be about $21 billion. This might be less than that required by other proposals (see below) but would clearly not provide any cost savings. The AMA proposal would increase access. In fact, physicians would benefit by having a larger pool of insured patients to treat. However, the proposal does exclude nonpoor nonworkers (Blendon & Edwards, 1991). The American Public Health Association gives the program moderately positive marks for quality control and efficiency, but poor evaluation for promoting health and preventing disease (American Public Health Association, 1991). The proposal must be regarded as relatively weak in its emphasis on improving health outcomes. Overall, the AMA proposal is not a strong one in terms of the three goals of cost containment, access, and improved outcomes.

The Pepper Commission

In September of 1990 a bipartisan commission on comprehensive health care examined the health care crisis in the United States. The inquiry, known as the Pepper Commission, was created by the Medicare Catastrophic Coverage Act of 1988. There were 12 representatives on the Commission, with 6 from the House and 6 from the Senate. In addition, there were 3 presidential appointees. The charge to the Commission was very general. The group was supposed to examine the problems of the American health care system and to develop recommendations for new legislation that would provide a remedy. The Commission conducted hearings in a variety of different locations and heard from numerous witnesses. They were given expert briefings and provided with a mass of information.

The Pepper Commission must be considered the most thorough investigation of health care problems in the United States. The Commissioner's final report to

Congress is a very important document that must be carefully considered by anyone proposing a potential remedy ("A Call for Action," 1990). The key elements of the Pepper Commission's "blueprint for reform" are summarized in Table 3.2.

The four components of the plan emphasize that health insurance must be available to all and that fundamental reform is required in order to achieve this objective. The Commission did not endorse a Canadian-like system and preferred that the large fundamental reform be some alteration of the current system. Further, the Commission recognized the importance of cost containment and pledged to coordinate expanded access with cost control (Rockefeller, 1991).

In order to accomplish these objectives, the Pepper Commission recommended that employers provide health insurance to all employees and dependents. There would be a grace period and tax credits for companies that employed fewer than 100 persons. The current Medicaid program would be disassembled and replaced with another public program that would cover all people who do not get health insurance through work or through Medicare. Several aspects of the plan are directed at containing costs. Cost controls would include copayments and deductibles. Individuals would pay more out of their pocket for health care but there would be adjustments based on income. Cost control would also be achieved through the encouragement of managed care and health maintenance organizations. This would be achieved by requiring that insurers offering managed care to large businesses also offer it to smaller businesses. Small businesses would be guaranteed state-mandated rates without facing the risk associated with having employees with preexisting conditions. The Commission recommended that small businesses be monitored for 4 to 5 years. If, after that period, they do not cover at least 80% of those who now lack insurance, the Commission recommends intervening and requiring small businesses to purchase insurance coverage as large businesses would be required to do.

The Pepper Commission recognized problems associated with health care quality. They recommended several programs that would assist consumers to become better consumers of health care. The Commission specifically recom-

---

TABLE 3.2

Key Findings of the Pepper Commission

1. Health insurance coverage must be universal.
2. Universal coverage cannot be achieved through modification of the existing Medicaid program.
3. Replacing the current system with a government-run national health insurer program is not practical.
4. Cost control must go hand in hand with expanded access.

mended outcomes research and the development of practice guidelines to help both public and private consumers make better choices.

The Pepper Commission also attempted to take working pieces from previous reforms. For example, the Commission recognized problems associated with malpractice but did not have a specific malpractice solution. Instead, they recommended that the Physician Payment Review Commission (PPRC) (Chapter Two) and the Prospective Payment Assessment Commission (PROPAC) (Chapter Two) take responsibility for overseeing cost containment. These commissions have proposed useful policies for Medicare recipients. Under the Pepper Commission plan these agencies would have authority to oversee all aspects of health care.

The supporters of the Pepper Commission plan believe that their proposal is affordable (Rockefeller, 1990). The Commission suggested that the plan could be enacted for less than 2% more than current expenditures on health care. The 1990 estimate was used to suggest that the nation's health care expenditures would rise from $647 billion to $659 billion—an increase of $12 billion. The largest share of these costs would be paid by employers and government. However, the Commission suggested that employers would save $13 billion because they would no longer have to pay the cost of double-insured dependents. The Commission also suggested that families and individuals would save $19 billion by transferring their expenditures to employers and government. Seven billion dollars in payments, the amount currently spent to cover the uninsured who are not in Medicaid, would be saved by the states. The extra costs would be made up by employers who are not currently offering health insurance. Revenues of $28 billion would be raised from these employers. The Commission has argued that this would only be about 4% of payroll taxes after employers received credits from taxes.

Do these numbers add up? Although legislation based on the Pepper Commission is being introduced, there are some serious critics. Even some of the Commission members could not stand behind cost estimates and many believe that the Commission does not offer a practical way to manage costs. The plan receives poor marks for affordability but good marks for access. With regard to accountability, the plan has potential for relating treatment to outcome. However, the specifics of how this might be accomplished were not provided. Thus, the rating for accountability remains neutral.

The Stark Proposal

One of the best developed plans has been offered by Representative Fortney (Pete) Stark. This California Democrat essentially proposed to extend the Medicare program to all individuals. Stark's plan, known as MediPlan, would go beyond Medicare by providing a single public insurance company that would provide basic benefits and long-term care for all individuals. Stark, recognizing the success of the Canadian plan, argues that only a single payer can assure that every American will get basic health care services. Two different bills have been introduced by Stark (HR 2530 and HR 651). One bill raises revenue by creating a

MediPlan Trust Fund of $1000 per person per year. These funds would be contributed by employers (80%) and by individuals (20%). The alternative bill raises revenues through a 2% tax of gross income. Stark argued that the plan recommended by the Pepper Commission did not go far enough. In particular, he voiced concern that too many people would be left out in employer-based systems. In the Stark plan accountability would be achieved through the control of the single payer. The system would impose cost controls on doctors and hospitals by refusing to pay inappropriate charges.

The Stark plan would significantly increase access. It would also improve accountability, but there is no specific provision that it would improve health outcomes. One of the major concerns with the Stark proposal is its cost. Early estimates suggest that the plan would require $120 billion to be gathered from new taxes. This high cost estimate makes its implementation somewhat unlikely.

Physicians Who Care Plan

In contrast to disassembling the insurance system, another physician-based plan attempts to keep the current insurance system intact. This plan, known as the Physicians Who Care Plan (Bronow et al., 1991), attempts to improve upon the current system of multiple insurers.

The Physicians Who Care Plan has five components. First, it would include universal employer-based insurance with high deductibles. There would be protection to keep rates down and to protect those with preexisting conditions from exclusion. The plan would also emphasize a high deductible as a mechanism for controlling costs. A second component of the plan is the development of "medisave" accounts. Workers would be able to pay into special accounts that could be used to pay for deductibles or for uncovered medical expenses. These accounts would be created from pre-tax dollars. The third component of the plan would increase Medicare funding. The mechanism for doing so would be unique. The plan calls for partially funding Medicare through Individual Retirement Accounts (IRAs). These IRAs would be a required purchase for each child during the first year of life. An IRA that costs $125 and earns 10% interest would produce $65,000 by the time a person reaches Medicare eligibility. The fourth component of the plan is to revamp Medicaid. The plan suggests that Medicaid will not cover long-term care (that would be covered elsewhere) but instead will focus on health care problems of the poor. The program would cover everyone below the poverty line with an opportunity for those just above the poverty level to purchase income-related health insurance. The final provision of the plan calls for the development of scientific guidelines for practice.

Although the plan is an interesting one, very few of the details have been worked through. Further, it is not certain that the requirement of an IRA purchase for infants is either practical or realistic. The plan fails to recognize that $125 invested at birth does not equal $65,000 in *real* dollars at Medicare age. This assumption ignores opportunity costs and does not take inflation into consideration. Further, the guaranteed 10% annual interest rate may not be realistic. Even if there was a mechanism for financing health care, the $65,000 would still be spent in other areas. Thus, the plan does not control costs.

Realistically the plan may do little to enhance access. The plan does consider mandatory insurance but apparently has few teeth to ensure that the IRAs and insurance will actually be purchased. One of the most serious concerns is with the accountability, although the plan does call for the development of practice guidelines. The group also emphasizes that only physicians can decide how medicine should be practiced. It provides no specific mechanism for creating guidelines and it emphasizes that there should be local validation in the implementation of practice protocols. This almost assures that there will be continuing small-area variation in the use of services. Overall, the Physicians Who Care Plan is interesting but unlikely to become a major health policy contender.

USHealth Act

The USHealth Act was first proposed by House of Representatives Congressman Edward R. Roybal in 1986. The goal of USHealth is to provide catastrophic and basic health protection for all Americans regardless of age, income, or health status. The plan would be administered by a new federal agency known as the USHealth Administration which would replace the current Health Care Financing Administration (HCFA). Under the plan, Medicare, Medicaid, and private insurance would be consolidated into a single system. The system would be funded by cost sharing, employer contributions, state assessments, and federal resources obtained from income taxes. In addition, premiums would be collected from beneficiaries. The plan makes good use of existing and established mechanisms. For example, much has been learned through the Medicare experience and US-Health would use these lessons to contain costs. The system would set fees based on DRGs and RBRVS, two mechanisms used to control costs. Patients would still have the privilege of seeing the providers of their choice.

The funding for the system comes from existing resources. Beneficiaries would also be required to pay a portion of the bills with exceptions for those who are poor or near poor. Some of the money would come from existing payroll taxes and from existing Medicaid funding. Another source of revenue would be an employer tax which would be equivalent to the amount that employers now pay for private insurance. Finally, there would be a tax surcharge to make up any revenue shortfalls.

The Roybal plan was the first proposed solution to the access problem. However, the effect on outcomes is less clear. Further, the impact of the plan on costs is uncertain. Although the Roybal plan has been an important contender for the last few years, several of the newer plans provide more specific details for cost containment and accountability.

Other Plans

In the previous section we reviewed several of the major proposals. A variety of other plans have also been proposed. For example, the Kansas Employer Coalition on Health (1991) advocated the development of a political consensus to resolve problems. However, the plan does not provide enough specific details to be evaluated. Others have proposed federal–state partnerships for universal health insurance and cost containment (Fein, 1991) or plans modeled after those used in the Netherlands and the Federal Republic of Germany (Kirkman-Liff, 1991). None of these ideas are developed well enough at this point to be given formal consideration. However, there are at least two major plans that deserve special consideration. These will be discussed in detail in the next section.

THE CURRENT MAJOR ALTERNATIVES

Among all of the alternatives, two proposals have gained the greatest recognition. These two approaches represent major trends in current thinking. The first is the Physicians for a National Health Program; the second is a proposal for Managed Competition.

Physicians for a National Health Program

The Physicians for a National Health Program is a group that advocates a Canadian-based system. The group (also known as NHP) is alarmed that there are currently 1500 insurers in the United States. The basic theory behind the NHP plan is that administrative costs are too high and that money devoted to administration and to insurance companies could be re-allocated to provide tens of billions of dollars for serving the uninsured. Under the NHP plan, hospitals, nursing homes, and clinics would be funded on a per capita basis. This would be comparable to how fire stations are currently funded in the United States. The hospitals would have the responsibilities of caring for patients without generating itemized bills. Under this system, hospitals would care for patients when appropriate but could deny services that are unnecessary. This would greatly reduce the need for hospital administrators, billing specialists, and insurance arbitrators.

Physicians would submit all claims to a single state-sponsored insurance company. The physicians would, through their professional organizations, negotiate a fee schedule. The health care providers could choose to work in private practices and bill the centralized payer or they could work for hospitals on a salary basis. The plan would provide access to all and, according to the proposal, reduce cost. Figure 3.2 summarizes the costs for the NHP by category of expenditure. Under the NHP, hospital expenditures would be about the same but physician expenditures would be somewhat higher. However, total costs would be lower because there would be a savings of about $18 billion in administrative costs and profits. In the future, the NHP spending would be indexed to the GNP with

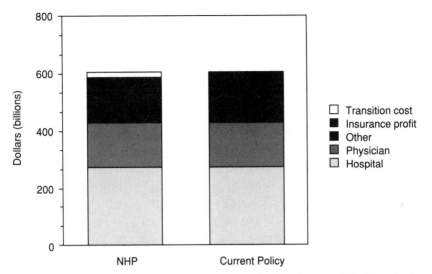

Figure 3.2 Comparison of costs of national health plan (NHP) and current. "Other" includes drugs, dental, and professional services. (Adapted from Grumbach *et al.,* 1991.)

adjustments for demographic and technological changes. Further, adjustments could be made for the outbreaks of expensive epidemics. The program would be financed with new health care taxes which would replace employer insurance premiums. Thus, the cost to the average consumer would not increase.

Arguments favoring Canadian-type national health insurance have an interesting political history. The current opponents of the system include insurance companies, organized medicine, and hospitals. The American Medical Association position has actually changed over the years. In 1917, the AMA encouraged the study of various approaches to health insurance. Indeed, it condemned blind opposition to "the rising tide of social development." In the early days, the pluralistic system of multiple insurers was endorsed by labor. Samuel Gompers, President of the American Federation of Labor (AFL) in the post-World War I era, regarded a single insurer system as "paternalistic." With his support, labor pressed for the right to have multiple, union-sponsored insurance systems (Gerber, 1992). By the late 1940s and early 1950s, the AMA had clearly changed its position. In that era, President Harry Truman launched a major effort to create a Canadian-like health insurance system. The Truman proposal kept physicians and hospitals as private and used a centralized single payer system to reimburse them. The Truman proposal was resoundingly challenged by organized medicine and by big business. The American Medical Association launched a multimedia blitz to persuade citizens that Truman was endorsing socialized medicine. Big business also opposed the proposal, suggesting that it would mark the destruction of free enterprise in the United States (Bernstein, 1989).

By 1990 most parties had changed their position. Labor, which had originally opposed a single payer system, had become one of its strongest advocates. The AFL–CIO had become one of the strongest supporters of a centralized system. Big business, which had opposed the Truman proposal in the late 1940s, had come to recognize that it could no longer afford the current system. Led by Lee Iacocca, Chairman of the Chrysler Corporation, many major businesses also began calling for major alterations in the system.

The NHP proposal is appealing for several reasons. First, it is among the few programs that may be capable of controlling costs. By channeling all payments through a single payer, fees can be set in a reasonable manner. The system has worked in Canada and other countries. There is evidence that the quality of physician services is high in Canada and that Canadians get a good buy for their investments. For instance, as Fuchs has suggested, Canadian physicians see more patients and deliver higher-quality services than U.S. physicians. The NHP has been criticized for endorsing aspects of the Canadian system that many Canadians dislike. For example, it has been argued that Canadians must wait in line for services and that many cross the border in order to obtain health care in the United States. The NHP advocates, however, do not propose reducing United States spending to Canadian levels. Instead, they suggest that we use Canadian efficiency to deliver more services to more people (Grumbach et al., 1991).

The NHP proposal has many important elements. It is simple, there is international evidence that it may work, and it takes the bite out of the administrators rather than the taxpayers. The proposal may address the spending problem and clearly addresses the access problem. The proposal does not address the accountability problem. Indeed, in the conclusion of the Grumbach *et al.* (1991) proposal, emphasis is placed on solving the cost and access problems. After all these problems have been resolved, the proposal suggests, we can begin to turn our attention toward identifying which services improve the quality of life. Overall, the NHP proposal is an important one that deserves serious consideration.

Managed Competition

The alternative major contender is based on the concept of "managed competition" (Enthoven & Kronick, 1991). According to Enthoven and Kronick, America has not yet tried competition as a mechanism for controlling costs and improving quality. The current fee-for-service system is open-ended and allows physicians to be paid more for doing more. The consumer is often unaware of this because sick patients must trust providers and patients are often blinded to the costs of bills paid by their insurance companies. The powerful incentives that shape the behavior of providers have propelled the system in the wrong direction. There are too many specialists, too many hospital beds, and too many procedures.

The Enthoven and Kronick proposal emphasizes "managed competition."

Under this plan, public sponsors would be created in each state. These sponsors, which would be quasipublic agencies like the Federal Reserve, would offer subsidized health coverage to those who are otherwise uninsured. The agencies would pay 80% of the cost of health insurance. There would be mandated employer-provided health insurance with premiums contributed by both employers and employees. The public sponsors would act as purchasing agents and there would be protection against excluding those who have preexisting conditions.

Employers would be required to pay an 8% payroll tax on the first $22,500 earned by each employee. This would extend to seasonal and hourly workers. Self-employed individuals would be required to pay the 8% contribution through an income tax system. Thus, there would be a variety of protections to ensure that everyone is covered. Small employers could participate through a public sponsor.

One of the provisions of the system is to change the tax law so that tax-free employer contributions are limited to 80% of the cost of the insurance. In 1991 that would be roughly $290 per family per month. This aspect of the plan has two advantages. First, it saves the federal government $11.2 billion by shifting some of the cost of health insurance from pre-tax to post-tax payment. Second, the major rationale for the limitation on tax-free contribution is that it forces consumers to be cost conscious.

Perhaps the most important part of the proposal is that there would be managed competition. The public sponsor and the employers must go beyond simply offering health insurance to their employees. In addition, employers would be required to offer the employee a choice among several alternative plans. The competition would force the plans to be efficient and attractive to consumers.

The Enthoven–Kronick plan has been analyzed in a variety of different studies. The Congressional Budget Office has suggested that the plan is neutral with regard to cost. It would require new revenues but these would be approximately equal to the amount the plan would save. It is likely that most individuals would end up in managed care programs. However, this is not necessarily bad since most patients like managed care and studies show that patient satisfaction with HMOs is usually high. There is the remaining concern that the plan does nothing about the excessive costs of health care administration (Woolhandler & Himmelstein, 1991). In response, Enthoven and Kronick have argued that managed competition will reduce administrative costs because plans will need to be efficient in order to succeed. Currently, some of the best options in managed care do not bill patients. Thus, some of the efficiencies in the Canadian system are realized in well-run health maintenance organizations. Over the course of the early competition, less efficient providers will be eliminated.

Overall, the managed competition proposal is neutral with regard to costs. It clearly achieves greater access and also provides considerable improvement in accountability. However, the proposal does not have a specific plan for improving patient outcomes. Managed competition has been very attractive because it includes elements that are appealing to different political philosophies. For instance, it is sympathetic to the underserved yet maintains an interest in a market system. The proposal has been endorsed by a variety of organizations and has been identified as the solution by several editorialists, including the *New York Times* and the *Wall Street Journal.*

SYNTHESIS

An editorial in the *Wall Street Journal* proclaimed that "self-interest reigns in the Health Care Reform" (Weinschrott, 1991). Physicians want fee for service with an expanded market and employers want insurance reform to reduce premiums. Large employers want legislation requiring small businesses to provide insurance to avoid cost shifting. Hospitals want guarantees that their bills will be paid while insurance companies want compensation for taking on high-risk groups.

Several organizations have reviewed the different proposals and have produced spreadsheets outlining the advantages and disadvantages of the many approaches. The spreadsheets differ in the criteria they use to evaluate the proposals. One important analysis was offered by the American Public Health Association (APHA) (1991). They reviewed 8 proposals based on 13 criteria. The evaluation categories were universal coverage, comprehensive benefits, elimination of financial barriers, equitable financing, organization and administration, quality and efficiency, payment mechanism, planning and evaluation, disease prevention and health promotion, education and training of health workers, affirmative action for health workers, nondiscrimination of service delivery, and consumer education. The absence of two categories in this analysis is notable. First, the APHA never mentions cost. Instead it considers "equitable financing" and gives higher marks to programs that are funded by government through progressive taxation. The second missing category in the APHA spreadsheet is health outcome. The proposals are not evaluated according to whether or not they will improve the public's health.

Using these criteria, it is not surprising that the most highly rated proposal is one developed by a closely related organization. A proposal introduced in 1988 by Milton Terris and his associates calls for a national medical care system financed by tax dollars (Terris, 1990). The proposal differs from some of the others because it requires a fixed percentage of expenditures to be spent on public health activities. In addition, the proposal includes provisions for consumer education, affirmative action for health workers, and nondiscrimination in service delivery. Although many of the proposals probably embrace these concepts, few formally address them. Thus, in the APHA evaluation, the Terris proposal receives many positive marks where other proposals receive only question marks. However, since its introduction, the Terris proposal has not been taken seriously enough to find its way into many other proposal comparisons.

Among proposals reviewed in this chapter, the APHA analysis gives high marks to the Physicians for a National Health Program proposal. The managed competition proposal was not well received by the APHA. The program was faulted because it does not provide "comprehensive" benefits. To obtain a high score in this category, APHA requires that the plan support all medical services, presumably including those that are not medically necessary. In another spreadsheet, developed by *Business Week* magazine, managed competition obtained the highest marks.

Another spreadsheet analysis was completed by the National Association of Retired Federal Employees (NARFE). This analysis focused on specific pieces of legislation and was non-evaluative with regard to most proposals. However, the categories upon which proposals were rated gave greater weight to retired people. For example, each offering was rated according to its provisions for public long-term care. Few of the proposals specifically address long-term care (Sheets, 1991). NARFE concluded that the difference between proposals is distinguished by their financial support—employer-based versus government. NARFE did not take a position on which approach was preferred. To provide another perspective, the American Psychological Association has also produced a spreadsheet. As might be expected, its analysis emphasized mental health benefits and effects of the program upon mental health providers. In summary, there have been several different analyses of the proposals. The conclusions of these analyses differ because different analysts use different criteria to evaluate the proposals. None of the spreadsheets considers outcome. As a result, few of the analyses consider the effect of the different proposals upon the health status of the nation. We believe the most important criteria are related to the three A's—affordability, access, and accountability.

Table 3.3 summarizes the performance of the various proposals in relation to the criteria of access, affordability, and accountability. As the table shows, most proposals do not control costs. Generally, the proposals do well with regard to increasing access. The most serious of the proposals (NHP and managed competition) both control costs and improve access. However, none of the proposals has a strong answer with regard to outcomes.

CURRENT ACTIVE PROPOSALS

The Bush Proposal

In February of 1992 President George Bush unveiled his proposed resolution for the health care crisis. Under the plan, poor families would receive tax credits and families with incomes up to $80,000 would be given tax deductions for the purchase of medical insurance. Further, the plan would call for risk pooling. Legislation would extend access to medical insurance to everyone at a reasonable cost. Medicare and Medicaid patients would be encouraged to use health maintenance organizations and other lower cost options. In the announcement of the plan, Bush suggested that his proposal preserved what worked in the current

TABLE 3.3

Comparison of Proposals with Regard to Affordability, Access, and Outcome[a]

Proposal	Description	Sponsor	Affordability	Access	Outcome
Heritage Foundation	Eliminate tax credits for health insurance		0	–	0
U.S. Chamber of Commerce	Incentive–competition		–	–	–
American Medical Association	Creates risk pools and expands Medicaid	Kennelly (D-CT)	–	+	0
Pepper Commission	Expand Medicaid with cost controls	Rockefeller (D-WV), S1177	–	+	+/0
Mediplan	Single payor	Stark (D-CA), HR 650/651	–	+	0
Physicians Who Care	Mandates IRA accounts for Medicare and employer-based insurance		–	0	0
USHealth Act	Consolidates Medicare, Medicaid, and private insurance into new USHealth Administration	Roybal (D-CA), HR 2980	0	+	0
Physicians for a National Health Program	Creates a Canadian-style single payor system	Saunders (I-VT)	0	+	0
Managed Competition	Mandates employers to offer multiple alternative insurance plans to employees or to pay into general pool		+	+	0

[a]+, improves problems; 0, has no effect; –, may have negative impact.

system and reforms aspects that do not work. Under the plan, a maximum credit or deduction for a single person would be $1250. A married couple without children would receive a maximum deduction of $2500 while a family with children could receive a deduction of $3750. The deductions would not apply to single individuals who earn more than $50,000, single parents with incomes in excess of $65,000, or married couples with incomes greater than $80,000. In addition, the tax deductions would not apply to those who currently receive either Medicaid or Medicare.

The highlights of the Bush proposal are summarized in Table 3.4. Two of the most interesting reforms are aspects of the law that outlaw skimming. Skimming is the practice of covering only low risk individuals and administratively excluding patients with chronic illnesses or risks for developing serious health problems. This would be accomplished by abolishing preexisting condition clauses for new employees. The risk pooling would be achieved by providing encouragement for small businesses to form coalitions that jointly could obtain lower individual rates.

Another interesting aspect of the Bush plan is the proposed change in the malpractice and antitrust laws. Under the Bush proposal, there would be limitations on what could be captured in a malpractice law suit. This aspect of the plan drew considerable attention. Clearly it was a politically important part of the proposal, even though its likelihood of controlling costs is small.

When introduced, the Bush plan drew immediate criticism. There were many important challenges. First, the program was vague on cost control. It provided few specifics on how to solve the access problem. For example, it was uncertain whether the tax credit would be attractive to low income people. Will people with

---

TABLE 3.4

Highlights of the Bush Proposal

- A voucher worth up to $3750 would be provided to poor families. The voucher could only be used to purchase health insurance.

- Families with incomes up to $70,000 would get a tax deduction of $4750. There would be a lower deduction for those with incomes from $70,000 to $80,000. Families with incomes higher than $80,000 would not be eligible for a deduction.

- Self-employed persons would receive full deductions of medical insurance premiums.

- Companies must provide coverage to any employee willing to pay for it. This includes employees with pre-existing medical conditions.

- Small businesses are encouraged to form coalitions for purchasing health insurance for their employees. This is designed to lower cost by spreading the risk.

- Medical malpractice and antitrust laws would be modified to reduce "defensive medicine."

- Health maintenance organizations in private plans, Medicare, and Medicaid, are encouraged through incentives.

an annual income of $8000 use up to $3750 for medical insurance in order to get a tax credit? The proposal may actually increase access among some of the working poor. Among low income people only about 45% are covered by Medicaid, and those who work for small businesses may be more likely to gain insurance. Nevertheless, it is unclear whether the plan will actually work in practice. One of the major problems is that some of the resources used to pay for the plan would come from new regulation of Medicaid and Medicare. These two programs currently cover about one-quarter of the nation's population. The plan was seen as inequitable since it encourages the use of private doctors for most citizens but reduces choice in the Medicaid and Medicare programs. Another problem is that the program does not include nursing homes and other long term care facilities. Even supporters of the traditional insurance industry are concerned about the Bush proposal. For example, the proposal requires uniform premiums for sick and healthy people. This represents a radical departure from risk appraisal that will require a restructuring of the insurance premium base. Although the proposal, in principle, recognizes the high administrative costs of health care, it does not specifically deal with elimination of paperwork. There would be less administrative costs if Medicaid and Medicare shifted toward HMOs. On the other hand, considerably more paperwork would be created in order to ascertain eligibility for tax credits.

Finally, the President was unable to say where the money would come from to pay for the new plan. He estimated that the plan would cost an additional $100 billion. In summary, the Bush plan does improve access although it certainly does not come close to solving the access problem. It increases cost and does not even mention outcome. Thus, the plan is unlikely to resolve all of the problems. As a practical matter, it is unlikely that the plan will ever be enacted since the Democratically controlled Congress favors distinctly different approaches to the problem (Wines, 1992).

State Proposals

Several states have proposed innovative new approaches to health care. Three representative approaches have either been implemented or proposed in Hawaii, Minnesota, and California.

Hawaii The state of Hawaii has one of the most successful approaches to expanded access. Hawaii uses a pay or play strategy in which all employers are required to purchase health insurance. Those who are not working can purchase insurance through a pooling mechanism. The state has only two major insurers: Blue Cross and Kaiser. Reports about Hawaii tend to be very positive. Use of emergency rooms tends to be low and consumers are satisfied with their options. There are some complaints from employers about the expense.

Minnesota In April, 1992, Minnesota passed innovative legislation to expand health care access. The new program expanded access to more than 15,000 people who had no health insurance. The program is financed through a 2% tax on fees charged by physicians and hospitals and a tax on cigarettes. In addition, the law creates a twenty-six-member commission to oversee health care spending.

California California has not yet adopted a universal health insurance proposal. However, John Garamendi, the state insurance commissioner, has urged universal coverage. This proposal, which was introduced in the spring of 1992, creates a Health Insurance Purchasing Corporation. This corporation, which would be quasi-public, would raise revenue through a 6.75% payroll tax on employers and a 1% tax from employee wages. The plan would maintain managed competition by allowing employees to select from among competing plans.

The Garamendi plan would cost $34 billion per year. However, there would also be significant savings. Many of these savings accrue because of savings through other aspects of insurance. For example, Garamendi's Department of Insurance estimates that about 20% of worker's compensation insurance costs are attributable to the cost of medical care. If there were universal health insurance, the cost of worker's compensation would be significantly reduced because the program would only be responsible for disability and vocational rehabilitation. In addition, there may be significant savings in automobile insurance. Automobile insurance costs are, in part, high because of the costs of litigation. Recovering medical expenses following an automobile accident is typically a complex process that involves lawyers and law suits. If everyone had health insurance these costs could be avoided.

The future of Garamendi's proposal is uncertain. The California legislature clearly rejected a similar plan that had a single payer. Garamendi's plan includes managed competition, thereby maintaining the interests of the powerful insurance lobbies. The California Medical Association has also proposed a ballot initiative modeled after the Hawaiian system. However, the medical association's proposal has very little capability of controlling costs because it does not attempt to regulate physician fees through either a central payer or managed competition.

In summary, there are many proposals. The proposals differ in how they are financed. Some proposals are financed through an individually mandated insurance. For example, the Heritage proposal requires individuals to purchase their own health insurance. Other options use a "pay or play" strategy. Under these proposals, employers must purchase insurance for their workers (play) or pay into a centralized insurance fund. The third option is public financing through tax dollars. The proposals also differ in their approach to cost controls. Some favor centralized cost controls while others favor market approaches through managed competition. The proposals all are similar in one respect. None of them attempt to use information on health outcomes and the effectiveness of services as part of the reform.

SUMMARY

In this chapter we have reviewed a wide variety of proposals for reforming the health care system. Many of these are currently being given active consideration by Congress. The proposals include those from politically conservative groups such as the Heritage Foundation. Conversely, some of the proposals identify the market system as the major source of difficulty and call for a major reform and a socialized system. None of the proposals explicitly considers health outcome. In the next chapter an outcomes-oriented proposal will be offered. This proposal could include provisions of the other proposals which consider increased access and reduced cost. However, the review of the literature suggests that a new paradigm is needed. Not only do we need to reduce cost and expand access, we also need to obtain value for money. We need a new approach to health care that will use our limited resources to make people healthier.

CHAPTER FOUR

A General Health Policy Model for Setting Priorities in Health Policy

This chapter offers a new solution to the health care crisis in the United States. The proposed solution is based on a General Health Policy Model (GHPM) that has been developed at the University of California over the last 20 years. The preceding three chapters have reviewed the emerging crisis in health care and have emphasized that the problem has three parts: affordability, access, and accountability. Several proposed solutions address affordability and access. However, none of the proposals wrestle with the difficult issues of health outcome. Health care may be the only major industry in the United States that is completely unaccountable for what it produces.

Until recently, American medicine seemed almost disinterested in how it affected people. It has long been known that most of what medicine attempts to accomplish is not well represented in the traditional measures of morbidity and mortality. We need new ways of thinking about outcomes in health care and new ways of comparing the alternatives. The traditional approach to reimbursement for health care services has been to allow physicians to select which procedures and tests are appropriate for their patients. Although decisions are supposed to be between a doctor and his or her patient, patients have been in a disadvantaged position. The patient may be in a compromised position because of illness, and patients may have limited knowledge to challenge a physician who, after all, is an expert in the field. Patients have also become less price conscious since the bills are often paid by a faceless insurance company.

The approach presented in this chapter is simple. It is suggested that available resources be used to produce the greatest benefit for the greatest number of people. It has been suggested that as much as 30 to 50% of expenditures in health care has no effect upon health outcome (Brook & Lohr, 1986). By denying coverage for these services and targeting those outcomes where treatment makes a difference, costs might be reduced or stabilized and the savings could be used to increase access. Most importantly, this is a new paradigm in which health outcomes are the pivotal dimension. The major challenge in executing this system is in defining what is meant by health benefit.

UTILITY

Utility is a condition or quality of usefulness. High-utility items are the most useful and those with lower utility are less useful. States of being are also associated with utility, and health is often identified as the highest utility asset. When Rokeach (1973) asked subjects to prioritize their values, he found no variability for the rank of health. It was always ranked first and, for this reason, was eventually removed from the Rokeach value scale. One of the purposes of this chapter is to define health and to offer a quantitative expression of health status.

Since good health is so highly valued, people will spend their energy and assets attempting to achieve it. Last year Americans spent $666 billion ($666,000,000,000) on health care services and a much larger amount on other products and services related to health. Although there is tremendous incentive to promote products and services as health enhancing, we typically are left with little information about the extent to which health outcome is affected by these investments. Thus, another purpose of this chapter is to explore changes in a quantitative expression of health in relation to investments.

IS MORE BETTER?

One of the basic objectives in health care is to deliver service. Indeed, many policy options are justified because they provide more services. We assume that expenditure is an accomplishment. The more money allocated to a program, the better the expected outcomes. It is often assumed that the states or countries that are achieving the best health outcomes are those spending the most money. Thus, it might be argued, Americans should have the world's best health profile because they spend the most per capita on health care.

Recently, substantial evidence has emerged suggesting that many unnecessary services are delivered by our health care system. Consider coronary artery bypass surgery. The United States Congress Office of Technology Assessment reported that in France there are 19 such operations per million members of the population. In Austria, there are 150 operations per million in the population. In the United States, there are nearly 800 operations per million (Rimm, 1985). Approximately 200,000 procedures were performed in the United States in 1985—nearly twice as many as had been performed in 1980 (National Center for Health Statistics, 1986). There are also large differences in the use of other expensive interventions. For example, the number of people with end-stage renal disease is believed to be approximately equal in western countries. Yet, in the United Kingdom, less than 1 case per 1000 was on renal dialysis in comparison to 39 cases per 1000 in the United States (Schroeder, 1987). As argued by a variety of analysts, there is no evidence that these regional variations in use of procedures have substantial effects on health outcomes. They do have systematic effects upon health care costs.

Policy analysts are faced with difficult choices because they hope to maximize health outcomes while maintaining control over costs. Western countries differ in the rate at which health care costs have escalated, with the United States leading the pack in expenditures. It is not clear that escalating expenditure has been associated with equal return in health status. Among European countries reporting data to the Organization for Economic Cooperation and Development the shortest life expectancies for men are in Ireland and the longest are in Greece. Among the reporting nations, Greece paradoxically spends the smallest percentage of its GNP on health care while Ireland spends the most. In fact, there is a rough negative relationship among the reporting nations between expenditures and life expectancy (Sick Health Services, 1988). Studies (reviewed by Voulgaropolous et al., 1989) have shown that many widely used and expensive procedures have essentially no health benefit.

In order to gain a better understanding of the alternatives in health care, we have proposed a General Health Policy Model (GHPM) that attempts to provide a comprehensive expression of the costs, risks, and benefits of competing alternatives in health care. Some of these choices are difficult without a model because comparing programs might be considered analogous to comparing apples to oranges.

APPLES VERSUS ORANGES

There are many alternative ways to spend money on health care. These range from complex, high-tech interventions such as liver transplantation, to rehabilitation, to primary prevention. Comparing these alternatives might be analogous to comparing apples to oranges. Further complicating the comparison is the fact that the benefits of each intervention are measured in quite different units. Liver transplantation might be evaluated in terms of extended life expectancy while a vaccination program might be evaluated by a reduction in school days missed. The successful procedure might be one in which the patient survives for 1 year. These procedures might require large expenditures for a single patient. The same amount of money might be spent to provide a different smaller benefit for a large number of people. Recently, for example, the state of Oregon was faced with a complex dilemma. They had a limited number of health care dollars and had to choose between high-technology transplantation surgery and other alternatives including prenatal care. Each liver transplant, for example, costs about $325,000. After deliberation, Oregon administrators decided to rank funding for prenatal care higher than for some organ transplantation programs. Many people argued that this was a foolish decision. Yet, the systematic comparison between the benefits was not possible because the outcomes of the services were measured in quite different units. How can we compare apples to oranges? In the following sections, models will be discussed for thinking about this problem. Ultimately, Oregon explored methods for quantifying health benefits, and the use of these models may serve to challenge many of our assumptions about health care (see Chapter Six). One of these assumptions is that we benefit from greater expenditures in health care.

Public policy makers are faced with complex decisions that often involve comparisons between very different alternatives. When these alternatives are measured or described using different scales, decisions can be difficult, if not impossible. Often, the confused decision maker gives in to the alternative with the most emotional appeal. In this chapter, it is argued that general measurement models, based on outcome measurement, can provide important new insights for policy makers. These models depend on very general conceptualizations of the expected benefits or consequences of health care decisions. The GHPM (Kaplan & Anderson, 1988a) quantitatively expresses the ultimate objectives of health care—to extend life expectancy and to improve quality of life. Central to this model is the quantification of health status.

MEASUREMENT OF HEALTH STATUS

The conceptualization and measurement of health status has interested scholars for many decades. Following the Eisenhower administration, a President's Commission on National Goals identified health status measurement as an important objective. Shortly after, John Kenneth Galbraith, in "The Affluent Society," described the need to measure the effect of the health care system on "quality of life." Recent years have seen many attempts to define and measure health status (Walker & Rosser, 1988; Wenger et al., 1984; Bergner, 1989). A general measure of health status is required in order to make comparisons between different investments in health care.

COMPARISONS ACROSS DIAGNOSES—THE
INCREMENTAL OUTCOME PROBLEM

In order to resolve health care cost problems, we need formal decision-making models. Mathematical models of decision making are now being proposed in a variety of health care systems. For example, these models have been suggested for use in European, Australian, and American health care systems. There is a growing recognition that health care resources are very limited. The United Kingdom National Health Service, for example, has recognized the need to prioritize competing demands on its very limited budgets (Maynard, 1991; Rosser, 1992). Yet prioritization schemes make little sense without some consideration of outcome.

The most important challenge in developing a formal model for resource allocation is in defining a common unit of health benefit. Typically, the value of each specific intervention in health care is determined by considering a measure specific to the intervention or the disease process. Treatments for hypertension, for example, are evaluated in terms of blood pressure, while those for diabetes are evaluated by blood glucose. Yet it is difficult to compare the relative value of investing in blood glucose versus blood pressure reduction. Traditional public health measures, such as life expectancy, are usually too crude to allow appropriate prioritization. However, we believe a general model of health outcome is both feasible and practical.

Cost/Utility versus Cost/Benefit

The terms *cost/utility, cost/effectiveness,* and *cost/benefit* are used inconsistently in the medical literature (Doubelet et al., 1986). Some economists have favored the assessment of cost/benefit. These approaches measure both program costs and treatment outcomes in dollar units. For example, treatment outcomes are evaluated in relation to changes in use of medical services, economic productivity, etc. Treatments are cost beneficial if the economic return exceeds treatment costs. Diabetic patients who are aggressively treated, for example, may need fewer medical services. The savings associated with decreased services might exceed treatment costs. Russell (1986) argued that the requirement that health care treatments reduce costs may be unrealistic. Patients are willing to pay for improvements in health status just as they are willing to pay for other desirable goods and services. We do not treat cancer in order to save money. Instead, treatments are given in order to achieve better health outcomes.

Cost/effectiveness is an alternative approach in which the unit of outcome is a reflection of treatment effect. In recent years, cost/effectiveness has gained considerable attention. Some approaches, such as those advocated by Yates and DeMuth (1981), emphasize simple, treatment-specific outcomes. For example, Yates considers the cost per pound lost as a measure of cost/effectiveness of weight loss programs. Public competitions, for example, achieve a lower cost-per-pound loss ratio than do traditional clinical interventions. The major difficulty with cost/effectiveness methodologies is that they do not allow for comparison across very different treatment interventions. For example, health care administrators often need to choose between investments in very different alternatives. They may need to decide between supporting liver transplantation for a few patients versus prenatal counseling for a large number of patients. For the same cost, they may achieve a large effect for a few people or a small effect for a large number of people. The treatment-specific outcomes used in cost/effectiveness studies do not permit these comparisons.

Cost/utility approaches use the expressed preference or utility of a treatment effect as the unit of outcome. As noted in World Health Organization documents (World Health Organization, 1984), the goals of health care are to add years to life and to add life to years. In other words, health care is designed to make people live longer (increase the life expectancy) and to live with a higher quality of life in the years prior to death. Cost/utility studies use outcome measures that combine mortality outcomes with quality-of-life measurements. The utilities are the expressed preferences for observable states of function on a continuum bounded by 0 for death and 1.0 for optimum function (Kaplan & Bush, 1982; Kaplan, 1985a,b; Kaplan & Anderson, 1988a,b). In recent years, cost/utility approaches have gained increasing acceptance as a method for comparing many diverse options in health care (Russell, 1986; Weinstein & Stason, 1977; Williams, 1988). Over the last two decades, a general cost/utility model has been developed at the University of California, San Diego. That model will now be presented.

A GENERAL HEALTH POLICY MODEL

In order to understand health outcomes, it is necessary to build a comprehensive theoretical model of health status. This model includes several components. The major aspects of the model include mortality (death) and morbidity (health-related quality of life). In several papers, we have suggested that diseases and disabilities are important for two reasons. First, illness may cause the life expectancy to be shortened. Second, illness may make life less desirable at times prior to death (health-related quality of life) (Kaplan & Anderson, 1988b, 1990).

Over the last two decades, a group of investigators at the University of California, San Diego, has developed a GHPM. Central to the GHPM is a general conceptualization of health status. The model separates aspects of health status into distinct components. These are life expectancy (mortality), functioning and symptoms (morbidity), preference for observed functional states (utility), and duration of stay in health states (prognosis).

Mortality

A model of health outcomes necessarily includes a component for mortality. Indeed, many public health statistics focus exclusively on mortality through estimations of crude mortality rates, age-adjusted mortality rates, and infant mortality rates. Death is an important outcome that must be included in any comprehensive conceptualization of health.

Morbidity

In addition to death, behavioral dysfunction is also an important outcome. The GHPM considers functioning in three areas: mobility, physical activity, and social activity. Descriptions of the measures of these aspects of function are given in many different publications (see Kaplan & Anderson, 1988a; 1990, for summaries). Most public health indicators are relatively insensitive to variations toward the well end of the continuum. Measures of infant mortality, to give an extreme example, ignore all individuals capable of reading this book since they have lived beyond 1 year following their births (we assume that no infants are reading the book). Disability measures often ignore those in relatively well states. For example, the RAND Health Insurance Study reported that about 80% of the general population has no dysfunction. Thus, they would estimate that 80% of the population is well. Our method asks about symptoms or problems in addition to behavioral dysfunction (Kaplan & Anderson, 1990). In these studies, only about 12% of the general population reports no symptoms on a particular day. In other words, health symptoms or problems are a very common aspect of the human experience. Some might argue that symptoms are unimportant because they are subjective and unobservable. However, symptoms are highly correlated with the demand for medical services, expenditures on health care, and motivations to alter lifestyles. Thus, we feel that the quantification of symptoms is very important.

Utility (Relative Importance)

Given that various components of morbidity and mortality can be tabulated, it is important to consider their relative importance. For example, it is possible to develop measures that detect very minor symptoms. Yet, because these symptoms are measurable does not necessarily mean they are important. A patient may experience side effects but be willing to tolerate them because the side effects are less important than the probable benefit of consuming the medication. Not all outcomes are equally important. A treatment in which 20 of 100 patients die is not equivalent to one in which 20 of 100 patients develop nausea. An important component of the GHPM attempts to scale the various health outcomes according to their relative importance. In the preceding example, the relative importance of dying would be weighted more than that of developing nausea. The weighting is accomplished by rating all states on a continuum ranging from 0 (for death) to 1.0 (for optimum functioning). These ratings are typically provided by independent judges who are representative of the general population. Using this system it is possible to express the relative importance of states in relation to the life–death continuum. A point halfway on the scale (0.5) is regarded as halfway between optimum function and death. The weighting system has been described in several different publications (Kaplan, 1982; Kaplan et al., 1976; 1978; 1979).

Prognosis

Another dimension of health status is the duration of a condition. A headache that lasts 1 hour is not equivalent to a headache that lasts 1 month. A cough that lasts 3 days is not equivalent to a cough that lasts 3 years. In considering the severity of illness, duration of the problem is central. As basic as this concept is, most contemporary models of health outcome measurement completely disregard the duration component. In the GHPM the term *prognosis* refers to the probability of transition among health states over the course of time. In addition to consideration of the duration of problems, the model considers the point at which the problem begins. A person may have no symptoms or dysfunctions currently but may have a high probability of health problems in the future. The prognosis component of the model takes these transitions into consideration and applies a discount rate for events that occur in the future.

The Quality of Well-Being Scale (QWB) is a method for estimating some components of the general model. The QWB questionnaire categorizes individuals according to functioning and symptoms. Other components of the model are obtained from other data sources (Kaplan & Anderson, 1990).

A mathematical model integrates components of the model to express outcomes in a common measurement unit. Using information on current functioning and duration, it is possible to express the health outcomes in terms of equivalents of well-years of life, or as some have described them, quality-adjusted life years (QALYs).

How This Model Differs from Traditional Conceptualizations

The two major differences between the GHPM and other approaches to health outcome measurement are (1) the attempt to express benefits and consequences of health in a common unit known as the well-year or quality-adjusted life year, and (2) emphasis on area under the curve rather than point-in-time measurement. We argue that the general approach to health outcome is, intuitively, what patients and consumers use as a guide. Their physicians may be more directed by a less comprehensive model that considers only a component of health outcome. For example, health care providers might focus on a component of health outcome such as blood pressure. Focusing on blood pressure might allow the provider to disregard all of the other effects blood pressure management has upon health outcome. Consumers must integrate various sources of information in their decision process. Intuitively they are directed toward maximization of health outcomes. However, sometimes these decision options become overwhelming and the use of a formal model may aid their decision process.

A basic objective for most people is to function without symptoms as long as possible. Clearly, early death contradicts this objective. Illness and disability during the interval between birth and death also reduce the total potential health status during a lifetime. Many approaches to health assessment consider only current functioning. We refer to these snapshots of health status as point-in-time measures. The GHPM considers outcome throughout the life cycle. This is what we characterize as the "area under the curve." The more wellness a person experiences throughout the life span, the greater is the area under the curve. Success of interventions is marked by expanded area.

The general nature of the model leads to some different conclusions than more traditional medical approaches. For example, the traditional medical model focuses on specific diseases and on pathophysiology. Characteristics of illness are quantified according to blood chemistry or in relation to problems in a specific organ system. Often, focus on disease-specific outcome measures leads to different conclusions than those evaluated using a more general outcome measure. For example, studies on the reduction of blood cholesterol have demonstrated reductions in deaths due to coronary heart disease. However, the same studies have failed to demonstrate reductions in total deaths from all causes combined (Lipid Research Clinics Coronary Prevention Trial Results, 1984). All studies in the published literature in which patients are assigned to cholesterol lowering through diet or medication, or to a control group, have revealed that reductions in cardiovascular mortality for those in the cholesterol-lowering group are compensated for by increases in mortality from other causes (Kaplan, 1984; 1985). A meta-analysis of these studies has demonstrated that the average statistical difference for increase in deaths from nonillness causes (i.e., accidents, murders, etc.) is larger than the average statistical difference for reduction in cardiovascular deaths (Mauldoon et al., 1990).

Similar results have been reported for reductions in cardiovascular deaths attributable to taking aspirin. The disease-specific approach focuses on deaths due to myocardial infarction because there is a biological model to describe why aspirin use should reduce heart attacks. Yet, in a controlled experiment in which physician subjects were randomly assigned to take aspirin or placebo, there was no difference in total deaths between the two groups (Kaplan, 1991a). Aspirin may reduce the chances of dying from a myocardial infarction, but it does not reduce the chance of dying (Steering Committee of the Physicians' Health Study Research Group, 1988; 1989). The traditional, diagnosis-specific medical model argues that there is a benefit of aspirin because it reduces heart attack, but the GHPM argues that there is no benefit of aspirin because there is no change in the chances of dying from all causes (Kaplan, 1990a).

This same line of reasoning applies to many other areas of health care. Many treatments produce benefits for a specific outcome but induce side effects that are often neglected in the analysis. Estimates of the benefits of surgery must take into consideration the fact that surgery causes dysfunction through wounds that must heal prior to any realization of the treatment benefits. Further, surgeries often create complications. The general approach to health status assessment attempts to gain a global picture of the net treatment benefits, taking into consideration treatment benefits, side effects, and estimates of their relative importance.

APPLYING THE MODEL: STEP BY STEP

Patrick & Erickson (1992) outlined the eight steps required to apply the GHPM. These steps are summarized in Table 4.1. The steps might be implemented as follows.

Step 1: Specify the Decisions

The first step in building a decision model is to clearly identify the question. Maynard suggests that many questions are phrased too generally. For example, the question "Does the AIDS drug AZT work?" is much too vague. We need to ask,

TABLE 4.1

Eight Steps in the Health Resource Allocation Model[a]

1. *Specify the health decision* by identifying
   - the sociocultural and health services context in which the decision is occurring,
   - alternative courses of action under consideration,
   - stakeholders for outcomes of alternatives,
   - values of stakeholders for outcomes of alternatives,
   - method of socioeconomic evaluation to be used, and
   - budgetary constraints to be considered.

2. *Classify health outcomes and health states* by identifying
   - all relevant concepts, domains, and indicators of health-related quality of life,
   - hypothesized relationships among concepts, domains, and indicators, and
   - select combination of domains to be included in the health state classification.

3. *Assign preferences to health states* by
   - identifying population of judges to assign preferences,
   - sampling health states to be assigned preference weights,
   - selecting a method of preference measurement, and
   - collecting preference judgments and assigning preference weights to health states.

4. *Measure health-related quality of life of target population* using primary data collection or secondary analysis to
   - classify individuals in target population into health states,
   - assign a preference weight to the health state of each individual, and
   - average scores of all individuals to obtain a point-in-time estimate of the target population's health-related quality of life.

5. *Estimate prognosis and years of health life* by
   - calculating expected duration of survival (life expectancy) of target population, and
   - calculating years of healthy life by adjusting duration of survival by the point-in-time estimate or observed differences in health-related quality of life.

6. *Estimate direct and indirect health care costs* by
   - identifying all organizing and operational costs attributed to each of the alternative courses of action, and
   - specifying out-of-pocket expenses and psychic costs incurred by the recipients of each alternative.

7. *Rank health care costs and outcomes* by
   - calculating the ratio of costs per year of healthy life for each alternative course of action,
   - ranking the ratios from low to high with the budget constraint included in this ranking, and
   - identifying ratios that are less than the budget constraint as cost effective.

8. *Revise rankings of costs and outcomes* by
   - reviewing rank-order of each alternative course of action with stakeholders in the decision,
   - adjusting the rank-order to reflect stakeholder values for these alternatives, and
   - recommending the final rank-order to the decision process.

[a]From Patrick & Erickson (1992).

"Is the treatment effective?" "At what cost?" and "For which patients?" We must also ask if the treatment is effective relative to competing alternatives. In evaluating treatments, it is important to establish the perspective. Is the treatment being evaluated from the perspective of society at large, or is it applied to individuals? Patrick & Erickson (1992) also emphasize the description of the stake holders. From the societal perspective, everyone has a stake. However, individual stake holders may have special interests. Neonatologists may have a special interest in the birth weight of children as do the parents of these infants.

The cost issue is very important. If resources were unlimited a resource allocation model would not be required. However, the debate is occurring because we do not have enough money to pay for all of the alternatives.

Step 2: Classify Health Outcome/States

The second step in applying the model is to classify health outcomes. Patrick and Erickson emphasize that this should be done by identifying all relevant concepts, domains, and indicators of health-related quality of life. The GHPM obtains this information using a QWB scale. This scale has evolved over the course of the last two decades. During the early phases of the project, a set of mutually exclusive and collectively exhaustive levels of functioning was defined. After an extensive, specialty-by-specialty review of medical reference works, we listed all of the ways that disease and injuries can affect behavior and role performance. Without considering etiology, it was possible to match a finite number of conditions to items appearing on standard health surveys, such as the Health Interview Survey (National Center for Health Statistics, 1986), the Survey of the Disabled (Social Security Administration), and several rehabilitation scales and ongoing community surveys. These items fit conceptually into three scales representing related but distinct aspects of daily functioning: mobility, physical activity, and social activity. The mobility and physical activity scales have three levels, while social activity has five distinct levels. Table 4.2 shows the steps from the three scales. Several investigators have used this function status classification (or a modified version of it) as an outcome measure for health program evaluation (Reynolds et al., 1974; Stewart et al., 1978). However, the development of a truly comprehensive health status indicator requires several more steps. In particular, the system requires that subjective symptoms and problems be classified.

There are many reasons a person may not be functioning at the optimum level. Subjective complaints are an important component of a general health measure because they relate dysfunction to a specific problem. Thus, in addition to function level classifications, an exhaustive list of symptoms and problems has been generated. Included in the list are 25 complexes of symptoms and problems representing all of the possible symptomatic complaints that might inhibit function. These symptoms and problems are shown in Table 4.3.

The method for obtaining information on functioning and symptoms differs according to the purpose and resources of the analyst. In some applications of the

TABLE 4.2

Quality of Well-Being/General Health Policy Model: Elements and Calculating Formulas (Function Scales with Step Definitions and Calculating Weights)

Step no.	Step definition	Weight
	Mobility scale (MOB)	
5	No limitations for health reasons	−.000
4	Did not drive a car, health related; did not ride in a car as usual for age (younger than 15 yr), health related, and/or did not use public transportation, health related; or had or would have used more help than usual for age to use public transportation, health related	−.062
2	In hospital, health related	−.090
	Physical activity scale (PAC)	
4	No limitations for health reasons	−.000
3	In wheelchair, moved or controlled movement of wheelchair without help from someone else; or had trouble or did not try to lift, stoop, bend over, or use stairs or inclines, health related; and/or limped, used a cane, crutches, or walker, health related; and/or had any other physical limitation in walking, or did not try to walk as far as or as fast as others the same age are able, health related	−.060
1	In wheelchair, did not move or control the movement of wheelchair without help from someone else, or in bed, chair, or couch for most or all of the day, health related	−.077
	Social activity scale (SAC)	
5	No limitations for health reasons	−.000
4	Limited in other (e.g., recreational) role activity, health related	−.061
3	Limited in major (primary) role activity, health related	−.061
2	Performed no major role activity, health related, but did perform self-care activities	−.106
1	Performed no major role activity, health related, and did not perform or had more help than usual in performance of one or more self-care activities, health related	−.106

model, estimates of treatment effect are obtained from clinical experts. There are several alternative methods for obtaining this information and these are discussed in more detail in Chapter Seven. The best method is to perform a randomized clinical trial in which patients are assigned to treatment or control conditions. Then, these individuals are followed over the course of time and the observed difference between treatment and control conditions is used to estimate treatment effectiveness. When clinical trials are not feasible or possible, expert judgment is an acceptable alternative.

The QWB scale is one of several systems for evaluating health outcome. There are other alternatives. For example, the health utility index (Torrance, 1987;

TABLE 4.3

Quality of Well-Being/General Health Policy Model: Symptom/Problem Complexes with Calculating Weights

Complex no.	Description of complex	Weight
1	Death (not on respondent's card)	−.727
2	Loss of consciousness such as seizure (fits), fainting, or coma (out cold or knocked out)	−.407
3	Burn over large areas of face, body, arms, or legs	−.387
4	Pain, bleeding, itching, or discharge (drainage) from sexual organs—does not include normal menstrual (monthly) bleeding	−.349
5	Trouble learning, remembering, or thinking clearly	−.340
6	Any combination of one or more hands, feet, arms, or legs either missing, deformed (crooked), paralyzed (unable to move), or broken—includes wearing artificial limbs or braces	−.333
7	Pain, stiffness, weakness, numbness, or other discomfort in chest, stomach (including hernia or rupture), side, neck, back, hips, or any joints or hands, feet, arms, or legs	−.299
8	Pain, burning, bleeding, itching, or other difficulty with rectum, bowel movements, or urination (passing water)	−.292
9	Sick or upset stomach, vomiting or loose bowel movement, with or without chills, or aching all over	−.290
10	General tiredness, weakness, or weight loss	−.259
11	Cough, wheezing, or shortness of breath, with or without fever, chills, or aching all over	−.257
12	Spells of feeling upset, being depressed, or crying	−.257
13	Headache, or dizziness, or ringing in ears, or spells of feeling hot, nervous, or shaky	−.244
14	Burning or itching rash on large areas of face, body, arms, or legs	−.240
15	Trouble talking, such as lisp, stuttering, hoarseness, or being unable to speak	−.237
16	Pain or discomfort in one or both eyes (such as burning or itching) or any trouble seeing after correction	−.230
17	Overweight for age and height or skin defect of face, body, arms, or legs, such as scars, pimples, warts, bruises or changes in color	−.188
18	Pain in ear, tooth, jaw throat, lips, tongue; several missing or crooked permanent teeth—includes wearing bridges or false teeth; stuffy, runny nose; or any trouble hearing—includes wearing a hearing aid	−.170
19	Taking medication or staying on a prescribed diet for health reasons	−1.44
20	Wears eyeglasses or contact lenses	−.101
21	Breathing smog or unpleasant air	−.101
22	No symptoms or problem (not on respondent's card)	−.000
23	Standard symptom/problem	−.257
X24	Trouble sleeping	−.257
X25	Intoxication	−.257
X26	Problems with sexual interest or performance	−.257
X27	Excessive worry or anxiety	−.257

Note: X means population weights are not currently available. A standard weight is used instead.

Drummond, Stoddard & Torrance, 1987) applies a very similar methodology. A group in the European community has also proposed a similar methodology which they call the EuroQol approach.

Step 3: Assign Preference Weights to Integrate the QWB Scale

We now have described the three scales of function and 25 symptom/problem complexes. With these, all we can do is compare populations in terms of frequencies of each scale step (and, if necessary, of each symptom/problem complex) as was done for the mobility scale in Table 4.4. Although comparisons of frequencies are common in health services research, our system offers a strategy for integrating the frequencies into a single comprehensive expression. If our intention is to say which of these distributions is "better" off and which "worse" off, simple frequently distributions may not be able to help much. Is Group 1, with 80 people limited in their mobility and 5 restricted to bed, worse off than Group 5, in which 85 can travel freely and 10 are restricted to bed, and by how much? Obviously, comparing frequency distributions is complex. And, this example uses only two scales. How can one make decisions when there are three scales and symptom/problem complexes to consider?

Another step is necessary to integrate the three scales and the symptom/problem complexes in a manner that will allow a single numerical expression to represent each combination of steps on the scales and symptom/problem complexes. The empirical means of accomplishing this is measured preferences for the health states. These might be regarded as "quality" judgments. As we noted earlier, the GHPM includes the impact of health conditions upon the quality of life. This requires that the desirability of health situations be evaluated on a continuum from death to completely well. An evaluation such as this is a matter of utility or preference, and thus, function level–symptom/problem combinations are scaled to represent precise degrees of relative importance.

Human judgment studies are needed to determine weights for the different states. We have asked random samples of citizens from the community to evaluate the relative desirability of a good number of health conditions. Random sample surveys were conducted in the San Diego community during two consecutive years. The probability sample included 867 respondents ethnically representative

TABLE 4.4

Comparison of Three Scales Using Only Frequency Information

Mobility step	Group 1	Group 2	Group 3	Group 4	Group 5
5	80	75	75	78	85
4	15	20	22	22	5
2	5	5	3	0	10

of the population. When necessary, interviews were conducted in Spanish. From a listing of all possible combinations of the scale (mobility, physical activity, social activity, and symptom/problem complexes), we drew a stratified random sample of 343 case descriptions (items) and divided them into eight sets of computer-generated booklets. An example of a case description is shown in Table 4.5. All respondents were assigned randomly to one of the eight booklets, creating eight subgroups of approximately 100 respondents each. The cases were rated on a scale of 0 to 10. The instructions for the rating task are shown in Table 4.6. In a series of studies, a mathematical model was developed to describe the consumer decision process. The validity of the model has been cross-validated with an R^2 of .94 (Kaplan et al., 1976). These weights, then, describe the relative desirability of all of the function states on a scale from 0 (for death) to 1.0 (for asymptomatic optimum function). Thus, a state with a weight of .50 is viewed by the members of the community as being about one-half as desirable as optimum function, or about halfway between optimum function and death.

Some critics have expressed concern that community rather than specific population weights are used. The advantage of community weights is that they are general (like the model) and do not bias policy analysis toward any interest group. More important, however, is that empirical studies consistently fail to show systematic differences between demographic groups (Kaplan et al., 1978), providers, students, and administrators, (Patrick et al., 1973b) and Americans versus British populations (Patrick et al., 1985). Relevant to the general versus disease-specific issue, Balaban and colleagues (1986) found that weights provided by rheumatoid arthritis patients are remarkably similar to those we obtained from members of the general population. We will return to this issue in Chapter Seven.

Using preference weights, one component of the general model of health is defined. This is the QWB scale, which is the point-in-time component of the GHPM (Kaplan & Anderson, 1990). The QWB score for any individual can be obtained from preferences or "quality" judgments associated with his or her function level, adjusted for symptom or problem.

The example in Table 4.7 describes a person classified on the three scales of

---

TABLE 4.5

Sample Case Description for Scaling Studies

Age	Older adult (65 years or over)
Mobility	Drove car and used bus or train without help
Physical activity	Walked with physical limitations
Social activity	Had help with self-care activities
Symptom/problem	Headache, or dizziness, or ringing in ears, or spells of feeling hot, nervous, or shaky

---

TABLE 4.6

Instructions for Category Scaling

Each page in this booklet (OPEN BOOKLET TO SAMPLE ITEM) tells how an imaginary person is affected by a health problem on one day of his or her life. I want you to look at each health situation and rate it on a ladder with steps numbered from 0 to 10. The information on each page tells (1) the person's age group, (2) whether the person could drive or use public transportation, (3) how well the person could walk, (4) how well the person could perform the activities usual for his or her age, and (5) what symptom or problem was bothering the person.

This sheet (HAND DEFINITION SHEET) tells what the lines mean. Please notice, for example, that the word *hospital* includes nursing homes, mental institutions, and similar places; that *special unit* means a restricted area of a hospital such as an operating room or intensive care unit; and that *self-care* means specifically bathing, dressing, eating, and using the bathroom.

Think about the day described on each page and rate it by choosing a step on the ladder from 0 to 10. All health situations can be placed on one of the steps. If the page describes someone who is completely well, then choose the top step, 10. If you think the situation described is about as bad as dying, then choose the bottom step, 0. If you think the person's situation was about halfway between being dead and being completely well, then choose step 5. Six is one step better than 5, 5 is one step better than 4, and so on. You can choose any of the steps from 0 to 10 depending on how bad or good you think *that day was.*

The problem on the bottom line of each page could be caused by many different diseases or injuries. The line does not tell how severe the problem was. You must judge that from how the problem affected his activities. Also, there is no way to tell for sure whether the problem will get much better or much worse on the next day. So just assume that the person was getting the best medical treatment possible on that day, and that he felt and performed as well as his condition or treatment would permit.

Read the situation, and when I call off the number of the page, tell me the step on the ladder that you choose. Give your opinion about the situation *on that one day only.* Don't worry about what tomorrow will be like. There are no right or wrong answers; this is simply your opinion. Are there any questions? (ANSWER ANY QUESTIONS) O.K. then, let's begin.

[a]From Kaplan et al. (1979).

---

observable function and on a symptom/problem. The table shows the adjustments for each of these components. Using these, a weight of .605 is obtained. By including symptom/problem adjustments, the index becomes very sensitive to minor "top-end" variations in health status. The adjustments for particular symptom/problem complexes for wearing eyeglasses, having a runny nose, or breathing polluted air. These symptom adjustments apply even if a person is in the top step in the other three scales. For example, a person with a runny nose receives a score of .83 on the QWB scale when he is at the highest function level (i.e., the top step on each scale shown in Table 4.2). Thus, the model can make fine as well as gross distinctions.

Several studies attest to the reliability (Kaplan et al., 1978; Kaplan, 1982) and

TABLE 4.7

Example Calculation for Patient with Chronic Obstructive Pulmonary Disease

Formula 1. Point-in-time well-being score for an individual (W):

$$W = 1 + (1.0 + wt_{CPX}) + (wt_{MOB}) + (wt_{PAC}) + (wt_{SAC})$$

where wt is the preference-weighted measure for each factor and CPX is symptom/problem complex. For example, the W score for a person with the following description profile may be calculated for 1 day as:

CPX-11	Cough, wheezing or shortness of breath, with or without fever, chills, or aching all over	.257
MOB-5	No limitations	−.000
PAC-1	In bed, chair, or couch for most or all of the day, health related	−.077
SAC-2	Performed no major role activity, health related, but did perform self-care	−.061

$$W = 1 + (−.257) + (−.000) + (−.077) + (−.061) = .605$$

Formula 2. Well-years (WY) as an output measure:

$$WY = [\text{No. of persons} \times (wt_{CPX} + wt_{MOB} + wt_{PAC} + wt_{SAC}) \times \text{Time}]$$

validity (Kaplan et al., 1976; 1984) of the QWB scale. For example, convergent evidence for validity is given by significant positive correlations with self-rated health and negative correlations with age, number of chronic illnesses, symptoms, and physician visits. However, none of these other indicators was able to make the fine discrimination between health states which characterize the QWB scale. These data support the convergent and discriminate validity of the scale (Kaplan et al., 1976).

Step 4: Measure Health-Related Quality of Life of Target Population

The next phase in the application of the model involves the primary data collection. In primary data analysis, questionnaires such as the QWB are administered to representatives of the population. As noted above, there are also secondary studies in which health outcomes for the target population are provided by experts. Each individual in the identified target population is classified into one set of health states with one symptom for a particular set of days. These are typically the 4 or 6 days preceding the interview. In clinical studies these observations are made on repeated occasions, typically after treatment and at specified follow-up periods.

Once people are classified into observable states, preference weights are attached. For example, consider the person who was described as follows:

In hospital.
In wheelchair. Moved or controlled movement of wheelchair without help from another party.
Limited in role activity.
Headache or dizziness.

This is a state that is actually observed. Applying the preferences to this state gives a utility weight of .545 (=1.0−.09−.06−.061−.244). This means that an individual in the state described would be rated by people in the community as being in a state slightly more desirable than halfway between death and optimum function. If this person remained in the same state for 1 year they would have lost the equivalent of .455 well-years of life.

Many authors have expressed concern about the sensitivity of health outcome measures. Two aspects of sensitivity must be considered. First, there is sensitivity in population studies. Second, sensitivity in clinical studies will be reviewed.

As we have suggested elsewhere (Erickson et al., 1989), about 85% of the respondents in national surveys report themselves to be unlimited in major activities. Further, 50% report themselves to be in excellent or very good health. As a result, current health indicators provide little information about "well" populations, or at least those unlimited in their major activity. In contrast, the QWB questionnaire finds very few people who score at the top of the 0 to 1.0 continuum. For instance, a 1976 survey of a random sample of San Diego residents revealed that only 12% were completely functional and had no symptom/problem on a particular day. The increased sensitivity is gained through the greater precision of the questions and through the inclusion of symptoms and problems. Thus, an individual who has itchy eyes, wears eyeglasses, or has a cough scores below the optimal level on the scale.

Defining clinical sensitivity is more difficult. Some investigators (Guyatt et al., 1987) suggest that measures be designed which maximize differences between treatment and control groups in experimental trials. The quality-of-life measures, according to these authors, should be evaluated by their ability to detect differences between groups of patients treated in different ways. However, a statistically significant difference between groups is not necessarily a clinically meaningful one (Feinstein, 1988). For example, in a very large clinical trial, with several thousand patients per condition, essentially trivial differences can be statistically significant. Conversely, relatively large differences in small trials may be statistically nonsignificant. The issue of clinical versus statistical significance has been debated for many years. One of the advantages of the QWB system is that it presents differences between groups in a well-defined unit. For example, a difference of .05 units means that the treated and the untreated groups differ by an amount that is equal to 5% of the difference between optimum function and death.

If this difference is maintained for 1 year, each patient will have gained .05 equivalents of a well-year. If the effect is maintained for 20 years, or if it accrues to 20 individuals, the treatment will have produced the equivalent of 1 year of life. Within the QWB system, levels of functioning and symptom/problem complexes have been evaluated such that they represent perceived meaningful differences along the death-to-well continuum. For example, in order to justify two separate levels of function, it was necessary that the perceived difference between them be statistically significant. When differences along the continuum from death to optimum function were too small to be detected by human judges, they were merged into a single level.

Policy analyses are rarely conducted for a particular individual. Typically, scores are averaged across individuals in a particular population or treatment group.

Step 5: Estimate Prognosis and Calculate the Well-Life Expectancy

The QWB scale is the point-in-time component of the model. A comprehensive measure of health status also requires an expression of prognosis or the probability of moving between health states over time. People who are well now want to remain well. Those who are at suboptimal levels want to become well, or at least not to get worse. A GHPM must consider both current functioning and probability of transition to other levels of functioning over the course of time. When transition is considered and documented in empirical studies, the consideration of a particular diagnosis is no longer needed. We fear diseases because they affect our current functioning or because they alter the probability that there will be a limitation in our functioning some time in the future. A person at high risk for heart disease may be functioning very well at present but may have a high probability of transition to a lower level (or death) in the future. Cancer would not be a concern if the disease did not affect current functioning or the probability that functioning will be affected at some future time.

When weights have been properly determined, health status can be expressed precisely as the expected value (product) of the preferences associated with the states of function at a point in time and the probabilities of transition to other states over the remainder of the life expectancy. Quality of well-being (W) is a static or time-specific measure of function, while the well-life expectancy (E) also includes the dynamic or prognostic dimension. E is the product of W times the expected duration of stay in each function level over a standard life period.

An example computation of E is shown in Table 4.8. Suppose that a group of individuals was in a well state for 65.2 years, in a state of nonbed disability for 4.5 years, and in a state of bed disability for 1.9 years before their deaths at the average age of 71.6 calendar years. In order to make adjustments for the diminished quality of life they suffered in the disability states, the duration of stay in each state is multiplied by the preference associated with the state. Thus, the 4.5 years of nonbed disability become 2.7 equivalents of well-years when we adjust

---

TABLE 4.8

Illustrative Computation of the Well-Life Expectancy

State	k	Y_k	W_k	$W_k Y_k$
Well	A	65.2	1.00	65.2
Nonbed disability	B	4.5	.59	2.7
Bed disability	C	1.9	.34	.6

Current life expectancy EY_k = 71.6 life years
Well-life expectancy $EW_k Y_k$ = 68.5 well-years

[a]From Kaplan & Bush (1982).

---

for the preferences associated with inhabiting that state. Overall, the E for this group is 68.5 years. In other words, disability has reduced the quality of their lives by an estimated 3.1 years.

Step 6: Estimate the Direct and Indirect Costs

The costs of the various treatment alternatives must be clearly identified, measured, and valued. The value of the treatment alternatives should be specified in current prices. Identifying the costs of treatments can sometimes be difficult. Charges that appear on hospital bills or physician's statements may be poor indicators of actual resources required to produce a benefit. Health care has many examples in which a single supplier has a monopoly and can legally control the costs. Similarly, there are situations in which a single purchaser (monopsony) can distort pricing. Costing strategies require identification of the operating costs as well as the out-of-pocket expenditures. The latter may include costs incurred by patients or their families such as time lost from work or leisure. These costs might also include secondary losses. For example, wages lost by a wife when she resigns her job in order to care for an ailing husband.

In estimating costs, it is important to take time preference into consideration. For example, when given the choice between $1000 today or the same amount in 5 years, most respondents would prefer the money now rather than the promise that it will be delivered in the future. However, if offered $1000 now or $3000 in 5 years, the decision may be more difficult. The discount rate is the rate at which the current offer needs to be inflated in order to make it of equal value when delivered in the future. Typically, the cost analysis involves the application of some discount rate. Most often the chosen rate is the rate of inflation. There is less agreement for well-years. For example, it is uncertain whether people would prefer to have good health now or to reserve it for some time in the future. Nevertheless, it has become common practice to discount health benefits at the same rate that financial resources are discounted.

Step 7: Rank Health Care Costs and Outcomes by Forming a Cost/Utility Ratio

In a variety of publications, we have suggested how the concept of a well-life expectancy can be used to evaluate the effectiveness of programs and health interventions (Bush et al., 1973; Epstein et al., 1981; Kaplan & Bush, 1982; Kaplan et al., 1988). The output of a program has been described in a variety of publications as quality-adjusted life years (Bush et al., 1972; 1973), well-years, equivalents of well-years, or discounted well-years (Kaplan et al., 1976; Patrick et al., 1973a; Patrick et al., 1973b). Weinstein (Weinstein & Feinberg, 1980; Weinstein & Stason, 1983) has popularized the concept and calls the same output quality-adjusted life years (QALY), which has also been adopted by the Office of Technology Assessment (1979). It is worth noting that the QALY terminology was originally introduced by Bush et al. (1973) but was later abandoned because it has surplus meaning. The term *wellness* or *well-years* implies a more direct linkage to health conditions. Whatever the term, the index shows the output of a program in years of life adjusted by the quality of life which has been lost because of diseases or disability.

Using the information on costs and outcomes, a cost/utility ratio can be formed. This is simply cost/well-years.

The model for point in time with quality of well-being is:

QWB = 1 – (observed morbidity × morbidity weight)
        – (observed physical activity × physical activity weight)
        – (observed social activity × social activity weight)
        – (observed symptom/problem × symptom/problem weight)

The net cost/utility ratio is defined as

$$\frac{\text{net cost}}{\text{net QWB} \times \text{duration in years}} = \frac{\text{cost of treatment} - \text{cost of alternative}}{(QWB_2 - QWB_1) \times \text{duration in years}}$$

where QWB_2 and QWB_1 are QWB scores obtained at times 2 and 1 respectively.

Consider, for example, a person who is in an objective state of functioning that is rated by community peers as 0.5 on a 0 to 1.0 scale. If the person remains in the state for 1 year, they have lost the equivalent of half of 1 year of life. So, for example, a person limited in activities who requires a cane or walker to get around the community might be hypothetically at 0.50. Over the course of an entire year, he or she would lose the equivalent of 1 year of life. A person who has the flu may also get 0.50, but the illness might only last 3 days. Thus, the total loss in well-years might be $3/365 \times 0.50 = 0.004$ well-years.

Net health effects are estimated as

$$\frac{C_w - C_{wo}}{W_w - W_{wo}}$$

where C_w is the cost with the treatment or program, C_{wo} is the cost without the treatment or program, W_w is the well-years with the treatment or program, and W_{wo} is the well-years of life without the treatment or program.

Using the cost/well-year ratio it is possible to rank-order various programs. Typically, potential programs are rank-ordered by how much they return for the invested dollar. Interpretation of a rank-order list must take available resources into consideration. If enough resources are available, all services can be covered. However, if resources are restricted, funding programs according to the ordering on the list will provide the most health to the population given the resources available.

Another way to evaluate outcomes is within "policy space." Various approaches to cost/benefit and cost/utility analysis occasionally produce different results. The output for cost/benefit analysis is in monetary terms—a program that produces cost savings. Cost/utility analysis focuses on the cost to produce a well-year of life. Anderson et al. (1986) integrated the concepts of well-years and net dollars returned within a common framework. This was accomplished by creating a two-dimensional policy space as illustrated in Fig. 4.1. The x axis in the figure represents net dollars returned per person. Returns are defined as benefits minus costs in dollar units. The y axis displays well-years lost or gained through a particular treatment program, clinical intervention, or policy change. The right half of the plane would be used to represent programs in which benefits exceed costs, while the left half would display situations in which costs exceed benefits. The upper half of the figure displays outcomes that have positive health effects in terms of well-years. The bottom half of the figure would be used to represent negative health outcomes in well-year units.

The two-dimensional space yields four quadrants. One quadrant, the lower

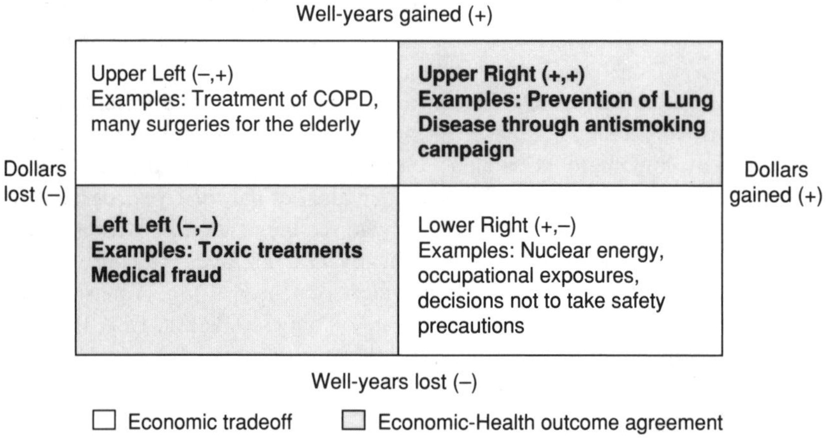

Figure 4.1 Two-dimensional policy space. The x axis represents net costs per person. The y axis displays well-years lost or gained through a particular program. (Adapted from Anderson et al., 1986).

left, represents unsuitable alternatives. In these cases, dollars are being spent and negative health consequences occur. Administration of a uniformly toxic treatment might be represented by this quadrant. The upper-right quadrant represents the most attractive alternatives. Here, well-year health benefits are gained and there are also economic benefits. Prevention of early heart disease might be an example. The upper-left quadrant shows well-year gains, but with more significant costs associated with these improvements. Transplantation surgery for the elderly might be described by this quadrant. Here, there are significant health benefits, but the recipients may not return to the productive economic sector.

The lower-right quadrant represents another level of economic tradeoff. Here, society may be willing to sacrifice some health benefits in exchange for cost savings. Anderson and colleagues suggested that these tradeoffs may be common in studies involving nuclear power; pollution control; occupational, environmental, and consumer product safety; highway speed limits, etc.

Step 8: Revise Rankings According to New Data

Decision analysis is an imprecise science. As a result, steps 1 through 7 may produce outcomes that are illogical or problematic. The imprecision of the model can be addressed in several ways. First, it is valuable to perform sensitivity analyses. These analyses take into consideration the imprecision of the data. In sensitivity analysis, the analysts recalculate the data for several values of important variables. For example, analysts might vary the incidence for a particular condition or the expected benefit of the treatment. Typically, the analysis considers assumptions that are both more pessimistic and more optimistic than the base case. For example, when evaluating the benefit of dietary intervention to prevent heart disease, we might establish a consensus base case from reviewing the literature. Then the analysis would be redone, assuming that the effective treatment is one standard deviation better than the base case and one standard deviation worse than the base case.

In decision analysis, there may be instances in which the base case looks suspicious. Careful scrutiny of any data that looks suspicious is encouraged. When newer observations are available, the model can be recalculated. The model should be dynamic, allowing for continual revision as new information becomes available.

Decision analysis is a guide for decision makers but does not necessarily provide restrictive rules. Ultimately, allocation of resources may take other factors into consideration. For instance, administrators for communities may have strong preferences for some programs that are not highly placed on the list. However, the model may help decision makers identify the most appropriate route for obtaining the greatest benefit for the most people.

SUMMARY

In this chapter we have offered a General Health Policy Model. The model is directed toward producing the best value for money. The major emphasis of the model is to identify how to produce the most health, given the financial constraints. The model is directly relevant to the problem of health care affordability and health care accountability. Although the model does not specifically address the issue of access, it can be applied in combination with many of the competing alternatives for national health insurance. For example, the GHPM could be applied by a single payer to establish which services should be funded. A centralized health insurance mechanism would allow the identification of maximum health benefit. The economic force of a single payer could be used to accomplish the prioritization process.

The GHPM could also work with managed competition. Competitors within the mix might use a GHPM in order to maximize health benefits within the limitations of their budgets. The model may be appealing to consumers because it uses the available resources to obtain the most effective health outcomes for beneficiaries.

The following chapters discuss applications of the model. Chapter Five presents several medical and public health problems that have been analyzed using this approach. Chapter Six reviews an attempt to apply the model by a Health Services Commission in the state of Oregon. The Oregon exercise identified methodological and ethical challenges. These problems will be reviewed in Chapter Seven. Chapter Eight summarizes the remaining research agenda.

Selected Applications of the General Health Policy Model

The notion that we should invest in health services that make people well seems straightforward. Yet, the application of this model is difficult. The major problem is that different programs in health care have different objectives. Some health care providers are trying to reduce the infant mortality rate. Rheumatologists strive to make their patients more functional, while primary care providers often focus on shortening the cycle of acute illness. All of these providers are attempting to improve the health of their patients. However, they all measure health in different ways. Comparing the productivity of a rheumatologist with that of an oncologist may be like comparing apples to oranges.

The diversity of outcomes in health care has led many analysts to focus on the simplest common ground. Typically, that is mortality or life expectancy. When mortality is studied, those who are alive are statistically coded as 1 while those who are dead are statistically coded as 0. Mortality allows the comparison between different diseases. For example, we can state the life expectancy for those who will eventually die of heart disease and compare it to the life expectancy of those who will eventually die of cancer. The difficulty is that everyone who remains alive is given the same score. A person confined to bed with an irreversible coma is alive and is counted the same as someone who is actively playing volleyball at a picnic. One purpose of the QWB scale is to quantify levels of wellness on the continuum between death and optimum function. Figure 5.1 shows a common comparison in survival analysis. The upper curve describes the probability of living to various ages, given that treatment is received. The lower curve describes the probability of living to these same ages in the absence of treatment. The difference in the area between the curves describes the impact of the intervention. Figure 5.2 shows a similar survival analysis that adjusts for quality of life. In other words, this figure rates the degree of dysfunction along this scale. The difference in the areas

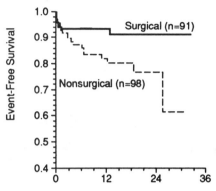

Figure 5.1 A comparison of two groups by survival analysis. The upper curve shows the probability of living to various ages for those who receive the treatment (in this case, surgery for occlusion of the carotid artery), while the lower curve shows the probability of living to these ages without treatment (Mayberg et al., 1991).

between the curves in Fig. 5.2 represents adjusted years of life. In other words, this is a survival analysis that adjusts for quality of life. The methods for making these adjustments were described in Chapter 4. This chapter reviews several applications of the model.

EXAMPLES OF CLINICAL PROBLEMS

There is growing pressure to make difficult health resource decisions. For example, the Department of Veteran Affairs (DVA) runs the largest chain of hospitals in the United States. These DVA medical centers once enjoyed substantial freedom in medication choices. Recently, however, budgets in the DVA have been constrained. The pharmacies have been asked to review alternatives and make formulary decisions about which products should be kept in stock. In response, the hospitals appointed formulary committees to help make these difficult decisions. One of the major difficulties is that the committees had very little data to guide their decisions. Further, the committees typically included physicians from competing medical specialties who are unable to find a common language that could be used to compare the different treatment alternatives. One application of the GHPM is to help with this type of decision.

Other applications of the model are more clinical. Treatments have side effects and they have benefits. When the outcome measures are highly focused, researchers may measure positive effects but ignore the negative. For example, treatments for hypertension have typically been evaluated in terms of reductions in blood pressure. However, these same treatments also produce headaches, dizzi-

Well

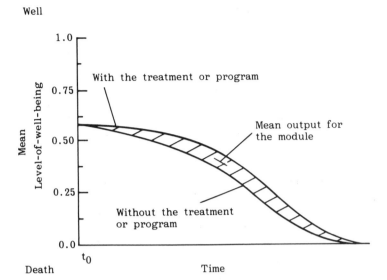

Figure 5.2 Survival analysis that adjusts for health-related quality of life. The area between the curves is the benefit of the program expressed in well-years of life.

ness, and impotence in males. For many years, researchers never even bothered to evaluate these side effects. Once documentation of side effects began, we were left with the difficult problem of knowing that the drugs did some good and some harm. Despite side effects, many drugs are worth using because the benefits outweigh the consequences. The challenge is to evaluate all the benefits and all the side effects and come to a comprehensive evaluation of treatment value. This chapter gives some examples of GHPM applications relevant to these different problems. The GHPM has now been used for a variety of different purposes. It would not be possible to review all of these applications here. Instead, some selected applications of the model will be presented.

The following sections provide several examples describing how this system might be used to evaluate medical technology or other health interventions. Examples describing the use of the system for the evaluation of health policy alternatives are given in the later sections of the chapter.

It is important to emphasize that the QWB scale is the measurement system for a GHPM. Ultimately, we hope that clinical trials will incorporate these measures so the estimates of treatment effects can be obtained in well-year units. Many of the analyses presented depend upon estimates of QWB scores rather than the actual measurements but are presented to emphasize the potential for utilizing quality-of-life measures for policy studies.

THE TIGHT CONTROL OF INSULIN-DEPENDENT
DIABETES MELLITUS

Several studies have suggested that the degree of hyperglycemia is associated with the long-term risk of diabetic complications (Tchobroutsky, 1978). However, there is no strong experimental evidence confirming that reduction in blood sugar leads to a parallel reduction in diabetic complications. The most frequently cited study purporting to show the benefits of the tight control of diabetes (Job et al., 1976) has been aggressively criticized because there were many therapeutic crossovers, data were incomplete, and the difference in blood glucose between experimental and control participants was not large (Schade et al., 1983). Other studies have failed to show reversals of microvascular diabetic complications with intensive therapy (Ballugooie et al., 1984).

The question of tight control of diabetes was considered ambiguous enough for the U.S. National Institutes of Health to begin a prospective clinical trial to evaluate the benefits of tight control versus ordinary care. The trial, known as the Diabetes Control and Complications Trial (DCCT), will include approximately 1400 subjects treated over a 10-year period. We will evaluate a portion of the DCCT subjects using the GHPM which may have substantial benefits for estimating treatment benefits. In addition to mortality, diabetes may be associated with poor outcomes in a variety of organ systems. For example, poor control might lead to differential rates of retinopathy, kidney failure, and foot infections. The difficulty is in finding one common expression for these outcomes. Some patients may have foot infections that result in amputations, while others have eye problems that result in blindness. One purpose of our system is to aggregate these outcomes with death to provide a single expression of the impact of poor control. Diabetic coma receives a score of approximately .32 on our scale while vision impairment that interferes with driving a car and work but does not interfere with self-care might receive a score of .610. This tells us that 2 days of diabetic coma add up to less than 1 day of vision impairment. However, a treatment that eliminates diabetic coma (averaged across the duration of the coma) might be considered more valuable than one that reduces vision impairment. The objective is to eliminate any sort of impairment. Our system does provide for some weighting of the very different outcomes assessed in the study.

The system also includes the capability of expressing side effects and benefits of treatments in the same unit. For example, suppose that the treatment reduces the probability of retinopathy by 25%. We will assume that 40% of the patients will eventually get serious retinopathy (Klein & Klein, 1985). Suppose further that the retinopathy begins at age 55 and continues until death at age 75. The weight associated with blindness or serious vision impairment might be .5. Our system might suggest that the chances of developing serious retinopathy (.4) multiplied by average decrease in well-being (.5) over 20 years, multiplied by the probability of reduction in severity resulting from treatment (.25) would equal 1.0 well-year

(.4 × .5 × 20 × .25 = 1.0. In other words, the improved treatment of diabetes might add up to the equivalent of one healthy year of life expectancy.

Now, we must consider the consequences or side effects of tight control. For the sake of argument, assume that the intensive treatment begins at age 30. One-third of the patients experience nausea and weakness associated with tight control on half of the days. So, let us assume that the duration is 75 – 30 = 45 years, multiplied by the proportion of days in which there are symptoms, .5 × 45 = 22.5 years, multiplied by the weight associated with the symptom of sick or upset stomach which is .75. The net side effects are .33 of all patients × 22.5 years × .25 average decrease in QWB = 1.87 years. In this example the side effects might cause a loss of the equivalent of 1.87 years while the benefits product a benefit of 1.0 years. However, the benefits for other aspects of treatment must also be considered. So, for example, we would also consider the altered probability of kidney disease, heart disease, etc. With these added in, the benefits would most likely outweigh the side effects.

Ultimately, the net effects of a treatment are expressed in these QALY units. The next question concerns determination of the costs to produce a quality-adjusted or well-year unit, from which comparison health care programs with very different specific objectives may be formed. These calculations have been completed for several treatments, including medication for arthritis.

AURANOFIN TREATMENT FOR PATIENTS WITH RHEUMATOID ARTHRITIS

Clinical trials for treatments of rheumatoid arthritis have considered a wide variety of end points. The traditional approach has been to review clinical outcomes such as degree of synovitis. This is typically assessed by measuring tenderness or swelling of joints, grip strength, time to walk 50 feet, or duration of stiffness upon rising in the morning. At an international conference on outcome measurement in arthritis, it was suggested that comprehensive assessments of quality-of-life outcomes were highly desirable (Bombardier et al., 1982). In a recent clinical trial involving 14 centers, more than 300 patients were randomly assigned to therapy with oral gold (auranofin) or a placebo. A wide variety of traditional and nontraditional measures were used to assess outcome, and among the nontraditional measures was the QWB Scale. The outcome using the QWB is shown graphically in Fig. 5.3. There was essentially no change in QWB function for the placebo group, while the group receiving auranofin showed a mean improvement of .023. This difference was statistically significant beyond the .005 level. Auranofin does not reach pharmacologically effective levels in blood until it has been used for about 2 months. It is interesting that QWB scores for the treatment and placebo groups begin to diverge at about 2 months. Considering the many measures used in the trial, the percentage of variance accounted for with the QWB measure was among the very most significant (see Fig. 5.4). Outcomes measures using tradi-

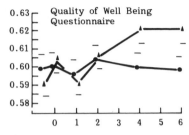

Figure 5.3 Comparison of rheumatoid arthritis patients treated with auranofin (▲) and placebo (●) using the QWB system (From Bombardier et al., 1986.)

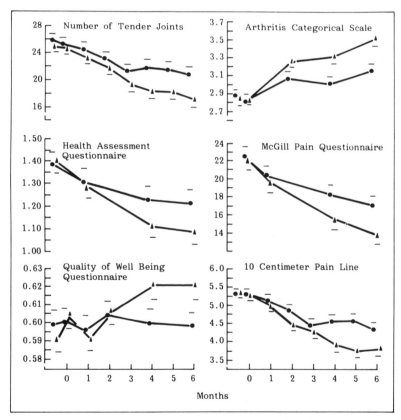

Figure 5.4 Comparison of QWB with 50-foot walk, duration of morning stiffness, and several other outcome measures in auranofin study. (From Bombardier et al., 1986.)

tional clinical measures, such as the 50-foot walk and the duration of morning stiffness, were not statistically significant, although they did favor the auranofin group. In addition, simple self-ratings by both patients and physicians failed to detect the significant effect. However, a significant network of associations emerged suggesting that the QWB was associated with other similar measures of general function (Bombardier et al., 1986).

It is important to consider the clinical importance of a difference of .023. Although this appears to be a small number, the QWB provides a direct translation into clinically meaningful units. A difference of .023 translates into 2.3 quality-adjusted life years for each 100 patients who maintain the difference for 1 year. Also, although .023 appears to be a small change, the entire continuum from death to optimal health is represented on the 0 to 1.0 scale. The differences observed in the auranofin trial are quire respectable in comparison to those obtained through other medical treatments.

One of the most important aspects of the QWB is its capability of quantifying side effects as well as benefits. Many of the specific scales used for the auranofin trial were not capable of detecting the general effect of the intervention upon health status. Yet gold preparations are known to cause significant adverse effects including diarrhea, headache, rashes, digestive problems, and abdominal pain. In fact, 59% of the auranofin-treated patients experienced diarrhea at some point in comparison to 19% of the placebo-treated group. The GHPM allowed these side effects to be integrated with benefits in order to provide a comprehensive expression of net treatment efficacy (Thompson et al., 1988). In comparison to control subjects, the costs associated with auranofin treatment were $788 per patient. The investigators estimated the cost/utility of auranofin therapy at just more than 10,000 U.S. dollars per well-year of life. This compares quite favorably to many alternatives in health care.

CORONARY ARTERY BYPASS GRAFTS

Despite some controversy (Braumwald, 1977; Hultgren et al., 1982; CASS Principle Investigators and Their Associates, 1983), coronary artery bypass graft (CABG) has become a major treatment for symptomatic coronary artery disease. The number of procedures performed in the United States has steadily grown to an estimated 332,000 in 1987 at an estimated cost of $35,000 per operation (Vital and Health Statistics, 1989). The significance of the procedure and the expenses associated with it led Weinstein & Stason (1982) to conduct a systematic evaluation of the literature on CABG using a cost/utility model with the data provided by clinical reports, systematic longitudinal data banks, and clinical trials including the major trials conducted by the European Coronary Surgery Study Group and the Veterans Administration (VA) Cooperative Study.

The analysis considered the benefit for a 55-year-old male population, since

55 years is approximately the median age for receipt of CABG. The analysis considered only those men who would be deemed operable by cardiologists on the basis of clinical characteristics and angiography and was done separately for men with obstruction (defined as 50% or more) of 1, 2, or 3 coronary arteries or with left main coronary artery disease. In each of these cases, ventricular function was good, with at least a 40% ejection fraction. The analysis for patients with poor ventricular function will not be considered here.

In order to calculate QALYs, Weinstein and Stason needed to integrate morbidity and mortality information. They used data about symptomatic relief from the European Coronary Surgery Study Group (1979, 1980) and from the Montreal Heart Institute (Campeau et al., 1979) and also simulated the benefit results using a variety of quality judgments for observed levels of functioning and symptomatic angina.

The approach used by Weinstein and Stason uses data from different sources. Data from the VA study and from the European trial differed in their evaluation of the benefits of surgery for one-vessel and two-vessel disease: The VA data suggest that surgery may be detrimental in these cases, while the European data indicate that there will be benefits. Results of these two trials and other data are merged to obtain central assumptions that are operative in the analysis, although the analysis can also consider differing assumptions and the impact these assumptions have upon quality-adjusted life expectancy. Under the assumption that the preference for life with angina is .7 (on a scale from 0 to 1), Weinstein and Stason estimated the benefits of surgical treatment over medical treatment for the various conditions. They found that the benefits in quality-adjusted life years would be .5, 1.1, 3.2, and 6.2 years for one vessel, two vessels, three vessels, and left main artery disease, respectively.

Next, Weinstein and Stason estimated the cost of the surgery and evaluated cost/utility under the central assumptions. Assuming that the surgery relieves severe angina, the estimates ranged from $30,000/well-year for one-vessel disease to $3,800/well-year for left main artery disease. Weinstein and Stason performed these analyses under a variety of assumptions and, in doing so, they revealed the impact of considering quality of life. One assumption ignored quality of life and considered only life expectancy. But the cost-effectiveness of bypass surgery for one-vessel disease with this assumption cannot be estimated since surgery has no effect upon survival. However, many of the benefits of surgery are directed toward the quality of life rather than survival. If the surgery is performed to relieve mild angina, the cost/utility for one vessel disease exceeds $500,000/well-year (1986 U.S. dollars). A model that did not integrate mortality and morbidity would have missed benefits for some types of surgery.

In summary, the Weinstein & Stason (1982) analysis demonstrates that the cost/utility of CABG differs by characteristic of disease state, but the cost/utility figures compare favorably with those from other widely advocated medical procedures and screening programs.

ADHERENCE TO ANTIHYPERTENSIVE
MEDICATIONS

Hypertension is a major public health problem because of its high prevalence and its association with heart disease and stroke. Many people are unaware that they have hypertension, and many of those who are aware are unwilling to take the necessary actions to control the condition.

Weinstein & Stason (1976) have calculated the cost/utility of screening programs for severe hypertension (diastolic > 105 mm Hg) to be $4850/well-year and the corresponding figure for mild hypertension screening programs (diastolic 95–104 mm Hg) to be $9800/well-year.

However, their analysis also considered a variety of factors that influence these cost/utility ratios. One of the most important factors is adherence to the prescribed medical regimen once cases have been detected. The figures given above assume full adherence to the regimen. Yet, substantial evidence reveals that full (100%) adherence is rare (DiMatteo & DiNicola, 1982). Compliance with antihypertensive medications is of particular interest because taking the medication does not relieve symptoms; in fact, medication adherence can increase rather than decrease somatic complaints. More studies have been devoted to compliance among hypertensive patients than to compliance in any other disease category, and some studies suggest that behavioral intervention can be very useful in increasing adherence to prescribed regimens (Haynes et al., 1976).

In their analysis, Weinstein and Stason considered the value of programs designed to increase adherence to antihypertensive medication. Two separate problems were considered. First, there are drop-outs from treatment and, second, there is failure to adhere to treatments that have been prescribed. The two cases may differ in their cost. One extreme is the patient who fails to see a physician and purchase medication; here the cost would be very low. The other extreme would be the patient who remains under medical care and purchases medications but does not take them. In this case, the costs would be high. Weinstein and Stason refer to these as the minimum-cost assumption and the maximum-cost assumption. Under the minimum-cost assumption, patients do not receive the full benefits of medication because of incomplete adherence, but they also do not spend money. Thus according to Weinstein and Stason, the cost/effectiveness under this assumption is very similar to full adherence in which patients receive the benefits of medication but make full expenditures. Under the maximum-cost assumption, the effect of incomplete adherence is substantial, particularly for those beginning therapy beyond the age of 50. Earlier it was noted that the costs to produce a well-year for a national sample (United States) were $4850 for those with pretreatment diastolic blood pressure greater than 105 mm Hg. With incomplete adherence, these values increase to $6400 under the minimum-cost assumption and $10,500 under the maximum-cost assumption. For mild hypertensive screening (diastolic blood pressure 95–104 mm Hg), the $9880 per well-year under the full-adherence assumption rose to $12,500 under the minimum-cost assumption and $20,400 under the maximum-cost assumption.

Since adherence under the maximum-cost assumption appears to have a strong effect upon cost/utility, it is interesting to consider the value of behavioral interventions to improve adherence. Several studies have shown the value of behavioral interventions and it is reasonable to assume that a successful behavioral intervention will improve adherence rates by 50% (Haynes et al., 1976). Weinstein and Stason considered the cost/utility of interventions that would improve adherence by 50% under the maximum-cost assumption. Their analysis of hypothetical programs that would reduce diastolic blood pressure from 110 to 90 mm Hg suggests a differential expected cost/utility for programs designed for males and for females. As the figure shows, the intervention would improve the cost/utility for both males and females and at each age of therapy reveals the finding from epidemiologic studies that blood pressure is better controlled in women than in men. In summary, the analysis demonstrates that even an expensive program can improve cost/utility because it produces substantial improvements in outcome relative to its costs.

In the Weinstein and Stason monograph, a variety of other hypothetical conditions were considered. Under the assumption that the program improves adherence by 50%, a significant benefit of the program remained under the maximum-cost assumption. However, under the minimum-cost assumption, the hypothetical adherence intervention would have a significant benefit if it increased adherence by 50% but no significant effect if it increased adherence by only 20%.

Other assumptions in the Weinstein and Stason analysis need to be considered. For example, they make (and discuss) many other assumptions about the relationship between hypertension and outcome, the linear relationship between adherence and outcome, and the effect of adherence programs. Some data support the reasonableness of each of these assumptions.

Figure 5.5 shows how very different programs can be compared using the system and summarizes the two Weinstein and Stason studies discussed above.

ACQUIRED IMMUNODEFICIENCY SYNDROME

The Acquired Immune Deficiency Syndrome (AIDS), resulting from infection with the human immunodeficiency virus (HIV), represents one of the most important threats to the world population in the 1990s. The Centers for Disease Control estimates that between one and two million Americans are currently infected with HIV (Centers for Disease Control, 1991). In April 1990 the CDC reported that 50,000 people had died from AIDS and that one million new cases were expected by 1992.

In addition to opportunistic infections and malignancies which define AIDS, HIV infection may cause a broad range of diseases. These conditions include persistent lymphadenopathy, thrombocytopenia, immune complex disease, wast-

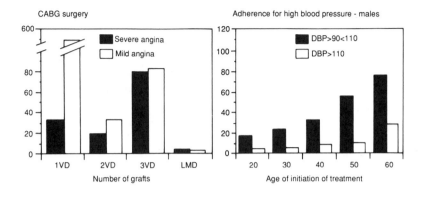

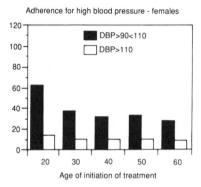

Figure 5.5 Comparison of the cost-effectiveness of blood pressure reduction strategies under several assumptions. (Adapted from Weinstein & Stason, 1976.)

ing, various constitutional symptoms, and HIV neurologic diseases. The impact of HIV infection on functioning is equally diverse. For example, HIV infection may result in fatigue, arthritis, blindness, memory loss, or paraplegia. Treatments for HIV infection should be designed to prevent early mortality and to reduce morbidity during periods before death. The diverse impacts of both HIV disease and its treatment require a general approach to assessment.

There have been several previous attempts to evaluate quality of life in HIV-infected patients. However, most of these have focused on psychological outcomes. Few studies have attempted to characterize the health status and economic impacts of HIV infection, and we are aware of only three studies that have applied general health-related quality-of-life scales.

Since September 1987, AZT has been available by prescription to treat patients with advanced HIV infection. This decision was based on the encouraging results of early clinical trials. In the multicenter phase II AZT trial, 19 of 137 placebo recipients died as compared to 1 of 145 AZT recipients. The incidence of opportunistic infections was also significantly reduced among AZT recipients. Thus, in certain groups of patients, AZT may profoundly lower both mortality and morbidity (Fischl et al., 1987). However, serious side effects are frequently associated with AZT, including anemia, neutropenia, nausea, myalgia, insomnia, and severe headache. Nearly one-third (31%) of patients who received AZT required blood transfusions for anemia (Richman et al., 1987).

In the San Diego arm of the multicenter AZT trial, Wu and colleagues obtained outcome data using the QWB and the Karnofsky Performance Status measure (Wu et al., 1990). The participants in the study were 31 patients (27 male, 4 female) with a clinical diagnosis of either AIDS or severe AIDS-related complex (ARC). They were randomly assigned to receive AZT treatment or placebo and were evaluated using the QWB before beginning the trial and at eight follow-up visits over the next 52 weeks. The value of the treatment was estimated using the repeated-measures analysis of variance (calculated using a general linear model).

The patients were divided into those with CD_4 cell (also known as T_4 lymphocytes or T-helper cells) counts less than or greater than 100×10^9. Patients in both groups were comparable at baseline with regard to age, CD_4 group, sex, diagnosis (AIDS or ARC), Karnofsky score, and QWB (t test and chi square, $p > .15$). In fact, mean initial CD_4 count was significantly higher in the AZT group ($t < .03$).

For the QWB measure, the repeated-measures ANOVA showed a significant effect of time and an interaction between group and time of testing. This interaction, illustrated in Fig. 5.6, is the crucial component in evaluating treatment effectiveness. It suggests that there was a differential rate of change between AZT-treated and control groups. As Fig. 5.6 demonstrates, QWB scores remained relatively constant over the course of time for the AZT group while they declined substantially for the placebo group.

These results suggest that the QWB can detect strong treatment effects associated with AZT. One advantage of the QWB system is that it allows the expression of program benefits in terms of well-year units and the comparison of treatment alternatives that are very different from one another. In the AZT trial, the placebo-treated group experienced substantial mortality and greater morbidity than the AZT group. Neither measures of mortality alone nor of morbidity alone were capable of detecting the potent treatment effect of this medication as could the QWB. Further, the comprehensive measure takes the side effects of AZT into account and expresses outcome as the net benefits minus the adverse effects (Kaplan, 1991).

THE NEONATAL CIRCUMCISION CONTROVERSY

There has been a long-standing debate about the medical indications for neonatal circumcision. In 1971, the American Academy of Pediatrics (1971) concluded that

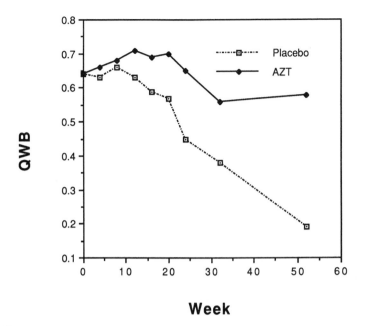

Figure 5.6   Comparison of patients treated with AZT and placebo using QWB scores.

there were no medically valid reasons for performing circumcisions on newborn males. This position was confirmed by the American College of Obstetrics and Gynecology in 1978 (Wallerstein, 1985). However, an important paper by Wiswell (Wiswell & Roscelli, 1986) suggested a tenfold increase in urinary tract infections for uncircumcised male infants. As a result of these data, new questions about an old controversy began to arise.

Recently a cost/utility analysis was performed in order to estimate the total health effects and the total costs of neonatal circumcision. The analysis considered the cost of the procedure, the pain associated with the procedure, the probability of urinary tract infections, and the risks of developing cancer of the penis. With the base assumptions, the net discounted lifetime U.S. dollar costs associated with neonatal circumcision were relatively low ($102/person). However, the discounted lifetime health costs were also quite low. Under the base assumptions, the expected health benefit is about 14 hours of well-life expectancy.

In cases such as the evaluation of neonatal circumcision, it is unlikely that a true randomized trial will ever be conducted. Therefore, the analysis typically considers outcomes under a variety of circumstances. However we are often uncertain about the accuracy of these assumptions. In order to deal with the uncertainty, the assumptions are varied. In the circumcision example, the base analysis assumed that the probability of developing cancer if uncircumcised is

.0001 while the probability for those who are circumcised is essentially 0.000. In the sensitivity analysis, it was assumed that the probability of developing cancer if uncircumcised is more severe. For example, it may be as high as 1/600 or 0.00167. The development of cancer may also have important cost implications. In the base case it was assumed that the work-up and treatment costs would be $25,000. The sensitivity analysis considered a lower estimate of $10,000 and a higher estimate of $100,000. Many variables are considered in the sensitivity analyses. For example, the cost of the procedure is considered to be 150 U.S. dollars in the base case while in the sensitivity analysis a lower cost of $50 was also included. The traditional method for comparing a value to be received in the future (e.g., medical expenses overted) with a value to be given at the present time (in this case the cost of the circumcision) is discounting. With the aim of looking at future gains and comparing them with the amount of money currently at hand, compound discount-rate multipliers are typically included in the analysis. In this analysis discount rates in the base case were 5% while a discount rate of 0% was considered for the sensitivity analysis. The discount-rate multipliers were also used with the number of well-years produced.

Under the base case assumptions, the costs of routine neonatal circumcision are $102,451 and the effects are an average loss of 1.61 well-years. Any program that damages health as a function of treatment is not advisable. However, under some assumptions, the analysis suggests more benefits. For example, in the case that a patient needs a second circumcision and experiences symptoms for 120 days prior to the second operation, the cost/utility ratio is $18,463/well-year. If the cost of the later circumcision is 5000 U.S. dollars, then the cost/utility ratio becomes $45,673/well-year. The base case assumes that the cost of circumcision is 150 U.S. dollars. Although the cost/utility of the procedure in the base case is questionable, reducing the cost of the procedure to 50 U.S. dollars makes the intervention look more worthwhile at $9054/well-year. The advantage is because money is saved, not because better health is achieved. Overall, the financial and medical advantages of neonatal circumcision cancel each other out. In this case cost/utility analysis helped clarify that the issue is not one of economics or medical outcome. Instead, the debate must be focused on personal preference and social custom (Ganiats et al., 1991).

SCREENING FOR BREAST CANCER

The need to formulate guidelines for public programs might best be illustrated by the case of screening for breast cancer. Breast cancer is a serious public health problem in the United States and most westernized countries. It is estimated that 150,900 new cases were detected in the United States during 1990. The American Cancer Society suggests that 1 in every 10 women will develop breast cancer at sometime during their lives and that the incidence of breast cancer has increased by 1% each year since the early 1970s (American Cancer Society, 1991).

As a result of concern about the breast cancer epidemic, many political groups have developed plans for action. Political pressure has motivated several new pieces of legislation and breast cancer has been declared an epidemic in several states. Part of the argument behind this political action is that all women are at risk and that all women need to be screened for breast cancer using mammography. Many advocates suggest that mammograms for all women should be reimbursed from public sources.

Breast cancer is a terrible disease and it would clearly be in the public's best interest to do everything possible to detect and eradicate this problem. Yet the analysis of cancer screening brings to light several important policy issues. One of the most complicated concerns is that breast cancer is an age-related condition. In 1991, we reviewed several popular women's magazines including *Women's Day, Self, RedBook,* and *Cosmopolitan.* Each of these magazines is oriented toward younger readers and each carried an article about the threat of breast cancer. The magazines all concluded that obtaining regular mammograms was an important way to prevent early death. The *Women's Day* article went on to suggest that breast tissue is much denser for younger women. Therefore, it was suggested that women not accept a negative mammogram as evidence that they were free of cancer. Instead, they were encouraged to continue seeking the exams.

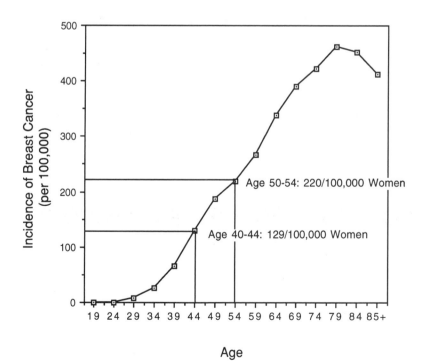

Figure 5.7 Relationship of age to breast cancer. (Data from National Cancer Institute, 1991.)

The relationship between age and breast cancer is illustrated in Fig. 5.7. For younger women, that is women less than 30 years of age, breast cancer is extremely rare. Thereafter, the incidence of the condition increases so that for women ages 40–44 the rate is about 129/100,000 women. One of the challenging questions from a public health perspective is to determine the cost per tumor detected. The reason this is important is that there is an opportunity cost associated with investing in breast cancer screening. Samuelson (1970) defines opportunity costs as foregone opportunities that result in doing one thing rather than another. For example, if we spend substantial amounts of public funds on mammography programs, we may have fewer resources to provide other programs for women or for other citizens. Imagine, for example, that we screen all 20-year-old women for breast cancer. If we assume that each test costs $100, it would cost $10,000,000 to detect a single case. Table 5.1 offers a summary of costs per tumor detected at various ages.

Of course, any amount of public funds spent to save lives is justifiable. The second question in evaluating mammography programs is whether or not screening results in favorable health outcomes. In other words, we must consider the relationship between finding tumors and the chances that women who are tested will live longer and/or better lives.

There is ample reason to believe that screening programs should result in longer life and improved quality of life. The American Cancer Society (1991) reports that the 5-year survival rate for localized breast cancer has improved from 78% in the 1940s to 90% today. In addition, they argued that breast cancer that is *in situ* (not invasive) can be cured through surgery in nearly 100% of the cases. However, if the cancer spreads to the local region the survival rate declines to 68% and for women with cancer spread to distant sites the survival rate is only 18%. These data clearly argue for the detection of tumors while they are localized.

Unfortunately, the evidence on the relationship between mammography screening programs and survival is less clear. Research consistently demonstrates that mammography programs are effective for women who are age 50 or above.

TABLE 5.1

Cost per Tumor Detected by Mammography as a Function of Age

Age	Cost/Tumor
20	10,000,000
30	416,666
40	112 ,000
50	54,000
60	38,167
70	31,645

To date, there is little evidence that women between the ages of 40 and 50 gain any health benefit from regular mammography. This evidence comes from clinical trials in which women are randomly assigned to receive regular mammograms or to a control group that does not receive the tests. Then both groups of women are followed to determine survival and cause of death. For women over the age of 50 at the beginning of the studies, there is evidence that getting regular mammograms leads to longer life and reduced chances of death from breast cancer. On the other hand, only one study shows the same benefit for women under the age of 50 and the effect was weak in this investigation. The study was conducted by the Health Insurance Plan of New York. When analyzed, separately, the benefit for women under 50 was not statistically significant. However, it was in the same direction as for older women and, when all age groups were added together, mammography saved lives. All of the other randomized experimental studies have shown that regular mammography increases the rate at which tumors are found in women less than 50 years. However, none of the other studies has found that women who get regular mammograms live longer or are less likely to die of breast cancer. To complicate matters further, there is at least some evidence that there is a negative effect. In other words, some studies have shown that women between the ages of 40 and 50 are *more* likely to die of breast cancer if they have regular mammography. This was most recently shown in a Canadian study in which women were randomly assigned to receive mammography on a regular basis to a control condition that was not offered mammography. The results of the study are summarized in Fig. 5.8. As might be expected, this study has created considerable controversy (Kopans, 1991).

Eddy (1989) has analyzed the expected benefits of breast cancer screening programs. In Eddy's analysis, the value of mammography in addition to clinical breast examination was considered. According to this analysis, an individual woman increases her life expectancy by about 20 days by receiving regular clinical breast examinations. Mammography may add an additional 28 days to the life expectancy. The probability that the average-risk woman would have a tumor detected if she were examined for 10 consecutive years beginning at age 40 is about 130/10,000. However, the probability of having an alarming false-positive test is about 2,500/10,000 for this 10-year interval. As these calculations suggest, there are some concerns about the regular screening of younger women. These tests may be costly and may provide only small advantages in terms of improving the woman's health outcome. Of course, these findings are extremely controversial and need to be the focus of continuing public debate.

Along with the controversy about mammography, we must also consider the problem of the breast cancer epidemic. Figure 5.9 shows the increase in the rates of breast cancer detection between 1973 and 1987. The incidence of detected breast cancer has increased significantly for both white and black women. An interesting feature of the graph is the increase in cases detected during 1973 and 1974. This corresponds to the identification of breast cancer in the wives of both

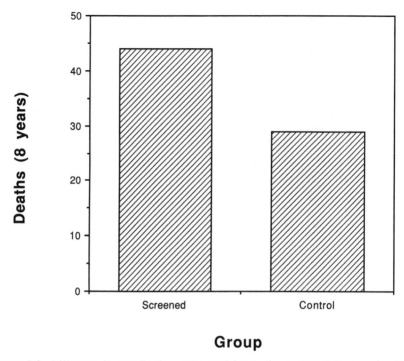

Figure 5.8 Differences in mortality for women receiving regular mammography or assigned to control group from Canadian study.

the President (Betty Ford) and the Vice President (Happy Rockefeller). Highly publicized cases of breast cancer led to a significant increase in the number of women who were screened. Figure 5.10 describes changes in breast cancer mortality between 1973 and 1987. As the figure shows, the death rate from cancers of the breast did not change at all over this interval. In fact, breast cancer death rates have remained relatively constant over the last 50 years. Figure 5.10 shows that these stable rates of breast cancer mortality have been unaffected by the war on cancer which began during the Nixon administration or by the increased use of mammography and breast self-examination (and the consequent increases in numbers of new cases detected early), and in spite of the reported breakthroughs in adjuvant chemotherapy for breast cancer.

This section was not intended to be negative with regard to secondary prevention of breast cancer. Studies clearly do show that mammography screening programs for women 50 years and older are of considerable value. Further, more research on the value of screening and early treatment is clearly required. However, political strategies designed to make breast cancer the exclusive focus of resource use for women may not be well directed. Using substantial resources to

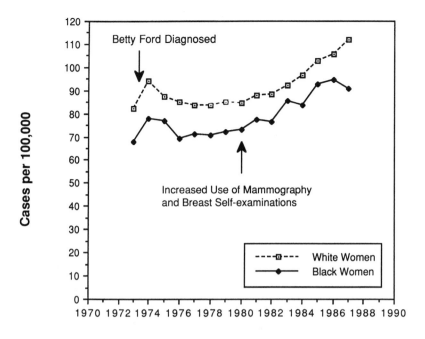

Figure 5.9   Increases in rates of breast cancer detection between 1973 and 1987.

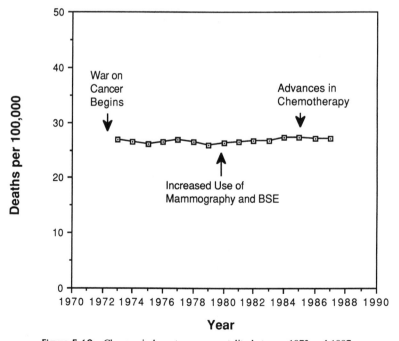

Figure 5.10   Changes in breast cancer mortality between 1973 and 1987.

screen for and treat breast cancer necessarily means that there will be fewer resources to address other problems affecting women or other citizens. Prenatal care, for example, is dramatically underfunded. Even within breast cancer, other areas of research deserve more attention. For example, Doll & Peto (1981) suggest that dietary factors may play an important role in the development of breast tumors. Figure 5.11 shows the relationship between dietary fat and breast cancer rates across a wide variety of cultures. Although this finding is debated, it certainly deserves further attention.

Finally, we must consider the correspondence between policies that promise screening for breast cancer and the known benefits of screening beginning at different ages. Table 5.2 summarizes these policies as developed in a variety of westernized countries. As the table shows, American organizations are somewhat atypical in their recommendation that women be screened at an early age. Most medical groups around the world that have evaluated this question have recommended screening women over the age of 50 and those who have familial risk factors for breast cancer. For example, women who have a mother or a sister who has suffered from the disease would be screened because they are at high risk. Women who have had no children or the first child after the age of 30 are also at higher risk and should be screened at younger ages. Similar conclusions were reached by the U.S. Preventive Services Task Force.

Table 5.2 does show that groups with a financial interest in early mammography are more likely to support it. For example, the American College of Radiologists and the American College of Obstetricians and Gynecologists recommend baseline mammograms at age 35 with screening beginning at age 40. These

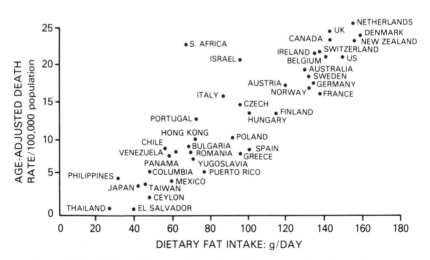

Figure 5.11   Relationship between dietary fat and breast cancer in various cultures.

TABLE 5.2

Comparison of Recommendations by Various National
and International Groups about Age for
Starting Mammography Screening

Group	Age
American	
American Medical Association	35, Baseline
American College of Radiology	40
National Cancer Institute	40
American College of OB/GYN	35, Baseline
American College of Physicians	50
U.S. Preventive Services Task Force	50
Foreign	
Finland	50
Sweden	40
Netherlands	50
United Kingdom	50

recommendations raise questions about the separation of scientific from financial interests in this screening test.

TOBACCO TAX

When asked how to improve health status, we typically think in terms of bio-medical treatment. However, there are many alternative approaches to improving the public health. Some years ago, we analyzed the cost effectiveness of several different programs. These programs ranged from acute medical care to prevention. The analysis demonstrated that the most efficient use of resources was not traditional medical, surgical, or public health programs. Instead, the best cost/utility ratio was associated with laws that required child automobile passengers to be in restraint seats and adults to be buckled in with seat belts (Kaplan, 1988). Expensive medical interventions are often justified because they save lives. However, stricter laws on seat belts also achieve this objective and they do so at a considerably lower cost. One of the advantages of the GHPM is that it allows for comparisons between very different types of programs. As an example, consider programs aimed at reducing the consumption of cigarettes. Substantial evidence suggests that cigarette smoking causes the largest number of preventable deaths each year (U.S. Surgeon General, 1989). Although cigarette smoking has declined in the United States and the United Kingdom within recent years, the worldwide trend is toward increased use of tobacco products. Peto (1990) projects that worldwide there will be 10 million tobacco-related deaths per year by the year

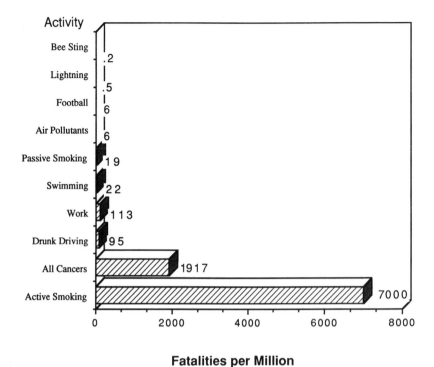

Fatalities per Million

Figure 5.12 Relationship between various activities and fatalities per million persons in the population. (Data from U.S. Surgeon General, 1989.)

2010. The importance of the cigarette smoking problem might be summarized in Fig. 5.12. This graph, based on data from the U.S. Surgeon General's report, compares the fatalities in the U.S. population associated with various causes. The public is very concerned about dramatic causes of death such as being struck by lightning, being killed by an accident at work, or being killed by a drunk driver. However, these are not common causes of death. For example, there are about 95 deaths per million persons in the population associated with drunk drivers. However, active smoking is associated with about 7000 deaths per million persons. For each person killed by a drunk driver, nearly 74 active smokers die prematurely.

There are many different approaches to the control of cigarette smoking. However, one of the best ways to control cigarette use may be to increase the price of these products. Economists use the term elasticity to refer to changes in demand that occur as a function of price. There has been some debate about whether or not demand for tobacco products is "elastic." The emerging consensus is that a significant proportion of the variation in tobacco use is responsive to price (Hu et al., 1991).

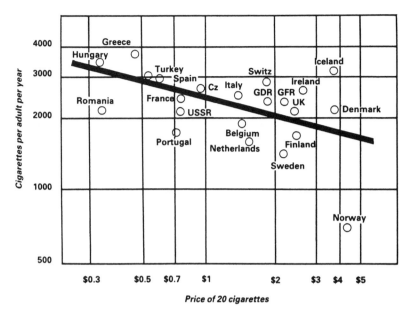

Figure 5.13 Relationship between price per pack of cigarettes and tobacco consumed in 22 European countries. (From World Health Organization, 1987.)

Figure 5.13 shows the relationship between price per pack of cigarettes and cigarettes consumed among 22 European countries. As the figure shows, there is a rough linear relationship between price and consumption. Countries charging more per pack tend to have lower rates of cigarette smoking, while countries charging less per pack tend to have higher rates. In order to evaluate the impact of tobacco taxes, we developed a series of computer simulations. The entire series of simulations will not be presented here. Instead, a summary of one set of simulations will be offered.

Tobacco taxes are appealing because there are multiple beneficiaries. The state benefits because increases in tax may increase revenues. Even if increases in tax reduce consumption, taxes can be raised to the point that there is a net benefit despite the reduced number of consumers. It has been argued that cigarette smokers also benefit from increased tobacco taxes. The reason for this is that about one-half of all cigarette smokers attempt to quit each year (Pierce et al., 1991). Increasing the tax provides extra incentives to reduce cigarette smoking and eventually increase health status. Public opinion polls in California have suggested that nonsmokers *and smokers* prefer increases in the tobacco tax (Pierce et al., 1991).

In order to estimate the impact of increasing the tobacco tax, we employed a series of different assumptions. Under the model presented here, we assumed an elasticity of −.26. Elasticity is defined as a change in the percentage demand divided by the change in the percentage price. The assumption used here suggests, for example, that if there is a 20% increase in price there will be approximately a 5% decrease in demand. The −.26 value was taken from the estimates of price elasticity for smokers of all ages as reported in the U.S. Surgeon General's report in 1989. These estimates are based on three studies by Lewit and colleagues (summarized in Lewit & Coate, 1982). The elasticity estimate is among the most conservative reported in the literature. The analysis also assumes that there are about 56 million smokers in the United States and that one in four of these smokers will eventually die of a tobacco-related disease. The simulation considers a tax increase of 20%.

The simulation uses Monte Carlo techniques. With these methods, a computer is used to generate data under various assumptions. Then, it simulates the expected distribution of outcome over thousands of trials and creates confidence intervals. This analysis considers the expected change in life expectancy for smokers and builds in a model of reduced quality of life for smokers beginning at age 50. The prevalence rate for reduced life expectancy and dysfunction is based on national estimates from the Health Interview Survey. The results of this analysis are summarized in Fig. 5.14. According to the analysis, there is a 50% chance that we could save 6,370,338 well-years of life in the United States by increasing tobacco taxes by 20%. The figure shows that there is a 90% chance of saving about three million well-years. The cost of the program would be very small. In fact, the program would pay for itself out of tax revenues. Such a program would benefit society by reducing the burden of disease and disability and may directly benefit

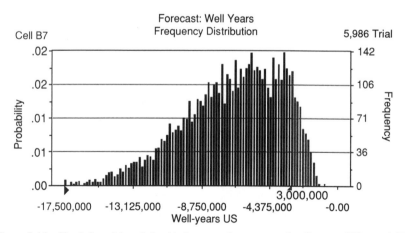

Figure 5.14 Simulation of the relationship between tobacco cost and well-years of life saved. The probability is .90 that the United States would save 3 million well-years of life by increasing the tobacco tax 20%.

TABLE 5.3

Summary of Cost/Well-Year Estimates for Selected Medical, Surgical, and Preventive Interventions[a]

Program	Reference	Cost/Well-Year
Seat belt laws	Kaplan (1988)	0
Ante-partum and anti-D injection[b]	Torrance & Zipursky (1984)	1,543
Pneumonococcal vaccine for the elderly	OTA (1979)	1,765
Post-partum and anti-D injection[b]	Torrance & Zipursky (1977)	2,109
Coronary artery bypass surgery for left main coronary	Weinstein (1982)	4,922
Neonatal intensive care, 1,000–14,999 g	Boyle et al. (1983)	5,473
Smoking cessation counseling	Schulman (1991)	6,463
T4 (thyroid) screening	Epstein et al. (1981)	7,595
PKU screening[c]	Bush et al. (1973)	8,498
Treatment of severe hypertension (diastolic > 105 mm Hg) in males age 40	Stason & Weinstein (1977)	10,896
Oral gold in rheumatoid arthritis	Thompson et al. (1987)	12,059
Dapsone for prophylaxis for PCP pneumonia[d]	Freedberg (1991)	13,400
Treatment of mild hypertension (diastolic 95–104 mm Hg) in males age 40	Weinstein & Stason (1976)	22,197
Oat bran for high cholesterol	Kinosian et al. (1988)	22,910
Rehabilitation in COPD[e]	Toevs et al. (1984)	28,320
Estrogen therapy for postmenopausal symptoms in women without a prior hysterectomy	Weinstein (1980)	32,057
Neonatal intensive care, 500–999 g	Boyle et al. (1983)	38,531
CABG (surgery) 2-vessel disease[f]	Weinstein & Stason (1982)	39,770
Hospital hemodialysis	Churchill et al. (1984)	40,200
Coronary artery bypass surgery for single-vessel disease with moderately severe occlusion	Weinstein (1981)	42,195
School tuberculin testing program	Bush et al. (1972)	43,250
Continuous ambulatory peritoneal dialysis	Churchill et al. (1984)	54,460
Cholestipol for high cholesterol	Kinosian et al. (1988)	92,467
Cholestyramine for high cholesterol	Kinosian et al. (1988)	153,105
Screening mammography	Eddy (1990)	167,850
Total hip replacement	Liang (1987)	293,029
CABG (surgery) 1-vessel heart disease[f]	Weinstein & Stason (1982)	662,835
Aerosolized pentamidine for prophylaxis of PCP pneumonia[d]	Freedberg (1991)	756,000

[a]All estimates adjusted to 1991 U.S. dollars; [b]treatment for Rh immunization; [c]PKU, phenylketonuria; [d]PCP, pneumocystic carinii pneumonia; [e]COPD, chronic obstructive pulmonary disease; [f]CABG, coronary artery bypass graft.

smokers by providing incentives to quit early. The losers in this scheme would be smokers who chose to continue their habit and the tobacco industry.

Overall, the analysis suggests that there is a public health advantage to raising tobacco taxes. Similar conclusions have been reached by several authors and have been summarized by Warner (1986). It is important to emphasize that this is one among several simulations we have conducted. However, even under the most conservative assumptions, the model appears to support the advantages of tobacco taxes in relation to the traditional public health programs.

COMPARISONS ACROSS DIFFERENT PROGRAMS

Table 5.3 summarizes the cost/well-year of life estimated for several medical, surgical, and preventive interventions. Using this system we can begin to rank-order the value for money for many interventions in health care. Among programs that have been analyzed, the most cost-effective option is not a medical procedure. Instead, it is a program that requires children to be in infant seats and adults to be in seat belts. Public health programs such as thyroid disease screening programs (T4), PKU screening, and screening for high blood pressure all compete very favorably. However, some screening programs such as mammography for younger women are less cost effective than other options. Some surgical options used for rescue, including coronary artery bypass surgery for one-vessel disease, produce less health for the dollar invested. Estimates such as those in Table 5.3 depend upon many assumptions and improved analysis is required before we can feel assured that the comparisons are correct. However, enough data are accumulated to begin making these comparisons.

SUMMARY

This chapter summarizes some of our current thinking on the potential for a general health policy model. We believe the system can be used as an aid for understanding clinical and public health problems. Several examples of the use of the QWB in clinical decision making are offered. Current research is often divided between measurement studies and policy analysis. The GHPM includes the measurement system described here. When taken in clinical studies, QWB measurements can be used directly in policy analysis. However, few clinical studies have taken QWB measures directly. The examples summarized in this chapter show how programs with very different objectives can be compared directly with one another. In Chapter Six, the application of this line of thinking to a state Medicaid program will be described.

CHAPTER SIX

The Oregon Experiment

The General Health Policy Model has not yet been tried as the method for resolving the problems of health care affordability, access and accountability. However, the state of Oregon attempted an innovative experiment that used many components of the model. This chapter provides an overview of the experience in Oregon. As we will see, Oregon had the right theory but unfortunately failed to adequately execute aspects of the model that would have achieved the state's objectives. Nevertheless, the exercise remains an important lesson in the political process.

HEALTH CARE ISSUES IN OREGON

Oregon is a relatively prosperous northwestern state that has problems much like many other states. Oregon is unique in its recognition of the seriousness of the health care problem. Health care expenditure became a public issue in 1987 when a young boy, Coby Howard, a sufferer of leukemia, needed a bone marrow transplant. At that time, the state did not reimburse for transplants under its Medicaid program. Reports to the state legislature indicated that 34 transplants to Medicaid patients during the period 1987–1989 used the same financial resources as prenatal care and delivery to 1500 pregnant women. When confronted with these issues, the Oregon legislature decided to use its limited resources to provide small benefits to large numbers of people rather than invest in expensive transplantation for a small number of beneficiaries.

Coby Howard died while this case was under appeal. However, the case attracted media attention and raised the issue of how health care resources were being used. Oregon citizens became much more aware that expenditures of high-technology medical care literally mean that many services for low-income people are eliminated. The debate was fueled by acknowledgments from many physicians that some expensive procedures had very limited value for extending life or for improving the quality of life.

The other major issue in Oregon is similar to the problem in essentially all other states. The costs of health care are expanding much more rapidly than are the budgets for Medicaid. The only alternative is to strip some individuals from the Medicaid rolls. Oregon also recognized that health care was not a two-tiered system, but rather a three-tiered system. There were people who had regular insurance and could pay for care, those in Medicaid, and a growing third tier of people who had no health insurance at all. In 1991 it was acknowledged that this third tier represented about one-fifth of the population in the state. In Oregon, that accounts for about 450,000 citizens. In addition, another 230,000 were under-insured. The trend indicated the number of uninsured and underinsured was steadily increasing. In 1989 Oregon citizens spent approximately $6 billion on health care, which is about 3 times what they spent in state income taxes.

Led by John Kitzhaber, the physician President of the State Senate, it was argued that Oregon (and most other states) were rationing health care. The problem is that the rationing was implicit and not always reasonable. Because of shortages of funding, people were being rationed rather than services. In other words, many individuals in need of care received none because they were in the wrong category. A young woman who was an hourly worker, for example, could have been ineligible for health care while a twin sister in the same category who became pregnant could receive care. Thus, the system created incentives to become pregnant in order to have a regular source of health care. The system allowed health care under Medicaid for poor families with young children but disallowed coverage for poor families with older children. Oregon, like many other states, defined Medicaid eligibility for the Aid to Families with Dependent Children (AFDC) as 50% of the poverty line. That policy set the criterion income at about $5700 per year for a family of three. A hard-working independent carpenter earning $11,000 might be completely excluded by the system even though he was at high risk for injury.

A study of health care allocation decisions in other states led the Oregon group to raise other challenging questions. In Illinois, for example, the State Legislature passed a bill that guaranteed reimbursement for organ transplantation up to $200,000. However, 60% of the black children in inner Chicago had not received preventive vaccines, allegedly because there were no public resources to pay for them (Kitzhaber, 1990). Public resources were being used to buy health care, but perhaps not in a way that would ultimately enhance health for the largest number.

Recognizing these problems, Kitzhaber and his associates argued for a new paradigm for health care reimbursement. Initially, his proposal looked remarkably similar to the GHPM. The overall goal of the Oregon plan was to expand Medicaid coverage to cover all citizens below the federal poverty line. This would raise the eligibility criterion from about $464/month to $928/month for a family of three. The second goal of the exercise was to mandate employer-based health insurance for full-time workers and their dependents by 1994. The third provision was to create an insurance "risk pool" to cover those with preexisting conditions. Overall, the plan had provisions to increase access, control cost, and improve accountability.

MECHANISM

In order to accomplish these goals, the Oregon State Legislature enacted three interconnected pieces of legislation. Together, these three bills have become known as the Oregon Basic Health Services Act. The bills are summarized by Fig. 6.1. Senate Bill 935 requires all employers in the state of Oregon to offer health insurance to their workers by 1994. In many respects, this bill is similar to the proposals for universal health insurance that were considered in Chapter Three. As all insurance mandates, there is a problem with those who are uninsurable or chronically ill. These individuals may be excluded because of preexisting health problems. Senate Bill 534 creates a risk pool for the coverage of these people. The risk pool would be subsidized by state resources. Together Senate Bills 935 and 534 address the problem of access. They are like other pieces of legislation directed toward universal health insurance. Neither Senate Bill 935 or Bill 534 directly attacks the problems of affordability or accountability. Those issues are considered in the most controversial portion of the package—Senate Bill 27. This bill mandated that health services be prioritized. The justification of the prioritization was to eliminate services that did not provide benefit. Specifically, the legislation requested

> A list of health services ranked by priority, from the most important to the least important, representing the comparative benefits of each service for the entire population to be served. [p. 3]

According to the report, the rank-ordering of procedures was to be based on the effectiveness of each procedure and upon surveys and the values of Oregon

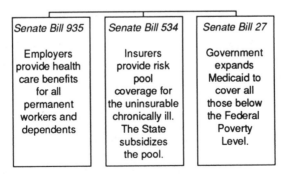

Senate Bill 935	Senate Bill 534	Senate Bill 27
Employers provide health care benefits for all permanent workers and dependents	Insurers provide risk pool coverage for the uninsurable chronically ill. The State subsidizes the pool.	Government expands Medicaid to cover all those below the Federal Poverty Level.

Figure 6.1   Summary of three bills covered by the Oregon plan.

citizens. These values would be determined by public processes. The purpose of the system was to identify those services that are least effective and least valued. Once these services were identified the system would make it less likely that these services would be funded. Conversely, the Commission intended to direct more of the resources toward services which were more effective and of more value.

Senate Bill 27 did not include all Medicaid recipients. Specifically, three groups of Medicaid recipients were excluded: (1) the aged, blind, and disabled, (2) adults who were in official custody or living in institutions, and (3) children who were wards of the court or in foster care.

HEALTH SERVICES COMMISSION

The major responsibility of the program was placed in the hands of an 11-member Health Services Commission, 5 members of which were physicians. The legislation specifically required that the participating physicians have experience in the general areas of obstetrics, prenatal care, pediatrics, adult medicine, geriatrics, or public health. The legislation also required that one of the physicians hold a degree in osteopathic medicine, and that the Commission include a public health nurse, a social worker, and four consumers of health care. These criteria were met and a description of the Commission is shown in Table 6.1.

The Commission began its task without specific expertise or theoretical experience in health services research. They reviewed a variety of resource allocation approaches, reviewed international health care systems, and considered earlier work done by the Oregon Priority Medicaid-Study Project. In addition, they reviewed a variety of different methods for prioritization. For example, they considered a classification system developed by David Hadorn from the University of Colorado. Initially, this approach was rejected because it did not incorporate public values. Similarly a method developed by the RAND Corporation was considered but rejected because it could not facilitate direct comparisons between different services. Two general approaches to estimating health benefits were reviewed. One was the Sickness Impact Profile (SIP) and the other was the Quality of Well-Being Scale (QWB). The Sickness Impact Profile requires responses to 136 health status items. Although the SIP considers the relative importance of aspects of a particular health state it does not provide a rating of overall health. Ultimately, the commission selected the QWB system for the analysis. The QWB is a component of the GHPM (see Chapter Four).

RANKING METHODOLOGY

The Health Services Commission used a variety of different procedures to create its list. In this chapter we consider two different approaches. Initially, the commission attempted a cost/utility analysis of a large number of cases. Later it simplified the process. Each of these stages will be reviewed below.

TABLE 6.1

Health Services Commission Member Biographies

Alan C. Bates, 44, of Eagle Point, is a family physician in Central Point. He is a member of the American Osteopathic Association. He attended Central Washington State University and received a D.O. degree from Kansas City College of Ostheo Medicine. Bates is a member of the Health Outcomes Subcommittee. His term expires in 1991.

Tina Castanares, 40, of Hood River, is a staff physician at La Clinica Del Carina and a health officer with Hood River County. She received the Distinguished Service Award from the U.S. Public Health Service in 1983. She received a bachelors degree from the University of California at Santa Cruz, and an M.D. from the University of Southern California School of Medicine. She is a member of the Social Values Subcommittee. Her term expires in 1993.

Donalda Dodson, 47, of Salem, is a nurse with the Marion County Health Department. She received her bachelor of science degree in nursing from the University of Oregon and her M.P.H. degree from the University of Washington. She is chairperson of the Mental Health, Chemical Dependency, and Substance Abuse Subcommittee. Her term will expire in 1992.

Sharon Gary-Smith, 40, of Portland, is a national health specialist with National Black Women's Health Project. From 1982 to 1984 she was clinic director for Carolyn Downs Family Medical Center in Seattle. Gary-Smith attended Oregon State University. She is a member of the Social Values Subcommittee. Her term expires in 1990.

Bill Gregory, 55, of Glendale, is owner and president of Gregory Forest Products, Inc. He received his bachelor of arts degree from the University of Washington and attended Harvard University of Washington and attended Harvard University, Graduate School of Business Administration. He is the chairperson of the Health Services Commission. His term expires in 1993.

Paul Kirk, 51, of Portland, is a professor and chairman of the department of obstetrics and gynecology at Oregon Health Sciences University. He is a member of the boards of Washington County Head Start program and Healthy Mothers/Healthy Babies Coalition. He attended the University of London where he received a bachelor of science and an M.D. degree. He serves on the Health Outcomes and Social Values Subcommittees. His term expires in 1993.

Amy Klare, 26, of Salem, is the research education director for the Oregon AFL–CIO. She worked for the Oregon Legislature as a legislative aide from 1986 to 1988. Klare received her bachelor of arts degree from Portland State University. She is a member of the Health Outcomes and Social Values Subcommittees. Her term expires in 1991.

Harvey Klevit, 58, of Portland, is chief of pediatrics and assistant regional medical director at Northwest Permanente. He won the Distinguished Service Award from the Oregon Health Sciences University Alumni in 1983 and "The Best and Brightest of Oregon's M.D.'s" from *Oregon Magazine* in 1981. He is the chairperson of the Health Outcomes Subcommittee. His term expires in 1990.

Yayoe Kuramitsu, 46, of Eugene, is director of the Medical Social Work Department at Sacred Heart General Hospital. She received her M.S.W. degree from Boston College School of Social Work in Massachusetts in 1970. She is the chairperson of the Social Values Subcommittee. Kuramitsu's term expires in 1991.

Ellen Lowe, 59, of Portland, is associate director of Ecumenical Ministries of Oregon. From 1972 to 1979 she served as a City of Salem Council member, and from 1976 to 1977 was president of the League of Oregon Cities. Lowe is a 1952 graduate of the University of Oregon. She replaces Minnie Zidell, who resigned. Her term will expire in 1992.

Richard Wopat, 40, of Lebanon, is a private practice family physician. He is president-elect of Western Oregon Independent Practice Association and senior medical advisor to Oregon Medical Professional Review Organization. He received a bachelor's degree from Northwestern University, an M.D. from the University of Wisconsin, and did his residency at the University of Oregon Health Sciences Center. Wopat is the chairperson of the Alternative Methodologies Subcommittee and a member of the Health Outcomes Subcommittee. His term expires in 1992.

There were at least five different steps to the prioritization process. Each of these will be reviewed as follows.

1. Condition–Treatment Pairs

The mission of creating a prioritized list of all health services is overwhelming. There are many different ways to divide up the task. One possibility is to prioritize the effectiveness of treatments while another is to prioritize the effectiveness of treating different conditions. Each creates difficulties. For example, some treatments are used for a wide variety of different conditions. Thus, the evaluation of a treatment such as "antibiotic medication" may be effective in some conditions but ineffective in others. Similarly, some conditions may be effectively treated by one type of intervention (for example, surgical) while not affected by another medical intervention. Recognizing these problems, the Commission decided to generate a list based on pairs of conditions and treatments. These came to be known as condition–treatment pairs or "CT" pairs. Examples of condition–treatment pairs are shown in Table 6.2. For example, a condition such as diabetes mellitus type I might be paired with medical treatment while injury to a blood vessel in the thoracic cavity would be paired with a surgical repair treatment. The treatment half of these pairs tended to be very general with about half of the treatments specified as either medical therapy or medical-plus-surgical treatment. Medical therapy included nontherapeutic activities as well. For example, office visits and usual ancillary care came under this category. In addition, some conditions were paired with more than one treatment. Thus, a particular condition may be listed and associated with medical or surgical interventions, or both.

2. Estimating Cost, Effects, and Duration

The second step in the process was to develop the net cost/benefit formula. The Commission mistakenly used the term *cost/benefit* instead of *cost/utility*. The Oregon formula is

$$\frac{C}{\Delta \text{QWB} \times D}$$

where C is the cost of treatment, ΔQWB is the expected difference between treated and untreated patients, and D is the ratio of the treatment benefit expressed in years.

The data for the cost component of the equation were obtained from the Oregon Medicaid Management Information System. This system was served by a commercial actuarial firm that imputed rates for usual care in managed-care settings. Typically, costs were presented in ranges and the midpoint of the range was used for the estimate. One of the important criticisms of the cost component is that the numerator of the equation represents treatment cost and not *incremental* cost. The bottom half of the equation represents incremental benefit. By in-

TABLE 6.2

Examples of Condition–Treatment Pairs

Condition	Treatment
Rectal prolapse	Partial colectomy
Osteoporosis	Medical therapy
Ophthalmic injury	Closure
Obesity	Nutritional and lifestyle counseling

cremental, we mean the difference between treated and untreated patients. The proposal has been criticized (Detsky & Naglie, 1990) for using incremental benefit and not incremental cost. The Commission had considered using net or incremental cost but rejected the idea because it felt the data were unavailable.

The QWB portion was estimated using clinical judgment. For each CT pair physicians estimated the QWB change for the average patient. A clinician panel placed patients into defined categories: into one step of mobility, physical activity, and social activity. In addition, clinicians were asked to identify which of the 23 symptoms or problems would be most likely at the beginning of treatment. Then, the clinicians were asked to repeat the exercise with their expectations for their average patient following treatment.

The initial task for providers was enormous. With more than 1600 condition–treatment pairs, the providers needed to be divided into many subgroups. Ultimately, 54 volunteer providers from many specialty groups participated. The groups included essentially all licensed practitioner associations in the state of Oregon and represented most medical subspecialties. In addition, the practitioner panels included chiropractors, acupuncturists, and massage therapists.

For each of the CT pairs, the providers were asked to evaluate the probability of individuals being in each of the five health states 5 years hence. Table 6.3 gives an example of these estimates. The clinical case is a combination of otitis media with replacement of Eustachian tubes/tonsillectomy and adenoidectomy/tympanoplasty. The calculation for otitis media is shown in Table 6.4. As the table suggests, a QWB value for being severely affected is .57 while that for being moderately affected is .78. For the severely affected person, the judges estimated that the affected person would be limited in usual activities and would have trouble learning, remembering, or thinking clearly (cpx 4). The mildly affected person would have no functional limitations but may experience cpx 17—having pain in ears or trouble hearing. The Oregon preferences associated with these states yield the QWB values. The exercise changes the probabilities that people would be in the two states. Using these probabilities, estimated treatment effects were generated as the sum of the probability times the QWB value.

TABLE 6.3

Example of Estimated Treatment Effect for Treatment of Otitis Media with Surgical Placement of External Tubes of Tonsillectomy/Adenoidectomy[a]

State	Without procedure	With procedure
Perfect health	.50	.91
Mildly affected	—	—
Moderately affected	.10	.03
Severely affected	.25	.05
Dead	.15	.01

[a]From Hewitt, Recker, & Sa'adah (1991).

3. The Oregon Weighting Study

Oregon citizens are proud of their state and their independent spirit. One of the problems in the exercise was that the only available preference weights had been obtained from citizens in San Diego, California. California preferences are clearly unfashionable in Oregon. Therefore, an independent preference assessment study was conducted in Oregon. A random digit dialing telephone survey was conducted with 1001 Oregon respondents. Although the scaling task was similar to the one that was used in California, some aspects were different. For example, the Oregon telephone respondents were asked to rate case descriptions on a scale from 0 which was "as bad as death" through 100 which represented "good health." The exact technique used for the rating tasks was also different.

In the telephone survey, the caller identified him or herself as from Oregon State University. After an introduction the interviewer said

> Because people have different ideas about how health problems affect their happiness or satisfaction with life, we would like to ask how *you* feel. In the next few minutes we will describe several health situations. We would like you to tell us how you feel about each one by giving it a score. If you feel the situation describes *good health*, give it a score of 100. If you feel it is as bad as *death*, give it a score of 0. If the situation is about halfway between death and good health give it a score of 50. You can use any of the numbers from 0 to 100, such as 0, 7, 18, 39, 63, 78, 89, 100, and so forth. Remember, you can use any number between 0 and 100. For each health situation, you should assume that you have no other problems than the ones described. Also, you should think of each health situation as *permanent*. OK?

As is customary in scaling experiments, the first case described is the best situation, while the second case describes the worst situation. This familiarizes respondents with the end points of the scale. Table 6.5 provides examples of some

TABLE 6.4

Calculating ΔQWB Using Example: "Chronic Otitis Media–Eustachian Tubes/Tonsillectomy and Adenoidectomy/Tympanoplasty; Medical Therapy"[a,b]

Health state	Without treatment					With treatment				
	P[c]	FL/S[d]	Weight[e]	QWB value[f]	(P × value)	P[c]	FL/S[d]	Weight[c]	QWB value[f]	(P × value)
Death	.15	—	-1.000	0.000	.0000	.01	—	-1.000	0.000	.0000
Severely affected	.25	S1	-0.062	0.571	.1428	.05	S1	-0.062	0.571	.0286
		H4	-0.367				H4	-0.367		
Moderately affected	.10	H17	-0.217	0.783	.0783	.03	H17	-0.210	0.783	.0235
Mildly affected	—	—	—	—	—	—	—	—	—	—
Perfect health	.50	—	0.000	1.000	.5000	.91	—	0.000	1.000	.9100
Δ (P × Score)					.7211					.9621

[a]The change in quality of well-being with and without treatment is the difference between the value of Δ(P × score) for patients with (.9621) and without (.7211) treatment. The change in quality of well-being for this condition is 0.2410.

[b]From Hewitt et al. (1991); OTA (1992).

[c]P = probability of being in health state.

[d]FL/S = functional limitation/symptom associated with health state.

[e]Weight = the weight the public assigns to the functional limitation/symptom. Can be interpreted as the amount taken away from perfect health (value as 1) because of the presence of a symptom.

[f]QWB Value = quality of well-being value = (1 + Weight). When there is more than one functional limitation or symptom assigned to the health state, weights are added before summing to 1. Can be interpreted as the value associated with the health state on a scale from 0 (death) to 1 (perfect health).

TABLE 6.5

Telephone Survey Used in Oregon Preference Assessment Study

REP: Phone No. _____

PAGE: Area No. _____

January 1990   OREGON STATE UNIVERSITY   Final

Hello, I'm _____. I'm calling from Oregon State University at Corvallis. First, I need to be sure I have dialed the right number. Is this (READ NUMBER)? We would like to speak to the adult who has had the most recent birthday if he or she is at home now. (IF R IS NOT AT HOME ASK): When would that person be home? (RECORD BELOW AND CALL BACK.)

(WHEN YOU HAVE CORRECT RESPONDENT, CONTINUE WITH): As I said, I'm calling for Oregon State University at Corvallis. Our interview contains several interesting topics about how people feel about their health and how their health affects the quality of their lives. The information is important, for it will help Oregon's Health Services Commission plan future health support programs for the state's citizens. All information that you give us is strictly confidential and the results are summarized for the state as a whole, not for any one person. Also, I want to assure you that the interview is voluntary, and if we should come to any question that you don't want to answer, just say so and we'll go on to the next question. If you have any questions after we have finished, we would be happy to have you call the study director at 737-3773 and he will answer them for you.

Because people have different ideas about how health problems affect their happiness or satisfaction with life, we would like to ask how *you* feel.

In the next few minutes, we will describe several health situations. We would like you to tell us how you feel about each one by giving it a score. If you feel the situation describes *good health*, give it a score of 100. If you feel it is as bad as *death*, give it a score of 0. If the situation is about halfway between death and good health, give it a score of 50. You can use any numbers from 0 to 100, such as 0, 7, 18, 39, 50, 63, 78, 89, 100, and so forth. Remember, you can use *any* number between 0 and 100.

For each health situation, you should assume you would have *no other problems* than the ones described. Also, you should think of each health situation as *permanent*. Okay?

The first description is the *best* health situation that you will be asked to rate; the second description is the *worst*. Here is the first one . . .

A. You can go anywhere, can move around freely wherever you are, have no restrictions on activity, and have *no health problems.* On a scale where 100 is *good health* and 0 is *death* what score would you give in this situation? . . . . SCORE ____
DK/NA. . 999

B. Now, here is the second. You have to stay at a hospital or nursing home, have to be in bed or in a wheelchair controlled by someone else, need help to eat or go to the bathroom, and have losses of consciousness from seizures, blackouts, or coma. Again, on a scale of 0 to 100, what score would you give in this situation? . . . . SCORE ____
DK/NA. . 999

C. Moving on to other situations, you have to stay at a hospital or nursing home, have to be in bed or in a wheelchair controlled by someone else, and need help to eat or go to the bathroom, but have no other health problems. . . . . SCORE ____
DK/NA. . 999

TABLE 6.5 (continued)

D. You can be taken anywhere, but have to be in bed or in a wheelchair controlled by someone else, need help to eat or go to the bathroom, but have no other health problems . . . . SCORE ____

DK/NA. . 999

E. You can be taken anywhere, but have to be in bed or in a wheelchair controlled by someone else. Otherwise, you have no restrictions on activity and have no other health problems . . . . SCORE ____

DK/NA. . 999

F. You cannot drive a car or use public transportation, you have to use a walker or wheelchair under your own control, and are limited in the recreational activities you may participate in. You have no other health problems . . . . SCORE ____

DK/NA. . 999

G. You can be taken anywhere but you have to use a walker or a wheelchair under your own control and are limited in the recreational activities you may perform, but have no other health problems . . . . SCORE ____

DK/NA. . 999

H. You can be taken anywhere, but you have to use a walker or a wheelchair under your own control. Otherwise, you have no restrictions on activity and have no other health problems . . . . SCORE ____

DK/NA. . 999

I. You can go anywhere and have no limitations on other activity, but wear glasses or contact lenses . . . . SCORE ____

DK/NA. . 999

Before we continue, I'd like to remind you that we are asking you to rate each health situation on a scale of 0 to 100, where 0 is *death* and 100 is *good health*. You may use any number from 0 to 100 for your rating.

J. You can go anywhere and have no limitations on physical or other activity, but have pain or discomfort in your eyes or vision problems that corrective lenses can't fix . . . . SCORE ____

DK/NA. . 999

K. You can go anywhere and have no limitations on physical or other activity, but have stomach aches, vomiting, or diarrhea . . . . SCORE ____

DK/NA. . 999

L. You can go anywhere and have no limitations on physical or other activity, but have trouble falling asleep or staying asleep . . . . SCORE ____

DK/NA. . 999

M. You can go anywhere and have no limitations on physical or other activity, but have a bad burn over large areas of your body . . . . SCORE ____

DK/NA. . 999

N. You can go anywhere and have no limitations on physical or other activity, but are on prescribed medicine or a prescribed diet for health reasons . . . . SCORE ____

DK/NA. . 999

	TABLE 6.5 (continued)	

O. You can go anywhere and have no limitations on physical or other activity, but have drainage from your sexual organs and discomfort or pain.. SCORE ____
DK/NA. . 999

P. You can go anywhere and have no limitations on physical or other activity, but have trouble with sexual interest or performance .... SCORE ____
DK/NA. . 999

Q. You can go anywhere and have no limitations on physical or other activity, but have pain in your ear or trouble hearing .... SCORE ____
DK/NA. . 999

R. You can go anywhere and have no limitations on physical or other activity, but have trouble learning, remembering or thinking clearly .. SCORE ____
DK/NA. . 999

S. You can go anywhere. You have difficulty walking, but no other limitations on activity .... SCORE ____
DK/NA. . 999

As we continue, please remember we are asking you to rate each health situation on a scale of 0 to 100, where 0 is death and 100 is good health. You may use any number from 0 to 100 in your ratings.

T. You can go anywhere. You have difficulty in walking because of a paralyzed or broken leg, but you have no other limitations on activity SCORE ____
DK/NA. . 999

U. You can go anywhere and have no limitations on physical or other activity, but you have trouble talking, such as a lisp, stuttering or hoarseness .... SCORE ____
DK/NA. . 999

V. You can go anywhere and have no limitations on physical, or other activity, but you can't stop worrying.......................... SCORE ____
DK/NA. . 999

W. You can go anywhere and have no limitations on physical or other activity, but you have a painful or weak condition of the back or joints SCORE ____
DK/NA. . 999

X. You can go anywhere and have no limitations on physical or other activity, but you have an itchy rash over large areas of your body ... SCORE ____
DK/NA. . 999

Y. You can go anywhere and have no limitations on your physical or other activity, but you have pain while you are urinating or having a bowel movement... SCORE ____
DK/NA. . 999

Z1. You can go anywhere and have no limitations on physical activity, but you have trouble with the use of drugs or alcohol................ SCORE ____
DK/NA. . 999

Z2. You can go anywhere and have no limitations on physical activity, but you have headaches or dizziness .... SCORE ____
DK/NA. . 999

TABLE 6.5 (continued)

Z3. You can go anywhere and have no limitations on physical or other activity, but you experience a lot of tiredness or weakness.......... SCORE ____
DK/NA. . 999

Z4. You can go anywhere and have no limitations on physical or other activity, but you are often depressed or upset..................... SCORE ____
DK/NA. . 999

Z5. You can go anywhere and have no limitations on physical or other activity, but you cough, wheeze, or have trouble breathing.......... SCORE ____
DK/NA. . 999

Z6. You can go anywhere and have no limitations on physical or other activity, but are overweight or have acne on your face............. SCORE ____
DK/NA. . 999

Thank you for your ratings. Next, I have here a list of medical conditions. As I read each one, will you please tell me if you have had or presently have the condition? (INT: START WITH RED-CHECKED ITEM AND WORK YOUR WAY THROUGH ALL 30.)

Condition	DK/NA	No not had	Yes: had or have	Yes month/year
1. You have been, at some time, unable to drive a car or use public transportation ...	1	2	3	____
2. You have used a walker or wheelchair under your own control..................	1	2	3	____
3. You have been limited in the recreational activities in which you participate	1	2	3	____
4. You have experienced difficulty in walking because of a paralyzed or broken leg	1	2	3	____
5. You have had stomach aches, vomiting, or diarrhea............................	1	2	3	____
6. You have had trouble falling asleep or staying asleep.......................	1	2	3	____
7. You have been overweight or have had acne on your face	1	2	3	____
8. You have experienced pain in your ear or have had trouble hearing..............	1	2	3	____
9. You have stayed in a hospital or in a nursing home	1	2	3	____
10. You have had trouble with the use of drugs or alcohol.....................	1	2	3	____
11. You have had drainage from your sexual organs and discomfort or pain	1	2	3	____
12. You have had headaches or dizziness	1	2	3	____
13. You have been in a bed or a wheelchair controlled by someone else.............	1	2	3	____

Condition	DK/NA	No not had	Yes: had or have	Yes month/year
14. You have often felt depressed or upset ...	1	2	3	____
15. You have had trouble learning, remembering, or thinking clearly	1	2	3	____
16. You have experienced pain while urinating or having a bowel movement	1	2	3	____
17. You have coughed, wheezed, or had trouble breathing	1	2	3	____
18. You have had pain or weakness in your back or joints......................	1	2	3	____
19. You have had an itchy rash over large areas of your body	1	2	3	____
20. You wear glasses or contact lenses	1	2	3	____
21. You have had trouble with sexual interest or performance.....................	1	2	3	____
22. You have had difficulty in walking	1	2	3	____
23. You have had trouble talking	1	2	3	____
24. You have been unable to stop worrying ..	1	2	3	____
25. You have experienced pain or discomfort in your eyes or had vision problems that corrective lenses can't fix	1	2	3	____
26. You have been on prescribed medicine or a prescribed diet for health reasons	1	2	3	____
27. You have had a bad burn over large areas of your body	1	2	3	____
28. You have experienced a lot of tiredness or weakness	1	2	3	____
29. You have needed help in eating or going to the bathroom	1	2	3	____
30. You have had loss in consciousness due to seizures, blackouts, or coma...........	1	2	3	____

TABLE 6.5 (continued)

of the items that were rated by the respondents. Using these preferences, weights for the QWB system were derived.

There were several differences between the Oregon and the San Diego procedure. In the San Diego studies, respondents rated case descriptions on an 11-point scale ranging from 0 (for death) to 1.0 (for optimum function). The Oregon preferences were obtained on a 0 to 100 scale and the results were slightly different. In particular, preferences at the high end of the continuum were closer to 1.0, while those at the lower end of the continuum were closer to 0. In the San Diego study, those completely functional but with a symptom as minor as wearing eye glasses receive a utility weight of about 0.90. This suggests that for each 10 years a person wears eye glasses, they give up the equivalent of 1 year of life. In the Oregon exercise, the same item produced preferences of .944. It might be argued that the finer-grain scale used in Oregon is more capable of detecting differences close to the top of the scale. For example, respondents in San Diego, recognizing that wearing eye glasses is not perfect health, may have given a utility judgment of 9 (translated into 0.90) because that was the next best option less than 10. The 100-point scale used in Oregon might have allowed more accurate expression of utility near the completely well end of the continuum. However, evidence from one recent investigation of this problem does not identify rating scale (0–10 versus 0–100) as a major explanatory factor. There are several other explanations for the differences between the Oregon and the San Diego utilities. For example, participants in the Oregon study were given a rationale that may have explicitly focused subjects on making tradeoffs, while the San Diego exercise requested ratings of cases for a particular day. In addition, the subject populations and settings were different in the Oregon and California studies. It is also worth noting that observed differences between San Diego and Oregon ratings were relatively minor. With the exception of three outliers, the relationship was linear and strong ($r = .92$).

With data on the preference weights, the only additional step needed to estimate treatment outcome was duration of benefit.

4. Duration of Benefit

The GHPM emphasizes the duration of benefit. A treatment gain that lasts 1 year should be given greater value than a treatment plan that lasts 1 week. Similarly, health conditions that last a long time must be evaluated more severely than health conditions that last a short time. A headache that lasts 1 hour is not the same as a headache that lasts 1 month. In order to estimate the duration of benefit, the medical consultants estimated how long the treatment would work. They assumed that life expectancy was 75 years. If the treatment had a lifetime benefit, it was assumed that the duration of the benefit was 75 years minus the age at which treatment was initiated. The 75-year mark differs from the standardized 100 years in the GHPM. One of the major difficulties with arbitrarily selecting 75 years is that it forces the system to discriminate against the elderly. In order to determine these benefits, the physician on the provider panel considers the median age at which a diagnosis was made. For a child with a condition such as otitis media, the average age of diagnosis might be 5 so that the duration of benefit could be as long as 70 years. For senior adults, the median age of diagnosis might be 64 so that the expected duration of benefit would be 11 years. Adults diagnosed at age 76 would receive no benefit.

Using the duration component, all of the elements are necessary to perform the calculations. Examples of applications of the formula are presented in Tables 6.6 and 6.7.

The steps described above are required by the GHPM. Although we would not have performed some of the steps in the same way, these represent a reasonable approach to the prioritization of health services. Essentially, this is what was done in the early phases of the Oregon exercise. However, the initial prioritization list

---

TABLE 6.6

Prioritization Using a Cost-Effectiveness Formula[a]

A "cost-effectiveness" formula was used to order a preliminary prioritized list in May 1990:

$$C/(NB \times D),$$

where C = treatment cost; NB = net benefit of treatment or the expected change in patients' "quality of life" with treatment; and D = expected duration of treatment benefit (years).

Treatment Costs
Estimates of the costs associated with a given CT pair (e.g., hospital, ancillary services, pharmacy, etc.) were based upon information from the Oregon Medicaid Management Information System (MMIS). Clinicians provided additional cost data as needed. Cost estimates were usually intended to include those anticipated over the remaining life of the patient. For treatments without a lifetime benefit, costs were estimated for the expected duration of the treatment benefit (e.g., hip replacements confer a benefit for about 10 years). Each CT pair was assigned one of 14 cost ranges.

Treatment Benefit
Expected change in "quality of life" was estimated using clinical prognostic data and public opinions about the desirability of experiencing a set of disabilities and symptoms.

Duration of Treatment Benefit
The duration of benefit is expressed in years. If the treatment has a lifetime benefit, the duration of benefit is the remaining life expectancy (life expectancy was set at 75 years). If the treatment is effective for a short duration, benefit is expressed as the period until the next treatment is required (e.g., hip replacements confer benefit for about 10 years). Provider panels estimated the median age range of diagnosis for each condition and the midpoints of the ranges were used in estimating duration of benefit.

Applying the cost-effectiveness formula
The cost-effectiveness formula values for the "chronic otitis media–eustachian tubes/ tonsillectomy and adenoidectomy/tympanoplasty" CT pair are as follows:

Formula terms	Formula values
Treatment cost (C)	$1500
Net benefit of treatment (NB)	.241
Duration of treatment benefit (D)	69 years

According to the formula, $C/(NB \times D)$, the value for this CT pair would be 90.20 (i.e., $1500 per 16.63 quality-adjusted life years). The value 90.20 can be interpreted as the cost of adding 1 quality year of life associated with procedures for chronic otitis media.

[a]From OTA (1992).

TABLE 6.7

Calculating Net Benefit Using Example: "Chronic Otitis Media–Eustachian Tubes/Tonsillectomy and Adenoidectomy/Tympanoplasty"[a]

Health state	Without treatment					With treatment				
	P[b]	FL/S[c]	Weight[d]	QoL value[e]	(P × value)	P[b]	FL/S[c]	Weight[d]	QoL value[e]	(P × value)
Death	.15	—	-1.000	0.000	.0000	.01	—	-1.000	0.000	.0000
Severely affected	.25	S1 H4	-0.062 -0.367	0.571	.1428	.05	S1 H4	-0.062 -0.367	0.571	.0286
Moderately affected	.10	H17	-0.217	0.783	.0783	.03	H17	-0.210	0.783	.0235
Mildly affected	—	—	—	—	—	—	—	—	—	—
Perfect health	.50	—	0.000	1.000	.5000	.91	—	0.000	1.000	.9100
Σ (P × value)					.7211					.9621

[a]Net benefit is the difference between the value of Σ (P × value) for patients with (.9621) and without (.7211) treatment, or 0.2410. From Office of Technology Assessment (1992) based on data from the Oregon Health Services Commission, March 15, 1991.

[b]P = probability of being in health state.

[c]FL/S = functional limitation/symptom associated with health state.

[d]Weight = the weight the public assigns to the functional limitation/symptom. Can be interpreted as the amount taken away from perfect health (valued as 1) associated with the presence of a symptom.

[e]QoL value = quality-of-life value = (1 + Weight). When there is more than one functional limitation or symptom assigned to the health state, weights are added before summing to 1. Can be interpreted as the value associated with the health state on a scale from 0 (death) to 1 (perfect health).

produced some counterintuitive findings. We will consider this issue of counter-intuitive findings again in Chapter Seven.

5. Community Meetings

The Oregon Health Services Commission also used a variety of other sources of information. One of these was the social values of Oregon citizens. As part of the early process the Commission hired a consulting firm, Oregon Health Decisions, to conduct 47 community meetings. These meetings were held throughout the state of Oregon. The purpose of the meetings was to determine which values were commonly held by members of the Oregon population. Oregon Health Decisions, in turn, trained 58 coordinators and facilitators. All of these were volunteers from local communities. The coordinators/facilitators were responsible for organizing and publicizing the meetings. The selected meeting locations were distributed along with information in both English and Spanish. A standard format was followed for the meetings. During each meeting the participants viewed a slide show that described the process and were told about potential changes that might occur as a function of the Oregon Basic Health Services Act.

During the second phase of the community meetings the participants completed a questionnaire concerning eight theoretical health situations. The situations are shown in Table 6.8. For each of the situations the participant was asked to place the situation into one of three categories: central, very important, and important. They were also asked to classify nine categories of care. These ranged from treatment of conditions where the health care is likely to extend life by more than 2 years or to improve quality of life, and "treatment not likely to extend life or make any improvement in quality of life" (see Table 6.8). The participants then took part in small group decisions that focused on these issues. On the basis of these discussions group consensus was estimated and results were recorded. The participants had the opportunity to send information to the facilitator after the meeting had ended. The facilitator was responsible for reporting the results of the meeting (Hasnain & Garland, 1990).

Community meetings were well attended. Groups ranged from small (7 participants) to fairly large (132 participants). An average of about 20 participants attended. Overall, the 47 meetings were attended by more than 1000 people. Nearly 64% of the participants were women. Few Medicaid recipients or medically uninsured or underinsured persons participated.

On the basis of the 47 town meetings, 13 community values emerged. These 13 values were grouped by the Commission into 3 attributes: values to society, value to an individual at risk of needing service, and essential to basic health care. The 13 values in relation to the three major categories are summarized in Table 6.9. Prevention was number one in all three categories. In other words, prevention was regarded as having the highest value to society, value to an individual, and essential to basic health care.

The input from the medical committee checked preferences for QWB states,

TABLE 6.8

Community Meeting Questionnaire Concerning Theoretical Health Situations[a]

Community meeting participants were asked to read and consider the following hypothetical health care situations:

A heavy user of crack cocaine wants help for drug addiction. Immediate treatment will stop use. A month of intensive in-hospital treatment and outpatient treatment for a year will help stop the alcohol and drug use for the long term.

A collapsed lung and internal bleeding have resulted from an accidental bullet wound through the chest. This person is conscious. Surgery to repair the lung and take care of the bleeding is likely to be successful; giving less treatment is likely to cause death or permanent damage.

A person wishes to have a facelift, saying that keeping the job absolutely depends on having a youthful appearance.

A person has advanced brain disease (Alzheimer's disease). Normal communication and function are impossible. The person has just started vomiting from a blocked intestine. Surgery to remove part of the intestine could help. The outlook is only fair to poor because of chronic bad health and nutrition.

A depressed parent of two preschool children is feeling hopeless and confused. The person is obsessed with thoughts of killing the children and him/herself. A week of hospital care and 6 months of outpatient treatment will allow the person to function as a parent and on the job.

A child needs routine immunizations which include polio, diptheria, and whooping cough. Without immunizations the child may become ill and spread the disease to others. Sometimes these illnesses cause death.

After three heart attacks, a patient is getting worse despite taking several medications daily. An operation to put in a pacemaker would probably help the heart's rhythm but not the general condition of the heart. The day-to-day activities of the patient may improve.

A severely mentally ill person is now unemployed and homeless. The person hears voices and feels threatened by "evil spirits." Regular treatment and medicine probably will help the person return to work and to a stable living situation.

Meeting participants were also asked to classify each of the health care categories below as "essential," "very important," or "important" by placing three categories in each classification. Participants were instructed that their rankings should be based on "beliefs and values about which categories are most important for [their] community as a whole."

Treatment of conditions which are fatal and can't be cured. The treatment will not extend the person's life for more than 5 years.

Treatment of conditions where the health care is likely to extend life by more than 2 years or to improve the person's quality of life.

Treatment for alcoholism or drug addiction.

Treatment of sudden or ongoing conditions where the person is likely to get well. If the person does not receive care, the length or quality of life will be reduced.

Treatment not likely to extend life or make any big improvement in quality of life.

Treatment of conditions where the health care is not likely to extend life by more than 2 years or to improve the quality of life.

Treatment provided in or out of the hospital for mental illness or emotional disturbance, which will restore the person's health.

Preventive care which definitely can prevent early death or a reduction in quality of life.

Treatment for chronic ongoing conditions where health care will improve quality of life for the person's remaining years.

[a]From Oregon Health Services Commission, 1991.

TABLE 6.9

Health Care Values Elicited as Community Meetings

Prevention. Preventive services such as prenatal care and childhood immunizations were unanimously agreed upon as essential.

Quality of life. Services that enhance emotional and physical well-being, as well as extend life, were generally thought to increase quality of life and should receive higher prioritization than those which only extend life.

Cost effectiveness. Cost-effective treatments were given high priority, although some community members disagreed that cost alone should be a primary determinant in prioritization.

Ability to function. The importance of independence and ability to perform daily activities was mentioned at three-fourths of the community meetings.

Equity. Equity was described as a fundamental belief that everyone should have equal access to adequate health care. Discussions of equity raised various objections to the prioritization process—many participants, for instance, thought that health care services should be available equally to all segments of society. There was support for increased federal funding for health care services, and some advocated establishment of a national health insurance plan. Other issues of equity included increasing access to treatment services in rural communities and universal access to health care for children.

Effectiveness of treatment. Treatments with proven efficacy and those that improve quality of life should be prioritized over those less likely to have successful outcomes.

Benefits many. Services that benefit many should receive higher priority than those for whom few benefit.

Mental health and chemical dependency. Prevention, including drug education, was more highly valued than treatment services. While mental health and chemical dependency services were frequently discussed at meetings, there was some ambivalence regarding society's obligation to provide substance abuse services. Some participants, for example, felt that treatment was appropriate only in cases where patients were "motivated to undergo treatment," and that recidivism needed to be considered in cases of "repeat offenders."

Personal choice. Some community members expressed a desire for increased choice of type of providers, while others wanted more patient and family autonomy in making medical treatment decisions.

Community compassion. Society is obligated to provide treatments and services that alleviate pain and suffering (e.g., hospice care).

Impact on society. Treatments for infectious diseases and for alcoholism or drug abuse are examples of services that yield societal as well as individual benefit (discussed at approximately half of the community meetings).

Length of life. Prolonging life was viewed as important, but a treatment's value is limited if extending life sacrificed quality of life.

Personal responsibility. Personal responsibility was viewed as the individual's obligation to society to seek appropriate health education and treatment services and to generally take responsibility for one's health. Individuals taking responsibility for their health should receive priority, and those whose illnesses are related to lifestyle, such as alcohol- and drug-related conditions, are low priority if health care services are rationed.

[a]From Hasnain & Garland (1990).

and the social values meetings formed the basic data collection. However, the Commission also held a series of 12 public hearings in various parts of the state. The hearings were conducted in Portland, Salem, Pendleton, Eugene, Bend, Coos Bay, and Medford. During these meetings, testimony was solicited from seniors, handicapped persons, mental health consumers, low-income Oregonians, and health care providers. A variety of grass roots organizations participated, providing publicity for the meeting and door-to-door shuttle service for those who had disabilities. On the basis of the testimony, the Commissioners concluded that the general public wanted coverage for services that may not be part of standard basic benefit packages. These services included dental care, prevention, mental health care, and chemical dependency services.

DEPARTURE FROM THE MODEL—ALTERNATIVE
METHODOLOGY SUBCOMMITTEE

The original publication of the list was troublesome for many of the Commissioners. They argued that cost/benefit ratios did not represent public values. In addition, there was concern that health services were difficult to rank because data about the effects of many medical services were not available. For instance, prevention and education were hard to evaluate against traditional medical services. Because of these problems, the Commission decided to add the personal judgment of its members to the net benefit and cost/benefit concept. The Commission created 17 categories of health service on the basis of its own judgment and other information it had obtained. These categories are shown in Table 6.10. Then each Commissioner gave a relative weight from 0 to 100 for three categories: value to society, value to an individual at risk of needing service, and essential to a basic health care package. These ratings took into consideration the preferences expressed in some of the community meetings. In addition to weighting the categories against each other, the Commissioners rated each of the 17 categories as relevant to each of the three attributes. These were each rated on a 1 to 10 scale where 1 was for least desirable and 10 was for most desirable. For example, a Commissioner could have assigned a 10 to infertility service based on "value to an individual." The same Commissioner could have given a 2 to the same condition based on the value to society and a 1 based on the centrality of the services for a basic health care package. A delphi method was used to obtain consensus among the Commissioners. On the basis of this exercise, the 17 categories were ranked and ordered. Categories 1 through 9 were regarded as essential, categories 10 through 13 were considered very important, and categories 14 through 17 were listed as valuable to certain individuals.

Using data on net benefit and placement among these categories the Commission ranked 709 condition–treatment pairs. The commissioners recommended to the Legislature that services in categories 1 through 9 be regarded as essential and covered for all people under the plan. Services described in categories 10 through

TABLE 6.10

Three Health Care Attributes[a]

Value to Society. This attribute takes into account the costs to society if a category of health service is not provided.

Prevention	Cost effectiveness
Benefits many	Community compassion
Impact on society	Mental health and chemical
Quality of life	dependency
Personal responsibility	

Value to an Individual at Risk of Needing the Service. Certain categories of services may be very important to a person seeking the service (e.g., services for infertility) but make very little difference on a societal level.

Prevention	Equity
Quality of life	Effectiveness of treatment
Ability to function	Personal choice
Length of life	Community compassion
Mental health and chemical	
dependency	

Essential to Basic Health Care. The categories of service essential are those, with respect to public input and expert testimony, below which no person shall fall.

Prevention	Cost effectiveness
Benefits many	Impact on society
Quality of life	

[a]From Oregon Health Services Commission (1991).

13 were considered "very important" and fundable to the extent that resources were available. Those in category 14 and below were rated as valuable to some individuals but less likely to be cost-effective or to produce long-term benefits. These categories would be less likely to be funded under the plan.

In their final list of 709 condition–treatment pairs, the Commission "used professional judgments of their interpretation of the community values to re-rank 'out-of-order' items on the draft list." The Commissioners explained that they used a "reasonableness" test to re-rank some of these procedures. In applying the reasonableness test, the Commissioners considered public health impact, cost, incidence and prevalence of the condition, treatment effectiveness, social costs, and costs of new treatments. The Commission was also troubled by the relatively low rankings of some preventive services. They stated "the commissioners also observed that it was not reasonable—logically or economically—to rank preventable or readily treatable conditions in relatively unfavorable positions. In other words, when either severe or exacerbated conditions were ranked in a relatively favorable condition compared to prevention of disease, disability or exacerbation, these occurrences were reversed" (p. 28).

In the final phase the state actuary costed out the various items on the list. On May 1, 1991 the funding line was drawn at condition–treatment pair 587.

WHAT WENT WRONG?

In the initial plan, the Oregon Health Services Commission proposed analyses that were very similar to the GHPM. The model is advantageous because it is positioned to provide the most benefits for the most people. Under the revised proposal, these objectives will not be met. In this section we focus on departures from the GHPM and how they may have adversely affected the objectives of the Oregon legislation.

Problems with the List

The major difficulty with the Oregon exercise was the attempt to prioritize a large number of services in a relatively short period of time. The initial publication of the list revealed many inconsistencies. In other words, replacement of some condition–treatment pairs was, in the opinion of the Commissioners, counterintuitive. There were many examples of counterintuitive placements. Almost certainly, these peculiar placements were based on faulty analysis. For example, treatment for thumb-sucking and acute headaches received higher rankings than treatment for AIDS or cystic fibrosis. The problem was not the method but rather the way data were generated by the medical committees. We should not fault the committees for doing a poor job. Indeed, tremendous personal effort went into estimation of treatment effectiveness. The difficulty was that the Commission attempted to do several decades of work within the confinement of a few months. Health policy analysts sometimes take 2 to 3 years to thoroughly analyze the expected benefits of a single condition–treatment pair. For example, Weinstein & Stason (1976) engaged in a several-year exercise to estimate the cost/utility of the screening and treatment for high blood pressure. A similar analysis might have been performed in a single meeting of the Oregon medical committee. Under this time pressure one could expect that some analyses would be poor.

CLINICAL CONTRADICTIONS

As part of their evaluation of the Oregon experiment, the Office of Technology Assessment (OTA) hired experienced clinicians to evaluate the list. Upon careful scrutiny, the clinicians identified several problems. For example, they found 21 condition–treatment pairs where the Oregon group had significantly underestimated the treatment effect. These included medical therapy and thymectomy for myasthenia gravis and medical therapy for chronic bronchitis. The clinicians also found at least 12 condition–treatment pairs where the Oregon group had overestimated the treatment effect. For example, the Oregon group had rated excision ganglion of tendon or joint as 495. The OTA reviewers felt that the condition was essentially trivial and needed no treatment. The Oregon group rated as 606 medical therapy for hepatorenal syndrome. Even with this low and unfundable ranking, the OTA reviewers commented that the ranking was too high since the treatment for this condition is regarded as futile. The clinicians were also concerned about some cases in which surgical therapy was higher on the list than medical therapy. The reviewers, who included an internist and a pediatrician, argued that medical therapy should always be tried before surgery is employed. Thus, medical therapy should typically rank higher than surgery.

One of the most serious concerns raised by the clinical reviewers was the inexplicable grouping of some condition–treatment pairs. For example, line 264 is for diseases of white blood cells. However, this category groups together some conditions which are quite trivial with others that are life threatening. Line 640 (testicular hyperfunction) combines a condition which may require no treatment with Schmidt's syndrome, which is likely to be fatal without treatment. Another medical concern was the problem of co-morbidity. Often in medical care it is difficult to assess the importance of a condition without knowing the other diseases or disabilities that go along with it. For example, medical therapy for problems in blood clotting is difficult to evaluate because it depends on whether the problem is caused by a transient infection or by a serious disease such as cancer. Sometimes it was difficult for the consultants to evaluate the condition–treatment pairs since identification of the problem requires treatment. An example includes surgery for peritoneal adhesions (line 508). The difficulty is that the diagnosis of this problem requires a surgical procedure or laparotomy. In addition to these problems, the consultants identified several problems of apparent miscoding or of mismatches between the international classification of disease (ICD-9) and the CPT code matches (Office of Technology Assessment, 1992).

Instead of focusing on problems with the analyses, the Commissioners decided to revamp the process. They did this by imposing a new structure. The new structure emphasized the 17 categories shown in Table 6.11. These categories represented the Commissioners' evaluation of a variety of different factors that emerged from public value studies, cost-effectiveness studies, and so on. For example, the public hearings had suggested that the state should be less sympathetic toward a person who obtained a spinal cord injury while riding a motorcycle without a helmet and under the influence of alcohol. The Commission took into consideration the preference for prevention, quality of life, and other community values.

Another of the major problem areas in the Commission's work was that it assessed community values without giving the community information on the effectiveness of treatment. In other words, the values discussed by community members were relatively global and vague. One of the major focuses of the GHPM approach is to reimburse services that work and withhold payment for services that

TABLE 6.11

Health Care Categories and Some Examples of Services in Each Category[a]

Essential

1. *Acute fatal,* treatment prevents death and allows full recovery: appendectomy for appendicitis; nonsurgical treatment for whooping cough, repair of deep, open wound in neck; nonsurgical treatment for infection of the heart muscle (myocarditis).
2. *Maternity care,* including most newborn disorders: obstetrical care for pregnancy; care of the newborn.
3. *Acute fatal,* treatment prevents death but does not allow full recovery: nonsurgical treatment for stroke; all treatment for burns; treatment for severe head injuries.
4. Preventive care for children: immunizations and well-child exams.
5. *Chronic fatal,* treatment improves life-span and quality of life: nonsurgical treatment for insulin-dependent diabetes; medical and surgical treatment for treatable cancer of the uterus; medical treatment for asthma; drug therapy for HIV disease.
6. *Reproductive services,* excludes maternity and infertility services: birth control and sterilization.
7. *Comfort care:* pain management and hospice care for the end stages of diseases such as cancer and AIDS.
8. *Preventive dental care,* adults and children: exams; cleaning and fluoride treatment.
9. *Proven effective preventive care for adults:* mammograms; blood pressure screening; Pap smears.

Very important

10. *Acute nonfatal,* treatment causes return to previous health: nonsurgical treatment for acute thyroiditis; medical treatment for vaginitis; fillings for cavities.
11. *Chronic nonfatal,* one-time treatment improves quality of life: hip replacement; corneal transplants for cataracts; rheumatic fever.
12. *Acute nonfatal,* treatment without return to previous health: relocation of dislocated elbow; repair of cut to cornea.
13. *Chronic nonfatal,* repetitive treatment improves quality of life: nonsurgical treatment for rheumatoid arthritis; gout; migraine headaches.

Valuable to certain individuals

14. *Acute nonfatal,* treatment speeds recovery: medical treatment for viral sore throat; diaper rash.
15. *Infertility services:* medical treatment for infertility; *in vitro* fertilization; artificial insemination.
16. *Less effective preventive care for adults:* routine screening for those people not otherwise at risk, such as diabetes screening if the person is under 40 years old and not pregnant.
17. *Fatal or nonfatal,* treatment causes minimal or no improvement in quality of life: aggressive treatment for end stages of diseases such as cancer and AIDS; medical treatment for nongenital viral warts.

[a]Each health service on the list is presumed to include necessary ancillary services such as hospital care, prescription drugs, and medical equipment and supplies necessary for successful treatment.

do not enhance health outcomes. Community members were never asked if they wanted policies that reimbursed providers for useless services. Information about the cost/utility of services may have refocused some of the discussion in the town meetings.

The Cost Problem

Another decision was to focus on net benefit without consideration of cost. This decision was largely influenced by David Hadorn. In a paper in the *Journal of the American Medical Association*, Hadorn (1991a) argued for the "rule of rescue." According to the rule of rescue, resources should be used to save lives regardless of cost. The rule of rescue represents a strong moral inclination. However, the current health care crisis does require consideration of cost. The issue of cost will be explored in more detail in Chapter Seven.

Duration

Another major issue in the assessment of health effects is the duration of benefit. A treatment effect that lasts 1 week is not the same as one that lasts 1 year. Similarly a health condition that is chronic must be considered more seriously than one that is acute. Formulas presented by the Oregon Health Services Commission recognize this and included duration. However, in the construction of the list, it appears that the duration component was neglected. Exclusion of duration may have been responsible for some of the counterintuitive results.

Commission Reshuffling

One of the most important concerns regarding Oregon's model is that the Commissioners took it upon themselves to reorganize the list. They argued that this was necessary because many of the rank-orders were illogical or in other ways inconsistent with the Commissioners' expectations.

In their final report, the Oregon Health Services Commission commented that changes in rankings were done rarely. However, a review of the February 1, 1991 versus the May 1, 1991 list suggests that changes in rankings were common. These changes were reviewed in detail by the OTA (Office of Technology Assessment, 1992). According to the Oregon Health Services Commission report, CT pairs were to be ranked by net benefit within category. For example, within the maternal and child health category, it would be expected that the condition with the highest net benefit would be ranked first while the condition with the next highest net benefit would be ranked second and so on. However, after the re-rankings, there was essentially no correlation between ranking and net benefit within some categories. Figure 6.2 shows a scatter plot comparing net benefit versus ranking within category two. As the figure shows, net benefit was not an important determiner of ranking for maternal and child health services. The Office of Technology Assessment (1992) analysis examined which services went up and which services went down as a function of the Commission review. Services that had

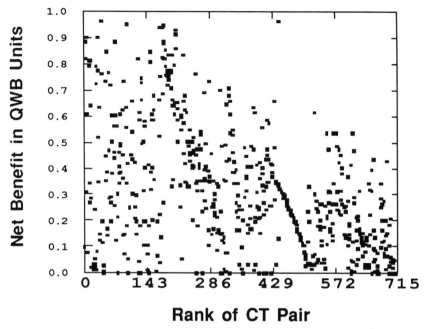

Figure 6.2   Scatter plot comparing net benefits versus ranking.

high benefit rarely moved far down the list (more than 100 lines). However, services that moved up the list more than 100 ranks were likely to be those that had few benefits.

Perhaps must disturbing is the nature of the services that moved up the list. Table 6.12 shows some of the services that moved up the most as a function of the Commissioners' inspection as well as the services that moved down the most. Those that moved up the most were maternal and child health services and care offered by general or family practitioners. Those that moved down the most tended to be complicated surgeries performed by surgical subspecialists. One of the major concerns is that the Health Services Commission included a variety of family doctors and primary care physicians who offered the types of services that moved up on the list most. Providers of services that moved down most tended not to be represented on the Commission.

SUMMARY

The Oregon experiment offered a unique opportunity to test particular aspects of the GHPM. Many features of the GHPM were emphasized in the early phases of the work. However, the initial analysis yielded some results that were counter-

TABLE 6.12

Services That Changed Positions on List after Commission Review

Examples of services moved from above to below the pay line after commissioner adjustment:
Limnectomy (surgery) for intervertebral disk disorder
Breast reconstruction following mastectomy
Lung transplantation for α-1-antitrypsin deficiencies
Stripping (surgery) for varicose veins
Medical therapy for food allergy

Examples of condition–treatment pairs moved from noncoverage to fundable levels by the commissioners:
Surgical treatment for cholesteatoma
Medical therapy for acute conjunctivitis
Medical therapy for lyme disease
Medical therapy for chronic otitis media
Medical or surgical therapy for endometriosis
Medical therapy for chronic sinusitis

intuitive for the Commissioners. This is likely to have happened because the analyses were not done thoroughly. Careful analysis could not have been expected given the time frame for creating the prioritization list.

The Commissioners responded by disassembling many of the important aspects of the GHPM. They eliminated the cost component, neglected the duration of benefit, and subjectively reprioritized many services. As a result of these changes, it is less likely that resource allocation would provide the most benefit for the most people.

The Oregon exercise should be regarded as an important learning experience. The challenge for the future will be to correct the problems that were observed in Oregon. For example, inconsistencies in the analyses suggest that those analyses need to be reexamined. Overall, development of a prioritized list is an iterative process. New data should continually reshape conclusions.

Another benefit of the Oregon exercise is that it identified a variety of ethical and practical criticisms of the GHPM. These issues will be addressed in Chapter 7.

CHAPTER SEVEN

Problems and Concerns

The proposed applications of the General Health Policy Model for use in Oregon stimulated considerable controversy. Ultimately, the Health Services Commission backed away from a genuine application of the procedures. However, the deliberations in Oregon identified a series of problems that deserve further consideration. This chapter explores some of these criticisms and assesses whether these concerns are valid. There are two major classes of criticisms. Concerning methodology, there have been concerns about the utility aspect of the model and about the way health outcomes are assessed. Several ethical concerns also surfaced and it was suggested that the plan is biased or unjustifiable on philosophical grounds. In the next sections we will examine some of these arguments.

TECHNICAL ISSUES

Several technical problems with the plan have been discussed both by opponents of the experiment and by neutral research methodologists. These include problems in utility assessment and difficulties in rating the outcome on clinical procedures.

Utility Assessment

The GHPM requires several different types of judgment. First, experts evaluate information that requires expertise. This includes the placement of individuals into different levels of health status and the expected benefit of treatment alternatives. These expert judgments are provided by physicians or other health care providers. The second type of judgment is the evaluation of specific health states. This is typically done by peers in the community. Critics of the system often get these two confused. Lay people do not provide judgments of treatment effectiveness. Instead, this is done by experts. A third and related type of judgment is the assessment of cost. This is typically done by health administrators who understand actuarial predictions. Many of the critics of the Oregon plan simply fail to understand that this information came from different data sources. Newspaper critics commonly emphasized that the assessment of medical treatments would be done in a completely subjective manner by persons with no understanding of contemporary medicine. These criticisms were even reflected in some sophisticated critiques of the Oregon plan. Mehlman (1990), a noted legal scholar, thought that preference data was used to prioritize the *effectiveness* of services.

Many of the criticisms of the use of utilities were based on the assumption that preferences differ. Thus, community preferences, it is argued, cannot be used to represent any individual. Further, the plan was designed to affect Medicaid recipients. Yet not all the people providing preferences were on Medicaid.

Choices between alternatives in health care necessarily involve preference judgment. For example, the inclusion of some services in a basic benefits package and the exclusion of others is an exercise in value, choice, or preference. There are many levels at which preference is expressed in the health care decision process. For example, an older man may decide to cope with the symptoms of urinary retention in order to avoid the ordeal and risks of prostate surgery. A physician may order expensive tests in order to ensure against the very low probability that a rare condition will be missed. Or an administrator may decide to put resources into prevention for large numbers of people instead of devoting the same resources to organ transplants for a smaller number.

In the GHPM, preferences are used to express the relative importance of various health outcomes. There is a subjective or qualitative component to health outcome. Whether we prefer a headache or an upset stomach caused by its remedy is a value judgment. Not all symptoms are of equal importance. Most patients would prefer a mild itch to vomiting. Yet providing a model of how well treatments work or a model that compares or ranks treatments implicitly includes these judgments. Models require a precise numerical expression of this preference. The GHPM explicitly includes a preference component to represent these issues.

The GHPM incorporates preferences from random samples of the general population. It is recognized that administrators ultimately choose between alternative programs. The GHPM asserts that these preferences should represent the will of the general public and not that of administrators. Yet there is considerable debate about technical aspects of preference assessment. Some of the debate has to do with whose preferences are considered. Another issue concerns the specific method used to obtain the preferences.

Whose Preference? Criticisms of the use of preferences abound. The naive critic typically assumes that preferences differ. For example, in most areas of preference assessment, it is easy to identify differences between different groups or different individuals. It might be argued that judgments about net health benefits for white Anglo men should not be applied to Hispanic men, who may give different weight to some symptoms. We all have different preferences for movies, clothing, or political candidates. Naive critics assume that these same differences must extend to health states. Thus, it is assumed that the entire analysis will be highly dependent upon the particular group that provided the preference data. In Oregon, for example, critics declared the whole process meaningless because the program was aimed at Medicaid recipients when the preferences came from both Medicaid recipients and nonrecipients (Daniels, 1991). Other analysts have suggested that preference weights from the general population cannot be applied to any particular patient group. Rather, patient preferences from every individual group must be obtained.

The difference between instrumental and terminal preferences (Rokeach, 1973) is important to understanding this debate. This difference is analogous to the difference between a means and an end. Instrumental preferences describe the means by which various assets are attained. For instance, socialists and capitalists hold different instrumental values with regard to the methods for achieving a fully functioning society. Different individuals may have different preferences for how they would like to achieve happiness, and evidence suggests that social and demographic groups vary considerably on instrumental values.

Terminal values are the ends or general states of being that individuals seek to achieve. The Rokeach (1973) classic study of values demonstrated that there is very little variability among social groups for terminal preferences. Within health states, there is less reason to believe that different social or ethnic groups will have different preferences for health outcomes. All groups agree that it is better to live free of pain than to experience pain. Freedom from disability is universally preferred over disability states. It is often suggested that individuals with particular disabilities have adapted to them. However, when asked, those with disabilities would prefer not having them. If disability states were preferred to nondisability states there would be no motivation to develop interventions to help those with problems causing the disabilities.

Although critics commonly assume substantial variability in preferences, the evidence for differential preference is weak at best. Our initial study demonstrated some significant, but very small, differences between social and ethnic groups on preferences (Kaplan et al., 1978). Studies have found little evidence for preference difference between patients and the general population. For example, Balaban and colleagues (1986) compared preference weights obtained from arthritis patients with those obtained from the general population in San Diego. They found remarkable correspondence for ratings of cases involving arthritis patients (see Fig. 7.1). Nerenz and colleagues (1990) performed a similar study with cancer patients. Again, they found that preference weights for these patients and the cognitive strategies used to evaluate these descriptions were remarkably similar to those from the general population.

There are very few differences by location. Patrick and his colleagues (1987) found essentially no differences between preference for another health status measure among those who live in the United Kingdom. and those who live in

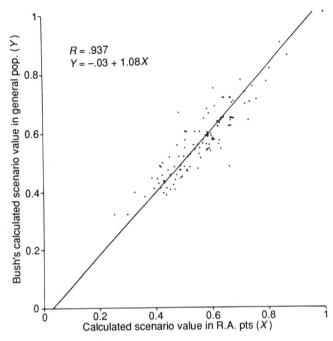

$R = .937$
$Y = -.03 + 1.08X$

Figure 7.1 Comparison between rheumatoid arthritic calculated scenario values and those obtained from the general population in San Diego. From Balaban *et al.* (1986).

Seattle. We have compared residents of the Navaho nation living in rural Arizona with the general population in San Diego and found few differences (Kaplan, 1991). The weights obtained by the Oregon Health Services Commission used a different scaling methodology and different wording in the case descriptions. Nevertheless, differences between San Diego citizens evaluated in the mid 1970s and Oregon citizens evaluated in the 1990s were remarkably small (Kaplan et al., 1991). A plot comparing California preferences to those obtained in Oregon is shown in Fig. 7.2. As the graph shows, there are remarkable similarities. It is also worth noting that observed differences between the San Diego and Oregon ratings were relatively minor. With the exception of three outliers (not shown), the relationship was linear and strong ($r = .92$). A similar scaling methodology was used by the EuroQol Group in a series of European communities. The data from those studies suggest that differences in preference among the European community are remarkably small and nonsignificant. We have used EuroQol scenarios and estimated approximate San Diego preferences for these cases. The results suggest that preferences are remarkably similar (see Fig. 7.3). We do recognize that there is considerable variability in estimating preferences for a particular case (Mulley, 1989). However, averaged across individuals, the mean preference for different cases in different groups is remarkably similar.

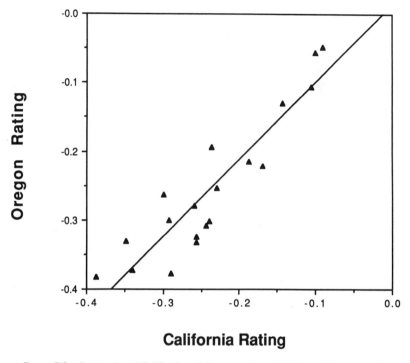

California Rating

Figure 7.2 Scatter plot of California and Oregon ratings with three outliers removed.

We should not leave the impression that there are never any mean differences in preference. For example, the original Kaplan *et al.* study (1978) did identify some significant differences between social groups. Further, the Oregon Health Services Commission did identify small, but observable, preference differences among those who had previously experienced a condition and those who had not. However, these differences were typically very small. Further analysis will be required in order to determine whether these small differences affect the conclusions of various analyses.

Measurement Method. In addition to the issue of whose preferences are obtained, we must also consider how preferences are measured. Economists and psychologists differ on their (preferred) approach to preference measurement. Economists favor approaches based on expected utility theory. The axioms of choice (von Neuman & Morganstern, 1944) depend upon certain assumptions about gambling or tradeoff. Thus, economists only acknowledge utility assessment methods that formally consider economic trades (Torrance, 1986). The advantage of these methods is that they clearly are linked to economic theory. However, there are also some important disadvantages. For example, Kahneman

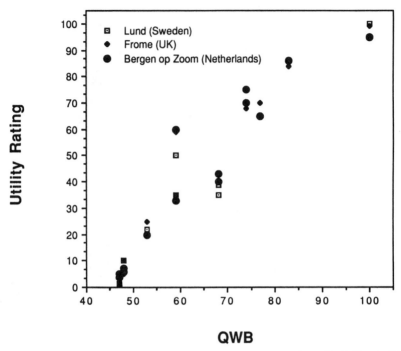

Figure 7.3 Comparison of preference ratings from three European sites with California QWB ratings.

& Tversky (1983) have shown empirically that many of the assumptions that underlie economic measurements of choice are incorrect. Human information processors do poorly at integrating complex probability information when making decisions that involve risk. Further, economic analysis assumes that choices accurately correspond to the way rational humans put information together. A substantial literature from experimental psychology questions these assumptions. In particular, Anderson (1979) has presented substantial evidence suggesting that methods commonly used for economic analysis do not represent the underlying true preference continuum. It seems that economists and psychologists have ignored one another's literatures.

In summary, we have considered the preference issue in some detail and we believe that preferences can be explicitly considered in a health policy model. A variety of studies have evaluated the generalizability (Kaplan *et al.*, 1978), the validity, and the reliability of the preference measures (Kaplan *et al.*, 1976; 1979). Methodological studies have tested some of the specific concerns about rating-scale methods (Kaplan, 1982; Kaplan & Ernest, 1983). We have little evidence that preferences differ across groups or that the small observed differences reported by others have much influence upon decisions in policy analysis. Having considered the evidence, we still believe that rating scales provide an appropriate method for utility assessment. However, we encourage continuing evaluations of these problems since they are expected to be important in the development of newer approaches to policy analysis.

Representativeness. There were two types of value studies in Oregon. The concerns reviewed above apply to the measurement of weights for the Quality of Well-Being scale. The other type of value study was the assessment of health care options in community meetings of Oregon citizens. These focus group discussions ultimately had an impact upon the placement of some items on the prioritized list. For example, the commissioners tended to place services for mothers and children higher on the list than would be expected on the basis of medical benefit alone. The rationale for this movement was justified by community preference as assessed in the town meeting. Critics were quick to point out that those who attended the community meetings were not representative of all Oregon citizens. For example, the experiment was designed to impact those with no medical insurance, and 91% of those who attended the meetings were themselves insured. More than a third of those who participated in the meetings had annual incomes in excess of $50,000 and two-thirds had graduated from college. Of the meeting participants, 1% were black (Office of Technology Assessment, 1992). As a result of this imbalance, there was concern that the process was biased in favor of procedures that would benefit the white, educated, and wealthy subpopulations of the society.

In response to these concerns, the Health Services Commission pointed out that it made extensive efforts to recruit all members of society and engaged in special outreach efforts for the poor. Clearly, the process would have been better if the town meeting participants had been more representative of the general population. However, public hearings are common components of public policy making. In this respect the meetings in Oregon were not different from the policy forums in nearly all levels of government. The fact that those who testify at public hearings are not representative of the general population has not stopped local, state, or federal governments from enacting legislation that they perceive to be the will of the people. If those participating in the town meetings were reckless in advocating policies to support their own self-interest, we would expect their opinions to be discrepant from those of the general public. The results of the town meetings indicated that the public wanted programs that benefit many, that emphasize prevention, and that improve quality of life. Is the suggestion that poor people are opposed to prevention and to equity in health care? Public opinion polls that include random samples from the general population show that the values expressed in the town meetings are very consistent with those of the general population (see Chapter One). Perhaps the strongest rebuttal is that nearly all states are currently rationing health care by changing the eligibility criteria and excluding categories of people. These rationing decisions are made with no or little public input whatsoever. The attempt in Oregon to gain public input represents a significant, although imperfect, improvement over the current system (Weiner, 1992).

Assessing Treatment Effectiveness

One of the most difficult problems encountered by the Oregon commissioners was in estimating the effects of treatment. Several questions have been raised about the estimates of treatment effects. Some have concerned the QWB method, while others are directed at the expert panels that generated the estimates of treatment effectiveness.

Technical Problems with the Method. Several critics have identified flaws in the method for evaluating health outcomes. In one important evaluation, published in the *Journal of the American Medical Association*, Eddy (1991) argued that the QWB system is too crude to evaluate medical outcomes. Many of Eddy's criticisms reflect basic misunderstandings of the QWB method. For example, Eddy emphasizes that the QWB has 24 health or functional states. These states are associated with preference weights that are used to reflect the quality of life associated with the symptom or problem. Apparently, Eddy thought that the symptom component of the QWB was the only aspect of patient classification. The QWB includes 24 symptoms or problems but these are only one component of the health status classification. In addition, the QWB includes a complex system for functional classification according to mobility, physical activity, and social activity. Overlooking this component of the QWB scale is quite serious. For example, one of Eddy's criticisms is that QWB states "do a poor job in registering differences in severity of symptoms" (p. 2138). Indeed, the symptom categories in the QWB are quite broad. However, the severity of the symptoms is determined by the degree to which they affect function. A cough, for example, might be relatively minor or it could be associated with more serious limitations. Simply reporting whether or not a person coughs provides relatively little information. However, the QWB system also determines whether the cough limits mobility, interferes with physical functioning, or disrupts role performance or self-care.

Eddy uses the example of "trouble speaking" which he claims could range from mild lisp to mutism. It is true that trouble speaking is a single symptom. However, we would that expect that mutism would be more likely associated with disruption in social role. Simply stated, a person with a mild lisp and one with mutism would score significantly differently on the QWB because the latter would need special assistance. In summary, Eddy was in error in his assessment of the QWB system. The problem he cited is actually well recognized and compensated for in the method.

Perhaps a more serious problem concerns the development of condition–

treatment (CT) pairs. In their evaluation, the OTA identified many problems with the CT pairs. For example, some of the CT pairs are made up of heterogeneous conditions. Pair 95, for example, includes several categories of heart failure (myocarditis, pericarditis, and endocarditis) which may require very different treatments. Other groupings of CT pairs were difficult to explain. For example, line 264 was for diseases of white blood cells. Some of these conditions might be of minor consequence while others can be life threatening. In other cases apparently different conditions were separated. Liver transplantation for alcoholic cirrhosis (line 690) was in a very different location than liver transplantation for nonalcoholic liver failure (line 366). In general, there was concern that CT pairs were defined so broadly that they included too many potential medical problems or treatments (Office of Technology Assessment, 1992).

Problems with Expert Judgment. The Commission used panels of experts to evaluate which aspects of treatment produce net health benefits. In order to estimate the incremental benefit of treatment, it is essential that the risks and benefits of all treatments be evaluated in the common measurement units described in Chapters 4 and 5. However, the methods for estimating these benefits have differed in different studies. There are at least three different approaches used to estimate health benefits in well-year or quality-adjusted life year units.

The first approach involves collection of prospective data using systematic medical experiments. For example, patients might be randomly assigned to treatment or to the control groups and then followed over the course of time. There are several randomized clinical trials that have used health status measurement strategies in an attempt to estimate well-years of life as a function of the treatment. For example, Toevs et al. (1983) randomly assigned chronic obstructive pulmonary diseases (COPD) patients to rehabilitation programs or to control conditions and evaluated the stream of outcomes over the course of 18 months. Their data suggested that rehabilitation does indeed produce benefits at a cost comparable to other widely advocated medical and surgical procedures. Kaplan et al. (1987) performed a similar experiment on weight loss for patients with noninsulin-dependent diabetes mellitus. A variety of other clinical trials using standardized health status measures are currently underway.

Clearly, the randomized clinical trial provides the best evidence for treatment effectiveness. Unfortunately, there are relatively few clinical trials that have gathered data using systematic experimental designs. Thus, for the vast majority of medical and surgical treatments we do not have data from systematic experimental studies. Further, there are problems with many experimental studies. For example, the external validity or the generalizability is not always optimal in randomized studies. It is becoming increasingly apparent that patients selected for randomized clinical trials may not be representative of patients cared for under usual circumstances. The inclusion criteria for many clinical trials often require that more than

90% of those screened for participation are excluded. Further, participants in clinical trials often are not representative of the general population in terms of age, sex, and ethnicity. A second concern about randomized clinical trials is that they are very expensive. It is extremely unlikely that we will have data from systematic clinical trials in all areas of medicine and surgery. Pharmaceutical companies and the National Institutes of Health are now beginning to include health-related quality-of-life measures in their clinical trials. Nevertheless, they are focusing on a small fraction of the potential therapeutic interventions and they often do not include the appropriate measures required for systematic outcomes assessment.

A final concern about clinical trials is that these medical experiments often take years to complete. Indeed, the best medical experiment would be one that follows patients long enough to estimate the full profile of treatment benefits and side effects. The difficulty is that we are witnessing rapid change in medical options. Therapeutic approaches are changing continually. By the time one approach is thoroughly evaluated in a clinical trial, a new therapeutic approach has taken its place. Thus, results from clinical trials are sometimes obsolete by the time the investigation is completed.

The second method for estimating treatment effects is to have experts perform systematic reviews of the literature. For example, Weinstein and Stason (1976) performed many detailed analyses on the effects of screening and treatment for hypertension. Their analyses carefully considered the medical literature and used the informed judgment of experts. Ultimately, they evaluated a variety of different public health approaches to the problem of high blood pressure treatment and control. Such analyses make use of data from clinical trials, observational studies, and computer simulation. Today, a substantial number of such analyses have been performed. For example, investigators have considered the cost/utility of pneumococcal vaccine for the elderly (Office of Technology Assessment, 1979), coronary artery bypass surgery (Weinstein & Stason, 1983), total hip replacement (Liang et al., 1990), and medical management of rheumatoid arthritis (Thompson et al., 1988). Although these analyses were performed by different analysts, they used a comparable methodology. Thus, it is possible to construct league tables across studies so that the costs/utilities of different interventions can be compared.

The third approach is to obtain judgment from panels of experts. This resembles the "science court" endorsed by Hadorn (1991b). The panel members may not necessarily be cost/utility analysts. Instead, panel members are typically experts who render judgment on the likely benefit of various treatments. For example, Bush, Chen, & Patrick (1973) estimated the cost/utility of PKU screening for the state of New York using delphi methods to obtain consensus from a panel of experts about the most likely outcomes of PKU given that the disease was not detected. The experts used their experience and knowledge of the literature to create simulations of outcomes under various scenarios. This process permitted the estimation of outcomes in the absence of any true experiment. A similar process was used by the Oregon Health Services Commission. This group of experts estimated the health benefits of 709 condition–treatment pairs.

The committee approach has the advantage of allowing the estimation of many health benefits in a relatively short period of time. It is the only approach that makes the implementation of guidelines feasible in the near term. The disadvantages of this approach are that physicians may overestimate the treatment benefits associated with services that they prefer to offer. As has been suggested (Mosteller, 1981), providers tend to be overly optimistic about the efficacy of their interventions. Indeed, Sachs, Chalmers, & Smith (1982) demonstrated that the likelihood that a medical or surgical treatment is effective declines as the source of evidence about treatment efficacy becomes more rigorous. Clinical judgment tends to provide the most optimistic view of likely treatment benefits. One of the concerns about the use of clinical judgment is the fear that some physicians will apply "gaming" strategies in order to obtain reimbursement for their specialty. For instance, there is clearly an incentive to provide optimistic estimates of treatment benefit. In a system such as the one proposed in Oregon, specialties that are pessimistic about their treatment efficacy risk putting themselves out of business. The model proposal calls for panels of physicians and nonphysicians to make these evaluations. However, the presence of nonphysicians does not assure a solution to the problem. In the absence of evidence nonphysicians are in an even poorer position to challenge clinical opinion.

Greely (1991) endorsed the use of expert committees for establishing the efficacy of treatments in a basic benefits package. He suggested that there be multiple panels and that the panels be privately funded. In endorsing panels, Greely implicitly accepts the fallibility of the process. However, the Greely proposal is an interesting one because competition among panels creates checks upon the system and may expose the effects of physician gaming. In addition, Greely proposed judicial review to prevent panels from becoming too autonomous. We believe that the use of panels is the only realistic solution for the near term.

The notion of a panel "grand jury" seems reasonable as long as it is recognized that the estimate of treatment effectiveness is an iterative process. We must expect that judgments of treatment efficacy will continually be revised as new data become available. This is not only good policy, it is good science. Panels should weight evidence by its quality. For example, randomized clinical trials should be given the most careful consideration in the judgment of treatment effectiveness. Panelists must also take into consideration biases associated with evaluation methods. For example, we know that treatments that have been evaluated in randomized clinical trials often appear less potent than the same treatments evaluated in nonrandomized studies (Sachs *et al.*, 1982). Thus, well-informed panels will need to consider these issues so that they do not create biases against those treatments that have been evaluated in the most systematic studies.

There have also been some proposals to avoid medical judgment altogether.

The framers of the Oregon plan clearly acknowledge that there may be alternative allocation methods. One such alternative was suggested by Fisher et al. (1992), who proposed that prioritization decisions be made by local hospitals. Most hospitals have excess capacity and there is considerable flexibility in discretionary admissions. When hospitals have too much capacity, they become inefficient. Resources must be used to maintain the infrastructure and to pay underutilized personnel. To remain active, hospitals may become more aggressive in their admission policies and they may be motivated to perform unnecessary services. This overuse of some hospital services drains resources that might be directed to the undeserved. Among 16 hospitals studied by Fisher and colleagues, discretionary medical admissions accounted for between 188 and 335 patient days per thousand admissions. Salem, Oregon, the state capitol, reports an average of 218 days per thousand. If Salem's rate was used as the ceiling, 238 beds could be closed in 20 hospital service areas. This would result in a savings of $47.3 million that could be used to support basic health services for all. This approach circumvents the process of denying coverage for specific services and it leaves the decision making in the hands of hospitals and providers.

ETHICAL CONCERNS

The Rule of Rescue

Plenty went wrong in the early applications of the GHPM to priority setting in Oregon. It first appeared that the formula misassigned many services. Hadorn (1991a,b) persuaded the Commission that they had ignored the ethical principles embraced by the "rule of rescue" (Jonsen, 1986). According to the rule of rescue, those in life-threatening situations must be saved. Many technologies may relieve pain or reduce disability but do not rescue people from imminent death. Somehow, there seems to be a moral obligation to invest in rescue if saving a life is a possibility.

Based on the rule of rescue argument, Hadorn persuaded the Commission to adopt a different strategy. Hadorn (1991a) describes the Commission as "stung by public criticism" and "dismayed by the intuitive unacceptability of the draft list's priority order" (p. 2220). The alternative was to develop a set of categories that described varying degrees of health benefit.

There are several problems with the abandonment of the GHPM in favor of a rule of rescue. One of the problems is mentioned in the analysis of the outcomes of the Oregon Health Services Commission. Table 7.1, taken from Hadorn's paper, underscores the problem. According to the table, tooth capping, which provides a very small benefit for a relatively short period of time is prioritized as very close to surgery for ectopic pregnancy. Yet surgery for ectopic pregnancy prevents death in 70% of the cases. How could it be that the cost/utility of these two procedures could be so similar? Similarly, splints for temporomandibular joint disorder (TMJ) are ranked at approximately the same level as appendectomy. Yet no one dies of

		TABLE 7.1			

Factors Producing the Priority Scores of Four Treatments in Oregon's Draft List[a]

Treatment	Expected net benefit from treatment[b]	Expected duration of benefit (years)	Cost ($)	Priority rating[c]	Priority ranking
Tooth capping	.08	4	38.10	117.6	371
Surgery for ectopic pregnancy	.71[d]	48	4015	117.8	372
Splints for temporomandibular joint disorder	.16	5	98.51	122.2	376
Appendectomy	.97	48	5744	122.5	377

[a]From Hadorn (1991a).
[b]Maximum achievable benefit = 1.0.
[c]Priority ratings were obtained using the following formula: priority rating = cost of treatment/(net expected benefit × duration of benefit). Ratings ranged from 1.45 (highest priority) to 999.998 (lowest priority).
[d]The net benefit is relatively low because Oregon's consultant physicians estimated that (only) 70% of patients with ectopic pregnancy would die if not operated on. Increasing the estimated net benefit from surgery to 1.0 would move this treatment to 326 on the draft priority list.

TMJ and, left alone, 97% of those with appendicitis would die without rapid treatment. Could this be correct?

At first glance, these analyses do seem peculiar. Yet reflection suggests otherwise. Let us have a closer look at dental capping. There are two issues that need to be explored in relation to this service: effects and costs. The effect of dental capping was estimated to be .08. That is a strong effect! It is about three times the effect that has been observed for the treatment of rheumatoid arthritis with oral gold medication. We do not know where the estimates of treatment effectiveness came from. The symptom for pain in the tooth or jaw including teeth missing, crooked, or replaced brings a weighting of −.17 on the QWB scale. It is possible that the expert panel halved this number and assumed the treatment effect would be about .08. However, this sort of analysis is difficult to evaluate. For example, it would assume that all of those who received dental capping would have pain in the tooth or jaw prior to the treatment or that without care they would end up with a tooth missing. The analysis also assumes that dental capping is the only alternative and that a less involved procedure (such as amalgam filling) would not suffice.

If people are in pain and the pain would continue without treatment, an estimated treatment effect of .08 may not be unrealistic. How much would you be willing to pay to eliminate a severe pain in the mouth that would not go away on its own? For those of us who have experienced dental pain there is little question that effective dental care is a valuable service. The issue is placing this service in the context of other health care opportunities.

Perhaps the most problematic aspect of the dental capping example is the cost. The Health Services Commission placed the cost of dental capping at $38 per tooth. There are two reasons that dental capping competes favorably with surgery for ectopic pregnancy. One is that it has a relatively large treatment effect and the other is that it is has a remarkably low cost. But is this cost figure correct? It appears that $38 for dental capping is a fantasy. If you present this price to a group of dentists you will be greeted with hearty laughter (I have tried it). Consider the resources required for dental capping. This procedure typically takes multiple dental visits. There is the initial diagnosis that requires X-rays. Then, the dentist must engage in several procedures. He or she must use anesthetics and cut the tooth. Then the dentist must use specialized material to form an impression. The impression is typically sent to a separate laboratory where the dental crown is prepared. The crown is then returned to the dentist and the patient comes for an additional appointment to fit the crown. Often there is a follow-up appointment to be certain that the crown is functioning properly. The materials used to make the dental caps are not inexpensive. For example, many crowns are made from gold.

Can this realistically be accomplished for $38? Our dental consultant suggested that the $38 figure may be less than one-tenth of what would be necessary. When the more realistic figure of $500 for dental capping is used, there is a profound impact on the comparison of this procedure with surgery for ectopic pregnancy. If we accept the estimated effectiveness of dental capping versus extraction or some other method (still somewhat questionable), the procedure still compares very favorably with many other procedures on the initial list. Nevertheless, there is now a profound separation of dental capping from ectopic pregnancy. The argument is not that dental procedures should not be included. Under almost all analyses, these turn out to be worthwhile investments of public resources. However, what appears to be an illogical ranking was probably based on a faulty estimate of either the costs or the effects of some procedures. The case of ectopic pregnancy also deserves reconsideration. Upon reexamination, it moved very high up on the list, ultimately resting at line 10. The model is not faulty—only the data that went into the calculations.

Hadorn's discussion of the rule of rescue has not escaped other criticisms. For example, Gillette (1991) wondered why it was necessary to remove cost from the equation. Eddy (1991) stated, "to remove cost from the definition of essential care . . . would separate the concept of a central care from the problem it is designed to solve." The unaffordability of health care is what created the problem in the first place and health care costs are continuing to go up.

Gillette (1991) also challenged the notion of a "rule" of rescue. In particular, he thought that the term *rule* was too strong since there are many places in the world where decisions are routinely made to withhold care because society is unwilling to pay. In the United Kingdom, for example, these decisions are made routinely and often without controversy (Aaron & Schwartz, 1990). It is understandable that the public would be upset by mass media accounts of children dying of treatable illnesses. Yet the emotional content of the media appeals does not necessarily make the process more rational.

MacLean (1991), another critic of Hadorn's paper, argued that the amount that we are willing to spend to save a particular life is finite rather than infinite. He cites other studies suggesting the specific number of dollars someone would be willing to spend to save a life and argues that, with adjustments, similar procedures could be used in Oregon. MacLean, a family physician, also supported the original plan since the rule of rescue tends to be biased in favor of physicians who perform emergency and rescue procedures. In doing so, the rule of rescue undervalues family physicians, who are the first line of defense in health care.

In defense, Hadorn argues that his proposal does not exclude costs, but rather makes cost a "meta-factor." Within equally effective services, cost will be considered. Further, any prioritization scheme will cut costs by eliminating procedures that have no effect at all. However, Hadorn argued that cost-effectiveness formulas will produce socially undesirable results because low-income people might be denied some life-saving services. In contrast, the wealthy would be able to attain any services that they chose. Hadorn fails to recognize that he is describing the system that we currently have. The wealthy can get nearly any service while the semi-poor (just above Medicaid eligibility) are denied everything. The cost-effectiveness formula attempts to provide basic services for all people, just as the Hadorn plan does. Hadorn denied that other westernized countries routinely withhold life-saving services on the basis of cost. Instead, services are withheld on the basis of expected benefit. However, despite Hadorn's argument, there is substantial evidence that cost has been a consideration in the development and application of some new technologies and therapeutics. For example, renal dialysis is not uniformily available in the United Kingdom and some expensive pharmaceuticals (such as AZT) have only recently been purchased by government health agencies in large countries such as Argentina. The rationale has been primarily financial.

Eddy (1991) argued that the rule of rescue is not in conflict with cost/utility analysis. For example, cost/utility analysis can be used to compare how many dental caps add up to one surgery for ectopic pregnancy. Further advances in the methodology might address other criticisms. As Eddy emphasizes, cost-effectiveness analysis is very flexible and can adapt to or incorporate many of the moral values embraced by a "rule of rescue." The major issue is in defining a measure of benefit correctly. The problem has less to do with the maturity of the method and more to do with the absence of appropriate data that can be used to properly estimate treatment effectiveness. Hopefully the new emphasis on outcomes research will help resolve some of these problems.

The debate over the rule of rescue is certain to continue. There is, however, a substantial group that contests whether the rule of rescue truly has more compelling moral force than does a system that attempts to provide the most benefit for the most people.

TARGETING THE POOR

One of the most severe criticisms of the Oregon plan is that it targets poor women and children. The program modifies payments under the Medicaid program. Medicaid funds a variety of different groups including the blind, the disabled, and families with dependent children. However, the other groups were excluded from the Oregon experiment. In Oregon, poor women and children make up about 75% of the Medicaid recipients. However, they only receive about 30% of the benefits. Most of the money goes to help elderly who have spent down to the poverty level. The rest goes to the blind and disabled. Many reviewers criticize the Oregon plan for focusing on poor women and children (Rosenbaum, 1991; Daniels, 1991). Even worse, the program had the appearance of being discriminatory because the blind, disabled, and elderly were predominantly white. However, minorities were much more commonly represented in low-income families.

Although these arguments are compelling, it is also important to consider the benefits the program provides for poor women and children. Currently, thousands of women and children have no coverage at all. The program will make funding available to an estimated 60,000 new women and children. Further, the prioritized list emphasizes services in child and maternity care. In fact, one of the new concerns about the plan (see Chapter Six) is that the Commission overemphasized non-technical preventive services. Essentially all services in category 2 will be covered and these interventions will focus almost exclusively on women and children. Figure 7.4 summarizes the number of people currently covered by the Oregon Medicaid program, the number covered under Senate Bill 27, and the number expected to be covered when all three pieces of legislation are in place. The benefits for children significantly increase rather than decrease under the new legislation.

The Children's Defense fund was dissatisfied with Senate Bill 27, because new Medicaid policy does extend benefits for children. In 1989 Medicaid developed the Early and Periodic Screening Diagnosis and Treatment Program (EPSDT) that entitled children to all medically necessary diagnostic and treatment services. Further, policy enacted in 1990 required states to expand coverage to all children below the poverty line. The policy will be phased in over the next 10 years. Since all children will get all services under the new policy, children can only be harmed by the Oregon program that restricts some services.

As compelling as the CDF arguments seem, counterarguments must also be considered. For example, the Oregon process ranked most procedures for children very high on the list. In fact very few items below the funding line would be expected to provide any health benefit for children, and some of the low-ranked services may do some harm. Further, the Oregon program will provide coverage to a broader range of children that could be accounted for by the EPSDT. Further, the greater resources devoted to children must come from either increased revenues or from reductions in other aspects of the program. As Wiener (1992) points out, uninsured adults also need some benefits. Overall, reallocation of the health care dollar should reduce the imbalance between the poor and the rest of society.

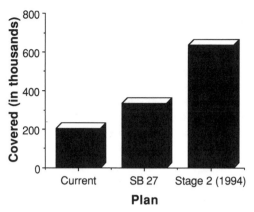

Figure 7.4 Number of people currently covered by the Oregon Medicaid program, the number covered under Senate Bill 27, and number covered under full implementations.

It is not technically true that the aged, blind, and disabled are completely excluded from the Oregon experiment. However, Oregon introduced innovative programs for these individuals who need ongoing long-term care. Further, many of the elderly already receive Medicare benefits over which the state has no control. In 1991 Oregon enacted legislation that would bring the aged, blind, and disabled into the experiment for services in mental health, physical medicine, and chemical dependency. The delayed strategy for these services is necessary because the Commission needed more time to deal with the complexities of integrating mental health and chemical dependency services with other health services.

The GHPM in no way discriminates against children. Indeed, services for children may fare better because they have the potential to produce many years of benefit. Indeed, many criticisms of the model have suggested that it discriminates *in favor* of children. For example, prevention of a birth defect may produce large numbers of well-years over the course of the life span. Lasting treatment effects are counted over and over again as the person ages.

WILL THE SYSTEM CHANGE THE WAY MEDICINE IS PRACTICED?

A variety of different arguments have suggested that the implementation of a general health policy model will destroy the way medicine is practiced. It is true that the system will change the way medicine is practiced, but whether or not this will be a negative result remains to be determined. Some groups have argued that providers will refuse to care for poor women and children as a result of the system. It is not clear where this argument is based. Providers may avoid performing ineffective procedures on women and children. However, they will be paid for offering services that produce health benefit. Further, the number of women and children they are able to care for will significantly increase. Screening and diagnostic procedures as well as a wide variety of preventive options will be candidates for reimbursement.

Another concern has been that cost to private insurers will go up because Medicaid will refuse to pay for expensive procedures. Thus, the system might ultimately increase medical care costs. In response to this argument, the Oregon Health Services Commission has suggested that avoidable emergency room use will be reduced because preventive services will be more available. The intent of the program is not to eliminate costly procedures but rather to eliminate procedures that are either ineffective or have little effect relative to their cost. Table 7.2 summarizes items that almost certainly will not be covered by the plan and items that have a high likelihood of being covered. As the table suggests, some very inexpensive procedures (medical therapy for scaly skin) will be denied coverage because they have no benefit. Items that are low on the list are not necessarily the expensive ones. The lists of items with high priority for funding and with low priority for funding include both expensive and inexpensive treatments.

Another concern is that providers will be caught in an impossible situation because they will not be able to discriminate between treatments that they should offer or not offer. In fact, the prioritized list should give providers a very clear understanding of what treatments that they should or should not make available.

TABLE 7.2

Sample Condition–Treatment Pairs and Their Rankings[a]

Examples of condition–treatment pairs ranked at or near the bottom of the prioritized list:

Line 685	Medical therapy for ichthyosis (scaly skin).
Line 694	Medical therapy for benign polyps of vocal cords.
Line 695	Medical therapy for acute upper respiratory infections and common cold.
Line 698	Hemorrhoidectomy for uncomplicated hemorrhoids.
Line 709	Life support for anencephalous and similar anomalies and reduction deformities of the brain.

Examples of condition–treatment pairs ranked at or near the top of the prioritized list:

Line 1	Medical treatment for pneumococcal pneumonia and other bacterial pneumonia.
Line 3	Medical and surgical treatment for peritonitis.
Line 10	Surgery for ectopic pregnancy.
Line 13	Medical and surgical treatment for acute pelvic inflammatory disease.
Line 18	Medical therapy for syphillis.
Line 22	Medical therapy for low-birth-weight babies (500 grams and over).

[a]From Oregon Department of Human Resources, July 10, 1991 (unpublished).

OTHER LEGAL AND ETHICAL CHALLENGES

The Children's Defense Fund has argued that there are both legal and ethical reasons not to proceed with the Oregon plan. For example, the CDF suggests that the plan creates a form of social experimentation in which women and children are forced to participate without consent. This may result in the denial of clinically effective care to socially disadvantaged groups. Among all of their arguments this may be the most peculiar. The Oregon Medicaid program now denies access to substantial numbers of women and children. These people are unable to get any medical service. Further, there are millions of women who are not pregnant or who do not have children who are denied any access to medical care. Apparently this situation is acceptable to CDF. In order to protect this system they will submit petitions to interfere with any attempts to broaden coverage for those who are currently excluded by the plan. The plan does not intend to take highly useful services away from current recipients. Instead, it attempts to cut expensive, non-useful services and use the savings to provide coverage for more people. According to the CDF reasoning, any legal chance or the development of any social program would, in effect, constitute "research." However, Federal Law [45, CFR, paragraph 46,102(E)] exempts research and development projects which evaluate public assistance programs.

Other legal challenges have been offered. For example, it has been suggested that the program violates federal civil rights laws, the Age Discrimination Act of 1974, Title XI of the 1964 Civil Rights Act, and Section 504 of the Rehabilitation Act of 1973. Analysis of these challenges by the Oregon Health Services Commission shows them to be without merit. For example, the program does not discriminate by race, sex, or age. Further, the disabled will continue to receive their current benefits until 1993, at which point Medicaid benefits for the disabled will be included in the plan. However, there is no evidence that the plan will provide specific discrimination against the disabled. Overall, there seems to be little merit in the legal challenges to the program.

CRITICISMS OF THE USE OF PREFERENCES

A substantial number of critics have challenged the use of preferences to make informed decisions about health care expenditures. A review of these criticisms will suggest that few of the critics actually understood how preferences are used in the GHPM. Most critics believe that people in the community prioritize which services should be funded. This would be a legitimate criticism if it were true. Most health care consumers do not have the medical knowledge required to determine whether or not procedures work. However, the GHPM is not an opinion contest. Instead, the model uses preference to quantify a health condition; the information on the effect of treatment, duration of benefit, and likelihood of treatment response is based on systematic data or informed clinical opinions.

TABLE 7.3

Summary of Views of Oregon's Medicaid Proposal[a]

Areas of concern	Advocates' points of view	Critics' point of view
Change in eligibility	Expands eligibility based on need and ability to pay rather than on current categories of beneficiaries (age, disease condition, employment status, marital status, income, family structure, disability)	Disproportionately affects children and women
		Affects only the entitlement of women and children to primary care services, but not that of the elderly and disabled, who account for a majority of program spending
	Guarantees that all "poor" people receive needed services (anyone with income below 100% of federal poverty level)	Results in federal cost sharing for newly defined Medicaid eligibles who are currently paid for entirely with state funds
Change in benefits	Provides same basic level of benefits to all state's citizens rather than current benefit system which varies by age and from one category of eligibility to another	Reduces benefit package for women and children while increasing both Medicaid eligibility and payment levels for providers
		Exempts the most expensive services—minimum benefits secured for aged, disabled, or nursing home beneficiaries
	Develops and guarantees a standard for adequate benefits plan and basic level of health care	Does not establish a floor of benefits thus potentially seriously reducing benefits covered by the Medicaid program—results in an inadequate benefit package and a denial of access to medically effective care
Effects on state budget	Attempts to spread limited Medicaid dollars to the services that will benefit the largest number of people	Shares portion of budget for mothers and children with new groups of eligibles
	Considers what Oregon can obtain most efficiently given level of spending	Provides no economic justification—does not curb either medical cost inflation in general or increases in Oregon's Medicaid budget
	Emphasizes a case management system to assist in containing costs	Does not control or reduce costs but rather eliminates services to needy women and children
	Mandates cuts in benefits only if insufficient resources are available	Generates insignificant savings since exempts most expensive populations and services
		Permits expansion of an adequate level of health care coverage to a significant number of uninsured with conceivable massive increases in spending

Significance of rationing	Stresses that rationing is a current practice which denies access to medically effective care to state residents	Does not prevent shifting of funds from aged and disabled social services and from general fund dollars
	Initiates an explicit resource allocation decision-making process to control increasing costs and to ration health care	Does not have an explicit implementation process for case management for which costs would be controlled
	Underscores that both the current and the proposed system are inadequate—Medicaid is currently a patchwork system and underfunded while the proposal allows for broader equity with a limit of depth of services	Does not consider costs of not providing health services nor the possible creation of incentives for overtreatment
		Constitutes rationing of health care to most vulnerable citizens and politically disenfranchised groups—ADC adults and children
		Should apply rationing to all members of society, not just to the poor
		Should eliminate waste from current system before rationing by addressing unnecessary services, overbedding, and oversupply of physicians rather than cutting services to poor
Implication on access	Provides equal and universal access to health care for the state's citizens (to a basic level of benefits) rather than a poor people's plan	Does not demonstrate universalization of program because of lack of imposing prioritization and rationing on its own employees, on privately insured, and on all Medicaid beneficiaries
	Increases access to services which effectively prevent health problems by providing expanded Medicaid eligibility to uninsured low-income families	Does not provide universal access to a basic health care package but rather to whatever level/amount of health care is funded biennially by the state
	Mandates "play or pay" employer health insurance	Does not improve access or health care by changing from who is covered to what is covered
	Expands state risk pool to create universal access	
Consequence of community participation	Creates a public rather than private decision-making process for rationing based on informed community content and active community participation in allocation decisions	Does not involve individuals affected by the program in the decision-making process
	Allocates health care resources to reflect experts' and provider community views on clinical effectiveness and citizen/public perception on social values	Encourages systematic biased selection because public aware in process that responses helped in deciding what services the states should provide to welfare recipients at taxpayers' expense

(continued)

TABLE 7.3 (continued)

Areas of concern	Advocates' points of view	Critics' point of view
Effect of prioritization methodology	Focuses on medical service prioritization model and outcomes Allows for emphasis on prevention and institutionalizes a skepticism about some high-technology interventions Highlights that services for aged, blind, and disabled have already been prioritized through a waiver for social services	Lacks specificity in defining treatments and conditions making it difficult to accurately estimate the extent of expected benefits from certain therapies Question accuracy of treatment outcome estimates by Commission to produce a reasonable and usable priority list Costs should be given equal weight with benefits/outcomes in determining the values of health care services
Implications on provider liability and patient choice	Stops defensive medicine and allows society, not the courts, to determine the level of care it wishes to guarantee to all citizens Increases payment to providers for essential health care services, thereby increasing the willingness to participate	Unjustly provides legal immunity to health providers who do not provide reasonable health care services to Medicaid recipients because the state refuses to pay for these services Runs counter to principles of informed consent and patient's own choice of services Potentially increases uncompensated care to certain providers or specialties Erodes freedom to choose a physician since patients locked into providers
Significance of legal process	Regards universal access and definition of essential health care services as a state issue in light of absence of effective federal action	Forfeits legal rights by eliminating or reducing standards and regulatory/legal protections for selected group (e.g., children, pregnant women, and caretaker relatives of children) Establishing universal access is not a state issue but federal for the provision for basic medical services for all citizens Does not include an appeals process

[a]From Office of Technology Assessment (1992).

The Children's Defense Fund has also argued that the town meetings in Oregon would have no meaning to those who are not allowed to participate. They contended that preferences expressed at these meetings involved "extraordinarily complex medical decisionmaking." In fact, the town meetings were used only to prioritize general health concepts such as prevention, quality of life, and so on. The complex medical decision making was left to trained medical professionals. Unfortunately, children are often not able to provide complex decisions. Thus, legal and social process allows parents to speak on behalf of children.

A variety of other arguments for or against the Oregon plan are summarized in Table 7.3. This table, taken from a report by the OTA, considers benefit, change in availability, effect on state budget, impact of rationing, and other community issues.

DEPARTMENT OF HEALTH AND HUMAN SERVICES REJECTION OF OREGON APPLICATION

In order to go forward with their proposal, Oregon needed a waiver from the U.S. Department of Health and Human Services (DHHS). Medicaid is funded jointly by states and the federal government. Since Oregon intended to revise trditional Medicaid policies, they needed a waiver in order to perform their demonstration experiment. Such experimentation had been widely promoted by President George Bush. However, in August of 1992, the Department of Health and Human Services rejected Oregon's application for a waiver that would have allowed them to go forward with the experiment. The rationale for this rejection was that the Oregon proposal violated the Americans with Disabilities Act which became law in July of 1992. Specifically, the Department stated that the Oregon preference survey on quality of life "quantified stereotypic assumptions about persons with disability." According to the statement, scholars have found that people without disability systematically undervalue the quality of life of those with disabilities. A discussion paper by David Hadorn and an analysis in the OTA (1992) report are cited to support this statement. However, the great bulk of the evidence summarized above is ignored. Most published studies show that differences between patients and nonpatients are small, and have relatively little if any impact on the policy analysis.

The DHHS decision fails to acknowledge that resource allocation designs necessarily require human judgment. Ultimately, decisions are made by patients, physicians, administrators, or their surrogates. Oregon clearly recognized this and attempted to separate aspects of human judgments. For example, when decisions required medical knowledge, they depended on a medical committee. When the decisions required in-depth understanding of human values, they depended on discussions held in open forums in Oregon towns. When the judgments involved an assessment of quality of life for those with either symptoms or disabilities, they depended on the preference of Oregon citizens. This exercise was unusual and all of these judgments were made publicly using methods that could be replicated by others.

The analysis underlying the rejection of the Oregon application was not only misinformed, it was incorrect. It assumed that there would be discrimination against persons with disabilities because treatment could not improve their chronic problems. However, this analysis makes a very serious conceptional error. Effectiveness of treatment is based on the estimated course of the illness with and without treatment. A treatment that sustains life, even without improvements in quality of life, produces very substantial benefits. For example, suppose a person is in an accident that leaves him or her in a state rated .5 on a 0 to 1.0 scale and the treatment will maintain them at this level while absence of treatment will result in death. According to the Oregon model, the treatment will produce .50 (calculated as .50–0) for each year the person remains in that state. That is a powerful treatment effect in comparison to most alternatives. The crucial element is that the treatment works. The system does attempt to exclude treatments that neither extend life nor make patients better. In other words, the targets for elimination are only treatments that use resources and do not make a difference.

DHHS also misrepresented the meaning of quality of life scores. They assumed that having a low quality of life score was discriminatory because people with disabilities and those without disabilities would not be rated the same. On the other hand, the statement is contradictory with the notion that people with disabilities need medical services. People who are at optimum health (1.0 on the QWB scale) may need fewer servics than those who occupy lower levels. Quantifying these differences allows us to set priorities for future resource allocation. If, for the sake of argument, we decide to score people with disabilities 1.0 it would follow that we should not provide any services for these individuals because they have already achieved the optimum level of wellness. Scores lower than 1.0 suggest that resources should be used to improve these conditions.

After several years of debate, intensive intellectual evaluation, and detailed bureaucratic scrutiny, the Oregon Experiment was ultimately denied on the basis of apparent misunderstanding of the methodology.

SUMMARY

The proposal in Oregon has attracted public comment. Many of the issues concern the use of preference information. Other criticisms concern the way judgments are made about the effect of treatment. Most of these issues can be addressed with existing data. A variety of ethical concerns have also been raised. For example, it has been argued that the rule of rescue must precede a prioritization scheme. Nevertheless, most of the ethical issues can be addressed. Our analysis suggests that a prioritization scheme using a GHPM is both desirable and feasible. Although there are important practical, ethical, and legal challenges, the consequences of continuing with our current system may be more severe.

CHAPTER EIGHT

Summary and Conclusions

This book provides a summary of the sorry state of affairs in contemporary health care. The current system represents a triple failure. Health care is unaffordable, it denies access to many of its citizens, and it has not been held accountable for what it produces. As a result of these failures, many new solutions have been proposed. Some solutions could not possibly work because they fail to recognize the complexity of the problems. Nationalizing health care, eliminating lawyers, reducing health care administration costs, or eliminating pre-tax status for health insurance have been suggested as solutions in various editorials. However, each of these, by themselves, would fall short of offering a comprehensive solution to the problem. Several important policy changes have focused on cost containment. However, most of these solutions apply only to the Medicare program, and all cost-cutting solutions must be simultaneously judged in relation to their impact upon access and outcome.

The solution to the problem cannot be simple. Among the dozens of suggestions, only three emerge as realistic competitors. Two of these are mutually exclusive of each other, while the third can work with either of the other two. The first solution is to adopt a Canadian-style single payer system as advocated by Grumbach and colleagues (1991). The alternative is a system of managed competition as advocated by Enthoven & Kronick (1989, 1991). Both of these systems improve access and there is a hope that each would control cost. However, neither of these proposals, nor any others in the current debate, have health outcome as a major component of the program.

In order to address these problems, we have proposed a General Health Policy Model (Kaplan & Anderson, 1990). Conceptually, this model was introduced by our group more than 20 years ago (Fanshel & Bush, 1970). Since that time, it has appeared in various formats in several other proposals (Weinstein & Stason, 1976; Drummond *et al.*, 1987; Patrick & Erickson, 1992). Although there are slight variations in concepts, most of the proposals are similar. The objective is to define a common unit of health benefit. Then, the model requires an estimate of the cost to obtain a unit of benefit. Using the model, various medical procedures are evaluated according to how much outcome they produce and how much cost is required. Outcomes are estimated according to the utility associated with the duration of life and quality of life produced by each procedure. Ultimately, a rank-ordering of procedures is created and available funds are used to produce the greatest benefit for the largest number of people.

Some editorialists believe that any alteration of the current system is politically unfeasible. The major problem is that some powerful group is likely to suffer. Under the universal payer proposal, insurance companies will be the major losers. Thus, insurance companies are major opponents of the single payer system. Interestingly, current proposals for a single payer system do not call for any reduction in total health care expenditures (Grumbach et al., 1991). Thus, funds now spent for administrative costs, which could approach $100 billion per year, would be redistributed in physician fees. This could make the proposal look appealing to physician groups. The managed competition alternative is more acceptable to the current establishment. However, its opponents suggest that it will result in inhumane care by HMO-like organizations that become overly focused on the bottom line. Perhaps people would suffer with either alternative. However, critics fail to acknowledge that substantial numbers of uninsured and underinsured people suffer under the current system. The new proposals spread the suffering to physicians, administrators, and insurance companies.

The GHPM recognizes that fundamental change must occur. However, the model can work with either the managed competition approach or the single payer system. A single payer might efficiently implement the model by clearly defining which services are covered and which are not. Similarly, managed competitions might provide alternatives that maximize health benefits. Plans in the competition could create prioritized lists for determining which services are covered and which services are denied. We recognize both single payer and managed competition as reasonable alternatives, and we encourage continued experimentation with each approach. Ultimately, the choice between these systems might hinge on both empirical and political considerations.

CAN AN OUTCOMES-ORIENTED APPROACH SUCCEED?

Even if a GHPM makes theoretical sense, many believe that the implementation would be impractical. There are at least three arguments against the application of these models. First, it has been suggested that this approach was tried and that it failed in Oregon. The second argument is that we do not have enough data to implement these models. The third argument is that the application of the GHPM is politically and ethically unacceptable. We will examine each of these briefly.

Did the Model Fail in Oregon?

Hadorn (1991a) argued that cost-effectiveness models came eyeball to eyeball with the "rule of rescue" in Oregon. When, nose to nose, cost-effectiveness blinked. Many of these problems were addressed in Chapter Six. There were problems with the implementation of the GHPM in Oregon including many technical difficulties in the execution of this ranking process. When the rank-ordering of services did not make intuitive sense, critics assumed that this was a flaw in the model rather than a fault in the way data were gathered. Beyond the methodological problems (see Chapter Six) there were many conceptual mis-understandings of the intent of the exercise. For example, critics failed to under-stand that the intent of the process was to improve health status. A basic mis-understanding of several critiques was the assumption that all medical care is worthwhile. Thus, denying coverage for some services was seen as damaging, even though there is no evidence that those services provide any benefit. The critics also failed to acknowledge that denying payment for these ineffective services would result in probable benefit for other people. An important point to emphasize is that the model is designed to provide the most help for the most people. It is indifferent to the amount of money providers or hospitals are making, the provider's credentials, or the socioeconomic status of the patients. The Oregon experiment was a bold and innovative attempt to use this system in a real policy context. Many important lessons were learned through the hard work of the Oregon Health Services Commission. However, we cannot consider Oregon to be a good test of the model.

Too Few Data

A second argument is that there are not enough clinical data to use the model in a reasonable way. We have surprisingly little information about the efficacy and effectiveness of medical and surgical procedures. As a result, any application of the model must depend upon educated guesses.

We must accept that our data are currently inadequate. However, that is no reason to stop making decisions. Clinicians make decisions every day, even though they do not have extensive clinical trial information for all of the treat-ments that they apply. Although clinical trial data are rarely available, there is typically some research base for most clinical treatments. We acknowledge that this information may be incorrect and that it may need to be revised as more information becomes available. Nevertheless, it seems reasonable to go forth with the best information available.

The GHPM may have a profound impact upon provider incomes. Thus, there is substantial concern about biases. However, peer review committees, as outlined in Chapter Seven, can be used to help oversee clinical judgments of treatment effectiveness to avoid bias. In time, with the appropriate support for research, ratings of treatment effectiveness and cost-effectiveness will be revised. It is also important to acknowledge that cost/utility rankings may create a competition that will help lower costs. Two variables affect the cost/utility ratio—treatment effectiveness and cost. It is conceivable that providers will lower their prices in order to place particular procedures in a more competitive place on the prioritization list.

Ethical Concerns

A variety of ethical questions have been raised about the prioritization process. It has been argued that the system discriminates against the poor, discriminates against the elderly, discriminates against children, or violates the rule of rescue. In Chapter Six, we challenged each of these assertions. If the application of the model became universal, it would not discriminate against the poor or against any other social group. The model would only consider how much benefit is obtained and how much it would cost to produce this benefit. Those with private resources could pay to obtain services that have a low priority in the ranking. However, the best evidence is that they would be wasting their money, since there would be little evidence that these procedures are valuable. There is the concern that some life-saving procedure would not be reimbursed because it is too expensive. Thus, the model would let some people die because they have a rare problem with a difficult or exotic treatment. Under the rule of rescue, these cases should always be given priority independent of the cost. When analyzed, however, nearly all highly effective treatments do well in the competition. Thus, under current analyses there is little evidence that any highly effective treatment would be denied coverage. Theoretically, effective but expensive treatments could be denied. In analyzing this possibility, we must recognize that resources are limited. Allocating funds for the one exotic case literally means denying services to many other people. Instead of letting one person die, we may let many people die.

When carefully analyzed, there is little evidence that the system discriminates against children. If anything, the system is biased toward children since saving a child produces many more years of benefit than saving an older adult. Further, completed analyses tend to show childhood intervention programs as very valuable (Berwick *et al.,* 1980). Similarly, it is assumed that programs for older adults will do poorly. Analyses show that some programs for the elderly do well and some do poorly. Pneumococcal vaccine for the elderly (Office of Technology Assessment, 1979) is among the most cost-effective interventions that has been analyzed. Rehabilitation programs for patients with chronic obstructive pulmonary disease (Toevs *et al.,* 1984) compete quite favorably with a variety of other medical and health care interventions. When analyzed carefully, this may be because treatments for older adults produce benefits in the near term. Since these individuals are often sick, treatment makes them better or at least slows their decline.

Perhaps most interestingly, the model helps identify interventions that people do not want. For example, heroic care at the end of life is very expensive and produces very few benefits. Even though treatment is ineffective, the rule of rescue argues that we must attempt to do everything possible. Recent evidence suggests that when patients are asked to sign an advance directive indicating whether or not they want futile care, very few are interested (Schneiderman et al., 1992). Patients want resources to be used for effective care. The model agrees with patient decisions to forego treatments that do not work.

Applications of a GHPM will continue to provoke ethical debates. We welcome the opportunity to participate in these discussions and we must emphasize the need to critically examine the implications of these methods. On the other hand, we must also recognize that our current health care system is ethically indefensible. It denies access for millions of people, it allows billions of dollars to change hands without high consumer satisfaction, and it allows logical inconsistencies in health care coverage. Presently, we see the ethical questions as challenging but not insurmountable.

WHERE DO WE GO FROM HERE?

This book has outlined a new paradigm for thinking about alternatives in health care. The proposed model is consistent with the thinking of several groups, including scholars in the U.S. (Weinstein & Stason, 1976; 1977; Office of Technology Assessment, 1979; Russell, 1986; 1987), the United Kingdom (Williams, 1988; Drummond et al., 1987; Maynard, 1991), Canada (Torrance, 1986) and Australia (Hall et al., 1992). Although the exact methodologies proposed by these different research groups vary slightly, the theory is nearly identical. Recently, Patrick & Erickson (1992) have detailed the methodological steps required to implement the system. Methods are now available to begin guiding policy decisions. However, our information base for the implementation of the model is still incomplete.

Three Needs for the Future: Data, Data, and More Data

This book has emphasized the crisis in contemporary health care. However, there is a second crisis—the crisis of ignorance. Our understanding of the effects of contemporary health care upon health outcomes is shameful. When new treatments are introduced we typically know something about the biological theory, the mechanism of action, and the effect of treatment upon some specific biologic outcome. However, the effects of treatment upon everyday functioning and quality of life are rarely evaluated. When the Oregon Health Services Commission began to prioritize health services, it recognized that there are no good information to help appraise the value of many current services. The U.S. Congress, in recognition of our ignorance about outcome, recently created the Agency for Health Care Policy and Research to focus on medical outcome studies. A recent emphasis on outcomes by the Food and Drug Administration has stimulated the measurement of health outcomes in the evaluation of pharmaceutical products. Further, the National Heart, Lung and Blood Institute now requires quality-of-life assessment in its clinical trials. Other NIH Institutes have also encouraged the measurement of health-related quality of life. New data are becoming available. Yet it may be several decades before we have enough information to apply the model with great confidence. Nevertheless, many steps toward the implementation of the model can be taken even while we await new information.

In the future, we will need at least three types of new data: information on the general population, outcome data, and cost data.

Health of the Population

With the failure of the current health care system, it is often argued that greater expenditures on health care in the U.S. have no effect upon common public health indicators. The indicator most commonly cited is infant mortality. Despite our higher expenditures on health care, it is not possible to demonstrate that the United States has a lower infant mortality rate than other westernized countries. The greater majority of services in health care have no effect on infant mortality. Any service for an individual older than 1 year of age is neglected by this indicator. The other indicator commonly cited is life expectancy. A substantial number of services have no effect on life expectancy. In effect, the value of investments in health care is being evaluated against incredibly crude measures. When the Department of Health and Human Services released the *Health Promotion Disease Prevention Objectives for the Nation, Year 2000,* it emphasized that the number one overall goal for the nation for the year 2000 was to increase the years of healthy life—a concept identical to well-years or quality-adjusted life years. Life expectancy in the United States was 73.7 years in 1980. It is estimated that about 11.7 years are lost to diseases and disabilities (see Fig. 8.1). Fries and colleagues (1989) argued that we may be reaching the point at which it is unlikely that we will be able to extend life expectancy. Once a human being reaches a certain age, he or she experiences multiple biological failures that are beyond remedy. However, Fries and colleagues have suggested that we may be able to make life better during these later years of life. These outcomes would be reflected in well-years of life but would not be captured with measures of life expectancy.

Because of the new interest in health-related quality of life, the National Center for Health Statistics is considering using the QWB scale (see Chapter Four) as part of the National Health Interview Survey. New data on well-years of life will greatly advance our understanding of the wellness of the population.

Outcome Data

As mentioned above, we know too little about the effects of medical care. Outcome data must be obtained from several sources. Ideally, the data will come from randomized clinical trials. However, as outlined in Chapter Four interim data can come from expert peer panels. In addition to outcome data, we need further information about preferences for various conditions and for health outcomes. Many of the analyses that are currently in the literature are based on weights from

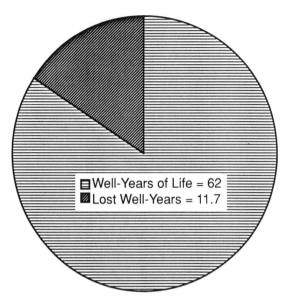

Figure 8.1 Life expectancy and well-life expectancy. From *Healthy People 2000.*

very small samples of subjects. For instance, a study of 867 individuals in San Diego, California, has been used in a variety of different analyses for people in different locations and from diverse social circumstances.

Cost Data

Finally, we need considerably more information on costs. Not only do we need to understand the variations in costs for procedures, but much more information is needed on the resources required to produce health outcomes. Currently, the resource base for most medical charges is poorly understood. The RBRVS system provides a start toward thinking about the resources required for physician services. Other resource-based costs are also required. The recent trend toward cost shifting in hospital charges makes cost accounting even more difficult.

CONCLUSIONS

The GHPM can contribute to the resolution of the current health care crisis. When properly applied, the model uses the best scientific information on costs, risks, and benefits of treatment. The model is directed toward using available resources to produce the greatest benefit for the largest number of people. Ethical challenges to the model are important but can be addressed. The greatest problem facing implementation of the model is lack of scientific data. We need considerably more research on the efficacy of clinical interventions. Until this information becomes available, we must recognize that the application of the model is an iterative process in which the best data available should be used. However, it is also important to recognize that we have limitations in our current understanding. Thus, evaluations must be continually modified as we learn more. Ultimately, policy science can contribute to the health and well-being of the population.

Oregon Prioritized Health Services*

A USER'S GUIDE FOR HEALTH SERVICES COMMISSION WORKING DOCUMENT

This appendix presents the current working document (List of Prioritized Health Services) of the Oregon Health Services Commission. The Commission voted on this document May 1, 1991 and all corrections have been made. Office of Medical Assistance Programs and the Health Services Commission have put together this "User's Guide" to explain some of the format of the working document, and to define some of the terms used.

What Are All Those Numbers?

The first thing you might notice is that most of what you are looking at is in numbers. That is because many people who work with the huge numbers of conditions and treatments that exist today use standard code numbers as a short-hand to describe the condition or treatment accurately. These standard codes are easy to use in a data base. There are two basic types of codes that you will see.

ICD-9 (International Classification of Diseases, 9th edition) are the codes used to describe the types of conditions or diseases which are to be treated. These codes are labeled as ICD-9 on the document and usually have the following format using numbers. (Example: 037.0 Tetanus)

CPT (Current Procedural Terminology, 4th edition.) These codes are used to accurately capture the exact procedure used to treat the condition. These are also expressed in number format and have 5 digits. Examples of CPT codes which you might see are 90050 (office visit), and 59400 (obstetrical care and delivery). On the other hand, CPT codes can be quite specific, for example 27754, (treatment of open tibial shaft fracture with uncomplicated soft tissue closure).

*Source: Oregon Health Services Commission, 1991.

The last set of numbers, you will notice, is the category number (e.g.: 15, 1, 16). Categories have been used by the Health Services Commission to organize the 700 plus condition/treatment pairs into manageable groups. The Commission applied values to the categories in order to rank them in order of most to least important. Additional values such as value to public health were applied to move the line items. You will notice, that many line items from the categories continue to be grouped together while others are scattered through the list, depending on the various additional considerations which Commissioners brought to bear in their final decision-making process. Categories are explained further below.

Why the Technical Language?

You will notice technical language in two places: condition descriptions and treatment descriptions.

Condition Descriptions: The technical descriptions that go with each line item have been simplified as much as possible without oversimplification. Sometimes there are ranges or families of diagnoses included (example: Fracture of shaft of bone, open). Sometimes conditions with similar symptoms, treatments and outcomes have been grouped together.

Treatment Descriptions: These descriptions have been consolidated as much as possible. The broad categories of medical treatment and surgical treatment include several types of interventions. These treatments are all treatments, rather than diagnostic visits, laboratory studies or other "Ancillary Services."

Categories

Each of the 700 plus condition/treatment pairs has been sorted first by the computer and then by the Commission into categories. The categories were developed in response to a need to organize the condition/treatment pairs into some kind of definable and manageable sized sub-lists. Many current methods of organization were unwieldy or required specialized medical knowledge.

The Commission used the categories to apply the public values. These were ranked from most important to least important and then the line items within them were ranked according to the quantitative data available as well as public values and Commissioner expertise.

You will notice that each line item includes a category number. We have enclosed a listing of the categories and their priority ranking so that you can understand roughly where each condition/treatment pair falls.

Why Do Many Services Appear More Than Once?

Each line in the document includes a diagnosis (ICD-9 code) and a procedure/ treatment (CPT-4 code). The same procedure/treatment is often provided for several diagnoses. For example, CPT-4 code 90050 stands for office visit, brief service; this is a very general sort of service which applies to many diagnoses.

Why Do Many Diagnoses Appear More Than Once?

A given diagnosis may be treatable with several treatment options. Each of these service options is listed, and the diagnosis appears in each listing.

Cost

The estimated per capita cost per month is shown at selected cut points. When these values are listed, they refer to the cost of all services on the list above the cut point.

PRIORITIZED HEALTH SERVICES LIST
OF MAY 1, 1991

Diagnosis: PNEUMOCOCCAL PNEU-
MONIA, OTHER BACTERIAL
PNEUMONIA, BRONCHO-
PNEUMONIA, INFLUENZA
WITH PNEUMONIA
Treatment: MEDICAL THERAPY
ICD-9: 020.3-.5,022.1,073,466,481-
483,485-486,487.1
CPT: 90000-99999
Line: 1   Category: 1

Diagnosis: TUBERCULOSIS
Treatment: MEDICAL THERAPY
ICD-9: 010-012
CPT: 90000-99999
Line: 2   Category: 5

Diagnosis: PERITONITIS
Treatment: MEDICAL AND SURGICAL
ICD-9: 567
CPT: 90000-99999
Line: 3   Category: 1

Diagnosis: FOREIGN BODY IN PHAR-
YNX, LARYNX, TRACHEA,
BRONCHUS & ESOPHAGUS
Treatment: REMOVAL OF FOREIGN
BODY
ICD-9: 933.0-.1,934.0-.1,935.1
CPT: 31635,40804
Line: 4   Category: 1

Diagnosis: APPENDICITIS
Treatment: APPENDECTOMY
ICD-9: 540-543
CPT: 44950,44900,44960
Line: 5   Category: 1

Diagnosis: RUPTURED INTESTINE
Treatment: REPAIR
ICD-9: 569.3
CPT: 44600-10
Line: 6   Category: 1

Diagnosis: HERNIA WITH OBSTRUCTION
AND/OR GANGRENE
Treatment: REPAIR
ICD-9: 550.0-.1,551-552
CPT: 39502-41,43330-31,43885,44050,
44346,49500-611,49000,51500,
55540
Line: 7   Category: 1

Diagnosis: CROUP SYNDROME, ACUTE
LARYNGOTRACHEITIS
Treatment: MEDICAL THERAPY, IN-
TUBATION, TRACHEOTOMY
ICD-9: 464.0-.4
CPT: 90000-99999,31500,31600
Line: 8   Category: 1

Diagnosis: ACUTE ORBITAL CELLULITIS
Treatment: MEDICAL THERAPY
ICD-9: 376.0

CPT: 90000-99999
Line: 9   Category: 1

Diagnosis: ECTOPIC PREGNANCY
Treatment: SURGERY
ICD-9: 633
CPT: 58700,58720,58770,58980,59135
Line: 10   Category: 1

Diagnosis: INJURY TO MAJOR BLOOD
VESSELS OF UPPER EX-
TREMITY
Treatment: LIGATION
ICD-9: 903
CPT: 37618
Line: 11   Category: 1

Diagnosis: RUPTURED SPLEEN
Treatment: REPAIR/SPLENECTOMY/
INCISION
ICD-9: 865.04
CPT: 38100,49000,38115
Line: 12   Category: 1

Diagnosis: ACUTE PELVIC INFLAM-
MATORY DISEASE
Treatment: MEDICAL AND SURGICAL
TREATMENT
ICD-9: 614.0,614.3,614.5,615.0
CPT: 11043,58150,58805,58925,58980,
90000-99999
Line: 13   Category: 1

Diagnosis: ACUTE PYELONEPHRITIS,
RENAL & PERINEPHRIC
ABSCESS
Treatment: MEDICAL AND SURGICAL
THERAPY
ICD-9: 590.1-.2
CPT: 50200,50220,90000-99999
Line: 14   Category: 1

Diagnosis: ANAPHYLACTIC SHOCK DUE
TO FOOD, DRUG OR OTHER
NON-VENOMOUS SOURCE
Treatment: MEDICAL THERAPY
ICD-9: 995.0,995.2
CPT: 90000-99999
Line: 15   Category: 1

Diagnosis: GALLSTONE WITH CHOLE-

CYSTITIS AND OTHER DIS-
ORDERS OF BILE DUCT
Treatment: CHOLECYSTECTOMY
ICD-9: 574.0-.1,574.3-.4,575.0-.5,576.1-.3
CPT: 47420-60,47480-90,47500-605,
49000
Line: 16   Category: 1

Diagnosis: RESPIRATORY OBSTRUC-
TION
Treatment: REPAIR OF CHOANAL
ATRESIA
ICD-9: 748.0
CPT: 30540
Line: 17   Category: 2

Diagnosis: SYPHILIS
Treatment: MEDICAL THERAPY
ICD-9: 090-097
CPT: 90000-99999
Line: 18   Category: 5

Diagnosis: HEMOLYTIC DISEASE DUE
TO ISOIMMUNIZATION,
LATE ANEMIA DUE TO ISO-
IMMUNIZATION, AND FETAL
AND NEONATAL JAUNDICE
Treatment: MEDICAL THERAPY
ICD-9: 773.0-.2,773.4-.5,774.0-.4,774.6-.7
CPT: 900000-99999
Line: 19   Category: 2

Diagnosis: POLYCYTHEMIA NEONA-
TORUM, SYMPTOMATIC
Treatment: MEDICAL THERAPY
ICD-9: 776.4
CPT: 36450,90000-99999
Line: 20   Category: 2

Diagnosis: PREGNANCY
Treatment: OBSTETRICAL CARE
ICD-9: 622.5,640-676,760-763,766,768,
772.0,772.3-.4,776.5,V22-V28,
V30-V39
CPT: 59000-59899,57700,90000-99999
Line: 21   Category: 2

Diagnosis: LOW BIRTH WEIGHT (500 GM
AND OVER)
Treatment: MEDICAL THERAPY
ICD-9: 765.12-.19,769,778.1

CPT: 90000-99999
Line: 22   Category: 2

Diagnosis: SYNDROME OF "INFANT OF
A DIABETIC MOTHER" AND
NEONATAL HYPOGLYCEMIA
Treatment: MEDICAL THERAPY
ICD-9: 775.0,775.6
CPT: 36510,36660,90000-99999
Line: 23   Category: 2

Diagnosis: OMPHALITIS OF THE NEW-
BORN AND NEONATAL
INFECTIVE MASTITIS
Treatment: MEDICAL THERAPY
ICD-9: 771.4-.5
CPT: 90000-99999
Line: 24   Category: 2

Diagnosis: GALACTOSEMIA
Treatment: MEDICAL THERAPY
ICD-9: 271.1,774.5
CPT: 90000-99999
Line: 25   Category: 2

Diagnosis: HYPOGLYCEMIC COMA;
HYPOGLYCEMIA
Treatment: MEDICAL THERAPY
ICD-9: 251.0-251.2
CPT: 90000-99999
Line: 26   Category: 3

Diagnosis: WHOOPING COUGH
Treatment: MEDICAL THERAPY
ICD-9: 032-033
CPT: 90000-99999
Line: 27   Category: 1

Diagnosis: PHENYLKETONURIA (PKU)
Treatment: MEDICAL THERAPY
ICD-9: 270.1
CPT: 90000-99999
Line: 28   Category: 4

Diagnosis: CONGENITAL
HYPOTHYROIDISM
Treatment: MEDICAL THERAPY
ICD-9: 243
CPT: 90000-99999
Line: 29   Category: 4

Diagnosis: ACUTE OSTEOMYELITIS
Treatment: MEDICAL AND SURGICAL
TREATMENT
ICD-9: 730.0
CPT: 90000-99999
Line: 30   Category: 1

Diagnosis: DEEP OPEN WOUND OF
NECK, INCLUDING LARYNX;
FRACTURE OF LARYNX OR
TRACHEA, OPEN
Treatment: REPAIR
ICD-9: 874,807.6
CPT: 12001-12007,13101,13131-50
Line: 31   Category: 1

Diagnosis: DISEASES OF PHARYNX IN-
CLUDING RETROPHARYN-
GEAL ABSCESS
Treatment: MEDICAL AND SURGICAL
TREATMENT
ICD-9: 478.21-.22,478.24
CPT: 42700-42999,90000-99999
Line: 32   Category: 1

Diagnosis: PNEUMOTHORAX AND
HEMOTHORAX
Treatment: TUBE THORACOSTOMY/
THORACOTOMY, MEDICAL
THERAPY
ICD-9: 512,860.2
CPT: 90000-99999,32020,32100,32500
Line: 33   Category: 1

Diagnosis: HYPOTENSION
Treatment: MEDICAL THERAPY
ICD-9: 458
CPT: 90000-99999
Line: 34   Category: 1

Diagnosis: FRACTURE OF SHAFT OF
BONE, OPEN
Treatment: REDUCTION
ICD-9: 812.3,813.3,813.9,818.1,
821.1.,823.3,823.9
CPT: 24500-15,25500-25575, 25610-
25620, 27500-06,27750-58,
27800-06
Line: 35   Category: 1

Diagnosis: PERIPHERAL NERVE INJURY

Treatment: NEUROPLASTY
ICD-9: 953.4-.9,955-956,957.9
CPT: 64413-50,64830,64787,64732-92,
64716-21,64830-76,64702-27
Line: 36 Category: 12

Diagnosis: PYOGENIC ARTHRITIS
Treatment: MEDICAL AND SURGICAL
TREATMENT
ICD-9: 711
CPT: 24000,25040,26070-80,27030,
27310,27610,29843,29871-72,
29894,90000-99999
Line: 37 Category: 1

Diagnosis: INTESTINAL OBSTRUCTION
W/O MENTION OF HERNIA
Treatment: EXCISION
ICD-9: 560.0,560.2,560.8-.9
CPT: 44005,44020,44050,44110-30,
44140-44
Line: 38 Category: 1

Diagnosis: PATENT DUCTUS ARTERI-
OSUS
Treatment: LIGATION
ICD-9: 747.0
CPT: 33820-22
Line: 39 Category: 2

Diagnosis: HEMATOLOGICAL DIS-
ORDERS OF FETUS AND
NEWBORN
Treatment: MEDICAL THERAPY
ICD-9: 776.0-.1,776.3
CPT: 90000-99999
Line: 40 Category: 2

Diagnosis: CONDITIONS INVOLVING
THE TEMPERATURE REGU-
LATION OF NEWBORNS
Treatment: MEDICAL THERAPY
ICD-9: 778.2-.4
CPT: 90000-99999
Line: 41 Category: 2

Diagnosis: BIRTH TRAUMA FOR BABY
Treatment: MEDICAL THERAPY
ICD-9: 767
CPT: 90000-99999
Line: 42 Category: 2
Diagnosis: HYPOCALCEMIA, HYPO-

MAGNESEMIA AND OTHER
ENDOCRINE AND META-
BOLIC DISTURBANCES SPE-
CIFIC TO THE FETUS AND
NEWBORN
Treatment: MEDICAL THERAPY
ICD-9: 775.4-.5,775.7-.9
CPT: 36510,36660,90000-99999
Line: 43 Category: 2

Diagnosis: PERINATAL DISORDERS OF
DIGESTIVE SYSTEM
Treatment: MEDICAL THERAPY
ICD-9: 777.1-.4
CPT: 90000-99999
Line: 44 Category: 2

Diagnosis: ANEMIA OF PREMATURITY
OR TRANSIENT NEONATAL
NEUTROPENIA
Treatment: MEDICAL THERAPY
ICD-9: 776.6-.9
CPT: 90000-99999
Line: 45 Category: 2

Diagnosis: HYDROPS FETALIS
Treatment: MEDICAL THERAPY
ICD-9: 778.0,773.3
CPT: 90000-99999
Line: 46 Category: 2

Diagnosis: ACUTE BACTERIAL MEN-
INGITIS
Treatment: MEDICAL THERAPY
ICD-9: 024,027.0,036,320
CPT: 90000-99999
Line: 47 Category: 3

Diagnosis: HYPOTHERMIA
Treatment: MEDICAL THERAPY
ICD-9: 991.6
CPT: 90000-99999
Line: 48 Category: 3

Diagnosis: BURN, PARTIAL THICKNESS
WITHOUT VITAL SITE,
10-30% OF BODY SURFACE
Treatment: FREE SKIN GRAFT, MEDICAL
THERAPY
ICD-9: 941.26-.27,.36-.37,942.20-.24,
.29-.34,.39,943.2-.3,944.20-.24,

.26-.34,.36-.38,945.20-.21,.23-.31,
.33-.39,946.2-.3,948,949.2-.3
CPT: 11000,11040-1,11960-70,14020,
14040-1,15000-15121, 15200,
15220,15240,15260,15350,15400,
15500-10,16000-16035,35206,
90000-99999
Line: 49   Category: 3

Diagnosis: ACUTE MYOCARDIAL
INFARCTION
Treatment: MEDICAL THERAPY
ICD-9: 410
CPT: 90000-99999
Line: 50   Category: 3

Diagnosis: ACUTE PULMONARY HEART
DISEASE AND PULMONARY
EMBOLI
Treatment: MEDICAL THERAPY
ICD-9: 415
CPT: 90000-99999
Line: 51   Category: 3

Diagnosis: THYROTOXICOSIS WITH OR
WITHOUT GOITER, ENDO-
CRINE EXOPHTHALMOS;
CHRONIC THYRODITIS
Treatment: MEDICAL AND SURGICAL
TREATMENT
ICD-9: 242,245.1-.9,246.8,376.2
CPT: 60245,67440,67599-67622,
90000-99999
Line: 52   Category: 5

Diagnosis: LIFE-THREATENING
ARRHYTHMIAS
Treatment: MEDICAL AND SURGICAL
TREATMENT
ICD-9: 427.1,427.4-.5,746.86,996.01
CPT: 33200-33208,33212,33820,
90000-99999
Line: 53   Category: 3

Diagnosis: FRACTURE OF RIBS AND
STERNUM, OPEN
Treatment: STABILIZE
ICD-9: 807.1,807.3
CPT: 21805,21810,21825
Line: 54   Category: 1

Diagnosis: FATAL RICKETTSIAL AND
OTHER ARTHROPOD-BORNE
DISEASES
Treatment: MEDICAL THERAPY
ICD-9: 080-083,085.0,085.5,085.9
CPT: 90000-99999
Line: 55   Category: 1

Diagnosis: POISONING BY INGESTION
AND INJECTION
Treatment: MEDICAL THERAPY
ICD-9: 960.2-.5,961.0,.3-.9,962.0,.2-.8,
963.0,.2-.9,964.5,.7-.8,965.5-.7,
966,968.0,968.5-.7,969.6,970.1,
971.0-.2,972.3,972.6,972.8,
974.0-.4,974.7,975.0-.1,975.7,
977.0, 978-985
CPT: 43235-47,90000-99999
Line: 56   Category: 1

Diagnosis: PERITONSILLAR ABSCESS
Treatment: INCISION AND DRAINAGE OF
ABSCESS, MEDICAL TREAT-
MENT
ICD-9: 475
CPT: 10160,42700,90000-99999
Line: 57   Category: 1

Diagnosis: RUPTURE BLADDER, NON-
TRAUMATIC
Treatment: CYSTORRHAPHY SUTURE
ICD-9: 596.6
CPT: 51860-51865
Line: 58   Category: 1

Diagnosis: FRACTURE OF FACE BONES
Treatment: SURGERY
ICD-9: 802
CPT: 21310-37,21454-5,21461,21462,
21360,21365,21385-6,21406,
21421-22,21470,30140,30520,
30620,31021
Line: 59   Category: 1

Diagnosis: LIFE-THREATENING
EPISTAXIS
Treatment: SEPTOPLASTY/REPAIR/
CONTROL HEMORRHAGE
ICD-9: 784.7
CPT: 30520-30999
Line: 60   Category: 1

Diagnosis: ACUTE MASTOIDITIS
Treatment: MASTOIDECTOMY, MEDICAL
THERAPY
ICD-9: 383.0
CPT: 69601-46,69670,90000-99999
Line: 61   Category: 1

Diagnosis: ACQUIRED DEFORMITY OF
HEAD AND COMPOUND/
DEPRESSED FRACTURES OF
SKULL
Treatment: CRANIOTOMY/
CRANIECTOMY
ICD-9: 738.01-.1,800,803,804
CPT: 21365,21395,61304-576,62000
Line: 62   Category: 1

Diagnosis: DISLOCATION OF ELBOW,
HAND, ANKLE, FOOT, CLAV-
ICLE AND SHOULDER, OPEN
Treatment: RELOCATION
ICD-9: 831.04,831.1,832.1,
833.1,837.1,838.1
CPT: 23520-52,23650-80,24600-35,
25660-95,26641-715,27840-48
Line: 63   Category: 1

Diagnosis: SEPTICEMIA
Treatment: MEDICAL THERAPY
ICD-9: 002,003.1,004.9,020.0-.2,020.8-.9,
021,022.3,024,027,036.2,038,
054.5,098.89,771.8,998.5,999.3
CPT: 90000-99999
Line: 64   Category: 1

Diagnosis: ERYSIPELAS
Treatment: MEDICAL THERAPY
ICD-9: 035
CPT: 90000-99999
Line: 65   Category: 1

Diagnosis: STEVENS-JOHNSON
SYNDROME
Treatment: MEDICAL THERAPY
ICD-9: 695.1
CPT: 90000-99999,11100-11101
Line: 66   Category: 1

Diagnosis: DISORDERS OF BILE DUCT
Treatment: EXCISION, REPAIR
ICD-9: 576.4-.9

CPT: 47420-60,47500-999
Line: 67   Category: 1

Diagnosis: RUPTURE LIVER
Treatment: SUTURE/REPAIR
ICD-9: 864.04
CPT: 47350,47360
Line: 68   Category: 1

Diagnosis: RESPIRATORY FAILURE
Treatment: MEDICAL THERAPY
ICD-9: 518.81
CPT: 31600,90000-99999
Line: 69   Category: 1

Diagnosis: LUNG CONTUSION OR
LACERATION
Treatment: MEDICAL THERAPY
ICD-9: 861.21,861.31
CPT: 90000-99999
Line: 70   Category: 1

Diagnosis: TRANSPLACENTAL
HEMORRHAGE
Treatment: MEDICAL THERAPY
ICD-9: 772.0,772.3-.4,776.5
CPT: 90000-99999
Line: 71   Category: 2

Diagnosis: NEONATAL THYROTOXICO-
SIS
Treatment: MEDICAL THERAPY
ICD-9: 775.3
CPT: 90000-99999
Line: 72   Category: 2

Diagnosis: DRUG REACTIONS &
INTOXICATIONS SPECIFIC
TO NEWBORN
Treatment: MEDICAL THERAPY
ICD-9: 779.4
CPT: 90000-99999
Line: 73   Category: 2

Diagnosis: NEONATAL MYASTHENIA
GRAVIS
Treatment: MEDICAL THERAPY
ICD-9: 775.2
CPT: 90000-99999
Line: 74   Category: 2

Diagnosis: CLEFT PALATE WITH AIR-
WAY OBSTRUCTION, PIERRE
ROBIN DEFORMITY
Treatment: LIP-TONGUE SUTURE, MED-
ICAL THERAPY
ICD-9: 749.0,519.8
CPT: 30140,30520,30620,41510,
90000-99999
Line: 75   Category: 2

Diagnosis: DRUG WITHDRAWAL SYN-
DROME IN NEWBORN
Treatment: MEDICAL THERAPY
ICD-9: 779.5
CPT: 90000-99999
Line: 76   Category: 2

Diagnosis: TOXIC EFFECT OF GASES,
FUMES, AND VAPORS RE-
QUIRING HYPERBARIC
OXYGEN
Treatment: HYPERBARIC OXYGEN
ICD-9: 986-987
CPT: 99180-99182
Line: 77   Category: 3

Diagnosis: PHLEBITIS & THROMBO-
PHLEBITIS, DEEP
Treatment: LIGATION AND DIVISION,
MEDICAL THERAPY
ICD-9: 451.0-.2,451.8
CPT: 11042,37720,37721,37735,37785,
90000-99999
Line: 78   Category: 3

Diagnosis: DISLOCATION KNEE & HIP,
OPEN
Treatment: RELOCATION
ICD-9: 835.1,836.4,836.6
CPT: 27250-55,27550-27557
Line: 79   Category: 3

Diagnosis: EMPYEMA AND ABSCESS OF
LUNG
Treatment: MEDICAL AND SURGICAL
TREATMENT
ICD-9: 510,513.0
CPT: 90000-99999,31622,32000-32100
Line: 80   Category: 3

Diagnosis: CERVICAL VERTEBRAL
DISLOCATIONS, OPEN
OR CLOSED; OTHER
VERTEBRAL DISLOCATIONS,
OPEN
Treatment: REPAIR/RECONSTRUCTION
ICD-9: 839.0-.1,839.3,839.5,839.7
CPT: 22315,22325-22327,22505,
22590-22650,22840-22855
Line: 81   Category: 3

Diagnosis: OPEN FRACTURE OF
EPIPHYSIS OF LOWER
EXTREMITIES
Treatment: REDUCTION
ICD-9: 820.11,821.32
CPT: 27516-27519
Line: 82   Category: 3

Diagnosis: SPINAL CORD INJURY WITH-
OUT EVIDENCE OF VERTE-
BRAL INJURY
Treatment: MEDICAL THERAPY
ICD-9: 952
CPT: 90000-99999
Line: 83   Category: 3

Diagnosis: ASPIRATION PNEUMONIA
Treatment: MEDICAL THERAPY
ICD-9: 507
CPT: 90000-99999,31645,31500
Line: 84   Category: 3

Diagnosis: ACUTE INFLAMMATION OF
THE HEART DUE TO
RHEUMATIC FEVER
Treatment: MEDICAL THERAPY
ICD-9: 391,392.0
CPT: 90000-99999
Line: 85   Category: 3

Diagnosis: FRACTURE AND OTHER
INJURY OF CERVICAL
VERTEBRA
Treatment: CERVICAL LAMINECTOMY,
MEDICAL THERAPY
ICD-9: 806.0-806.1,805.0-805.1,952.0
CPT: 22315,22326,22845,63250,63265,
63270,63275,63280,63285,63001,
63015,63020,63035-40,63045,
63048,63075-76,63081-82,63300,

63196,63198,90000-99999
Line: 86   Category: 3

Diagnosis: FRACTURE OF HIP, CLOSED
Treatment: REDUCTION
ICD-9: 820.00,820.02-.09,820.2,820.8
CPT: 27230-27232,27235-27240,
27242-27248
Line: 87   Category: 3

Diagnosis: SUBARACHNOID AND
INTERCEREBRAL HEMOR-
RHAGE/HEMATOMA
Treatment: BURR HOLES, CRANI-
ECTOMY/CRANIOTOMY
ICD-9: 430-432,852-853
CPT: 22640,61120-61151,61154,61210,
61304,61314-61315,61522-61712,
62223
Line: 88   Category: 3

Diagnosis: ACUTE PANCREATITIS
Treatment: MEDICAL THERAPY
ICD-9: 577.0
CPT: 90000-99999
Line: 89   Category: 3

Diagnosis: HYDATIDIFORM MOLE
Treatment: D & C, HYSTERECTOMY
ICD-9: 630
CPT: 58120,58150-200
Line: 90   Category: 1

Diagnosis: THROMBOCYTOPENIA
Treatment: MEDICAL THERAPY
ICD-9: 287
CPT: 90000-99999
Line: 91   Category: 1

Diagnosis: TOXIC EFFECT OF VENOM
Treatment: MEDICAL THERAPY
ICD-9: 989.5
CPT: 90000-99999
Line: 92   Category: 1

Diagnosis: CANCRUM ORIS
Treatment: MEDICAL THERAPY
ICD-9: 528.1
CPT: 90000-99999
Line: 93   Category: 1

Diagnosis: CANDIDIASIS OF LUNG, DIS-
SEMINATED CANDIDIASIS,
CANDIDAL ENDOCARDITIS
AND MENINGITIS
Treatment: MEDICAL THERAPY
ICD-9: 112.4-.5,112.81,112.83
CPT: 90000-99999
Line: 94   Category: 1

Diagnosis: MYOCARDITIS, PERICAR-
DITIS AND ENDOCARDITIS
Treatment: MEDICAL THERAPY
ICD-9: 420-423
CPT: 90000-99999
Line: 95   Category: 1

Diagnosis: RUPTURE OF ESOPHAGUS
Treatment: SURGERY
ICD-9: 530.4
CPT: 43100-01,43110-43235,43330-31
Line: 96   Category: 1

Diagnosis: TOXIC EPIDERMAL NE-
CROLYSIS AND STAPHYLO-
COCCAL SCALDED SKIN
SYNDROME
Treatment: MEDICAL THERAPY
ICD-9: 695.1
CPT: 90000-99999,11100-11101
Line: 97   Category: 1

Diagnosis: CHOLERA, RAT-BITE FEVER
AND TOXIC EFFECTS OF
MUSHROOMS, FISH,
BERRIES, ETC.
Treatment: MEDICAL THERAPY
ICD-9: 001,026,988
CPT: 90000-99999
Line: 98   Category: 1

Diagnosis: DELIRIUM: AMPHETAMINE,
COCAINE, OR OTHER
PSYCHOACTIVE SUBSTANCE
Treatment: MEDICAL THERAPY
ICD-9: 292.81,293.00
CPT: 90220
Line: 99   Category: 1

Diagnosis: INJURY TO BLOOD VESSELS
OF THE THORACIC CAVITY
Treatment: REPAIR

ICD-9: 901
CPT: 37616
Line: 100   Category: 1

Diagnosis: NECROTIZING ENTERO-
COLITIS IN FETUS OR NEW-
BORN AND PERINATAL
INTESTINAL PERFORATION
Treatment: MEDICAL AND SURGICAL
TREATMENT
ICD-9: 777.5-.6
CPT: 36510,36660,90000-99999
Line: 101   Category: 2

Diagnosis: DISSEMINATED INTRA-
VASCULAR COAGULATION
Treatment: MEDICAL THERAPY
ICD-9: 286.6,776.2
CPT: 90000-99999
Line: 102   Category: 2

Diagnosis: CEREBRAL DEPRESSION,
COMA, & OTHER ABNOR-
MAL CEREBRAL SIGNS OF
NEWBORN
Treatment: MEDICAL THERAPY
ICD-9: 779.2
CPT: 36510,36660,90000-99999
Line: 103   Category: 2

Diagnosis: TORSION OF OVARY
Treatment: OOPHORECTOMY, OVARIAN
CYSTECTOMY
ICD-9: 620.5
CPT: 58925,58940-43,59120-26
Line: 104   Category: 1

Diagnosis: SPONTANEOUS ABORTION
COMPLICATED BY INFEC-
TION AND/OR HEMORRHAGE
Treatment: MEDICAL AND SURGICAL
TREATMENT
ICD-9: 634.0-.1
CPT: 59820-21,90000-99999
Line: 105   Category: 1

Diagnosis: OTHER RESPIRATORY CON-
DITIONS OF FETUS AND
NEWBORN
Treatment: MEDICAL THERAPY
ICD-9: 770.0-.6,770.8-.9

CPT: 90000-99999
Line: 106   Category: 2

Diagnosis: OTHER NONINFECTIOUS
GASTROENTERITIS AND
COLITIS
Treatment: MEDICAL THERAPY
ICD-9: 558
CPT: 90000-99999
Line: 107   Category: 3

Diagnosis: UNSPECIFIED DISEASES DUE
TO MYCOBACTERIA, ACTI-
NOMYCOTIC INFECTIONS,
AND TOXOPLASMOSIS
Treatment: MEDICAL THERAPY
ICD-9: 031.9,039,130
CPT: 90000-99999
Line: 108   Category: 3

Diagnosis: BOTULISM
Treatment: MEDICAL THERAPY
ICD-9: 005.1
CPT: 90000-99999
Line: 109   Category: 3

Diagnosis: FRACTURE OF JOINT, OPEN
Treatment: REDUCTION
ICD-9: 810.1,811.1,812.1,812.5,813.1,
813.5,820.10,820.12-.19,820.3,
820.9,821.30-.31,831.33-39,822.1,
823.1,824.1,.3,.5,.7,.9,825.1,.3,
826.1,828.1,814.1,815.1,816.1,
817.1,819.1
CPT: 23500-15,23570-630,24530-88,
24650-85,25600-50,26600-15,
26720-85,27230-48,27409,27420,
27508-14,27520-40,27610,
27764-66,27780-92,27806,23,
27846-8,28400-530,28730,29874-
9
Line: 110   Category: 3

Diagnosis: ABSCESS OF INTESTINE
Treatment: DRAIN ABSCESS, MEDICAL
THERAPY
ICD-9: 569.5
CPT: 90000-99999,45355,45386,
45310-45315
Line: 111   Category: 3

Diagnosis: ADULT RESPIRATORY DIS-
TRESS SYNDROME
Treatment: MEDICAL THERAPY
ICD-9: 518.4-.5
CPT: 90000-99999
Line: 112   Category: 3

Diagnosis: HERPETIC ENCEPHALITIS
Treatment: MEDICAL THERAPY
ICD-9: 054.3
CPT: 90000-99999
Line: 113   Category: 3

Diagnosis: ARTHROPOD-BORNE VIRAL
DISEASES
Treatment: MEDICAL THERAPY
ICD-9: 060-066
CPT: 90000-99999
Line: 114   Category: 3

Diagnosis: BURN, PARTIAL THICKNESS
WITH VITAL SITE; FULL
THICKNESS WITH VITAL
SITE, LESS THAN 10% OF
BODY SURFACE
Treatment: FREE SKIN GRAFT, MEDICAL
THERAPY
ICD-9: 941.20-.25,.28-.35,.38-.39,942.25,
.35,944.25,.35,945.22,.32,946.2-.3,
948,949.2-.3
CPT: 11000,11040-2,11970,14020,
14040-1,15000-15121,15200,
15220,15240,15260,15350,
15500-10,15400-10,15505,15770,
16000-16035,35206,90000-99999
Line: 115   Category: 3

Diagnosis: FRACTURE OF PELVIS, OPEN
AND CLOSED
Treatment: REDUCTION
ICD-9: 808
CPT: 27033,27210-27225
Line: 116   Category: 3

Diagnosis: BURN FULL THICKNESS
GREATER THAN 10% OF
BODY SURFACE
Treatment: FREE SKIN GRAFT, MEDICAL
THERAPY
ICD-9: 940,941.30.-35,941.4-.5,942.35,
.4-.5,943.4-.5,944.35,.4-.5,945.32,

.4-.5,946.3-.5,947,948.11-.19,.
21-29,.31-.39,.41-.49,.51-.59,
.61-.69,.71-.79,.81-.89,
.91-.99.949.4-.5
CPT: 11000,11040-1,11960-70,14020,
14040-1,15000-15121,15200,
15220,15240,15260,15350,15400,
15500-10,15770,16000-16035,
20550,35206,90000-99999
Line: 117   Category: 3

Diagnosis: SUBACUTE MENINGITIS (EG.
TUBERCULOSIS, CRYPTO-
COCCOSIS)
Treatment: MEDICAL THERAPY
ICD-9: 013,054.72,117.5,117.9,123.1,
130.8,321-322
CPT: 90000-99999
Line: 118   Category: 3

Diagnosis: CRUSH INJURIES: TRUNK,
UPPER LIMBS, LOWER LIMB
INCLUDING BLOOD VESSELS
Treatment: SURGICAL TX
ICD-9: 900,902,926.11-.12,927.03,
927.2-.9,927.10,928,925,927.00,
927.01
CPT: 15220,24495,25020,27600-27602,
29105-29131,29240-29280,
29345-29440,29520-29580,
37615-18
Line: 119   Category: 3

Diagnosis: ACUTE GLOMERULONEPHRI-
TIS AND OTHER ACUTE RE-
NAL FAILURE
Treatment: MEDICAL THERAPY INCLUD-
ING DIALYSIS
ICD-9: 580.0,580.8-.9,584
CPT: 90000-99999
Line: 120   Category: 3

Diagnosis: ACCIDENTS INVOLVING EX-
POSURE TO NATURAL ELE-
MENTS (EG. LIGHTNING
STRIKE, HEATSTROKE)
Treatment: MEDICAL THERAPY
ICD-9: 991.0-.5,992.0,993.2,994.0-.1,
994.4-.9
CPT: 90000-99999
Line: 121   Category: 1

Diagnosis: DISSECTING OR RUPTURED
ANEURYSM
Treatment: SURGICAL TREATMENT
ICD-9: 441.0-.1,441.3,441.5
CPT: 33860-77,35081-103,35301-11,
35331-51,35450-515,35526-31,
35536-52,35560-63,35601-16,
35626-46,35651,35663
Line: 122   Category: 1

Diagnosis: ARTERIAL EMBOLISM/
THROMBOSIS: ABDOMINAL
AORTA, THORACIC AORTA
Treatment: SURGICAL TREATMENT
ICD-9: 444.0-.1,.8
CPT: 34101,34201,35081,35363,35381,
35536-51
Line: 123   Category: 3

Diagnosis: CONGENITAL ANOMALIES
OF DIGESTIVE SYSTEM EX-
CLUDING NECROSIS
Treatment: MEDICAL AND SURGICAL
THERAPY
ICD-9: 751
CPT: 44050,45100,45120-21,46070,
46080
Line: 124   Category: 2

Diagnosis: CONVULSIONS AND OTHER
CEREBRAL IRRITABILITY IN
NEWBORN
Treatment: MEDICAL THERAPY
ICD-9: 779.0-.1
CPT: 90000-99999
Line: 125   Category: 2

Diagnosis: ACUTE NECROSIS OF LIVER
Treatment: MEDICAL THERAPY
ICD-9: 570
CPT: 90000-99999
Line: 126   Category: 3

Diagnosis: COCCIDIOIDOMYCOSIS,
HISTOPLASMOSIS, BLASTO-
MYCOTIC INFECTION,
OPPORTUNISTIC AND OTHER
MYCOSES
Treatment: MEDICAL THERAPY
ICD-9: 114-118
CPT: 90000-99999

Line: 127   Category: 3

Diagnosis: INTRASPINAL AND
INTRACRANIAL ABSCESS
Treatment: MEDICAL AND SURGICAL
TREATMENT
ICD-9: 324
CPT: 63127-63173,63266-63273,
90000-99999
Line: 128   Category: 3

Diagnosis: ANEURYSM OF PULMONARY
ARTERY
Treatment: SURGICAL TREATMENT
ICD-9: 417.1
CPT: 33910-33915
Line: 129   Category: 3

Diagnosis: FLAIL CHEST
Treatment: MEDICAL AND SURGICAL
TREATMENT
ICD-9: 807.4
CPT: 21800-25,90000-99999
Line: 130   Category: 3

Diagnosis: SEVERE HEAD INJURY:
HEMATOMA/EDEMA W/
MODERATE/PROLONGED
LOSS OF CONSCIOUSNESS
Treatment: SURGICAL TREATMENT
ICD-9: 851.03,851.13,851.83,851.93,
851.43,851.53
CPT: 61108,61314-14,62140-41
Line: 131   Category: 3

Diagnosis: RUPTURE OF PAPILLARY
MUSCLE
Treatment: MEDICAL AND SURGICAL
TREATMENT
ICD-9: 529.5-.6
CPT: 33542,90000-99999
Line: 132   Category: 3

Diagnosis: ANAEROBIC INFECTIONS
REQUIRING HYPERBARIC
OXYGEN
Treatment: HYPERBARIC OXYGEN
ICD-9: 611.3,639.0,639.6,670.2670.4,
673.0,709.3,729.4,785.4,958.0,
996.52,996.6-.7,998.8,999.1
CPT: 99180-99182

Line: 133   Category: 3

Diagnosis: TRAUMATIC AMPUTATION
OF ARM(S) & HAND(S)
(COMPLETE)(PARTIAL) W &
W/O COMPLICATION
Treatment: REPLANTATION/AMPUTATE
ICD-9: 887.0-.3,887.5-.7
CPT: 20802,20804,20805,20806,23900,
23920,23921,24900,24920,24920,
24925,24930,24931,24935,24940,
25900-9
Line: 134   Category: 3

Diagnosis: ACUTE VASCULAR
INSUFFICIENCY OF
INTESTINE
Treatment: COLECTOMY
ICD-9: 557.0
CPT: 44140,44120-25,44141,44143,
34151,34421,34451
Line: 135   Category: 3

Diagnosis: BURN, PARTIAL THICKNESS
GREATER THAN 30% OF
BODY SURFACE
Treatment: FREE SKIN GRAFT, MEDICAL
THERAPY
ICD-9: 941.26-.27,942.20-.24,.29,943.2,
944.20-.24,.26-.28,945.20-.21,.
23-.29,946.2,948.30,.40,.50,.60,
.70,.80,.90,949.2
CPT: 11000,11040-1,11960-70,14020,
14040-1,15000-15121,15200,
15220,15240,15260,15350,15400,
15500-10,15770,90200,
16000-16035,35206,
90000-99999
Line: 136   Category: 3

Diagnosis: ACUTE GLOMERULONE-
PHRITIS: WITH LESION OF
RAPIDLY PROGRESSIVE
GLOMERULONEPHRITIS
Treatment: MEDICAL THERAPY INCLUD-
ING DIALYSIS
ICD-9: 580.4
CPT: 90000-99999
Line: 137   Category: 3

Diagnosis: IRON DEFICIENCY ANEMIA
AND OTHER NUTRITIONAL
DEFICIENCIES
Treatment: MEDICAL THERAPY
ICD-9: 260-268,269.0-.3,280
CPT: 90000-99999
Line: 138   Category: 5

Diagnosis: TETANUS NEONATORUM
Treatment: MEDICAL THERAPY
ICD-9: 771.3
CPT: 90000-99999
Line: 139   Category: 2

Diagnosis: TRAUMATIC AMPUTATION
OF LEG(S) (COMPLETE) (PAR-
TIAL) W/ & W/O COMPLICA-
TION
Treatment: REPLANTATION/AMPUTATE
ICD-9: 897.0-.3,897.6-.7
CPT: 20832,20834,27290-27598,
27880-27889,27880-84,27886-89
Line: 140   Category: 3

Diagnosis: TRAUMATIC AMPUTATION
OF FOOT/FEET (COMPLETE)
(PARTIAL) W/ & W/O COM-
PLICATION
Treatment: REPLANTATION/AMPUTATE
ICD-9: 896,897.6-.7
CPT: 20838,20840,27888,28800-28805
Line: 141   Category: 3

Diagnosis: ALCOHOL WITHDRAWAL
DELIRIUM: ALCOHOL
HALLUCINOSIS; UNCOM-
PLICATED ALCOHOL WITH-
DRAWAL; WITHDRAWAL
FROM AMPHETAMINES, CO-
CAINE, OPIOID, SEDATIVES,
HYPNOTICS, ETC.
Treatment: MEDICAL THERAPY
ICD-9: 291.00,291.30,291.80
CPT: 90220,90844
Line: 142   Category: 1

Diagnosis: PREVENTIVE SERVICES,
CHILDREN
Treatment: MEDICAL THERAPY
ICD-9: V01-V06,V20-V21,V40-V41,
V60-V62.3-.4,V70.0,V77,V79
CPT: 90000-99999

Line: 143   Category: 4

Diagnosis: STREPTOCOCCAL SORE
THROAT AND SCARLET
FEVER
Treatment: MEDICAL THERAPY
ICD-9: 034
CPT: 90000-99999
Line: 144   Category: 10

Diagnosis: RHEUMATIC FEVER
Treatment: MEDICAL THERAPY
ICD-9: 390
CPT: 90000-99999
Line: 145   Category: 10

Diagnosis: CONGENITAL ANOMALIES
OF UPPER ALIMENTARY
TRACT, EXCLUDING TONGUE
Treatment: MEDICAL AND SURGICAL
THERAPY
ICD-9: 750.2-.9
CPT: 43300-52,90000-99999
Line: 146   Category: 2
HYPERTENSION AND HYPER-
Diagnosis: TENSIVE DISEASE
Treatment: MEDICAL THERAPY
ICD-9: 401,402.01
CPT: 90000-99999
Line: 147   Category: 5

Diagnosis: HYPERTENSIVE HEART AND
RENAL DISEASE
Treatment: MEDICAL THERAPY
ICD-9: 404
CPT: 90000-99999
Line: 148   Category: 5

Diagnosis: ACUTE AND SUBACUTE
ISCHEMIC HEART DISEASE
Treatment: SURGICAL TREATMENT
ICD-9: 411.1,996.03
CPT: 92950-93799,33510-
16,33210,33570
Line: 149   Category: 3

Diagnosis: DIABETES MELLITUS, TYPE I
Treatment: MEDICAL THERAPY
ICD-9: 250.01,250.1-250.3,250.6,251.3,
775.1
CPT: 10060,10100,11000,11042,
11050-1,11400-2,11420,11700-1,

11710-1,11730,11740,12001,
17002,17100,17110,17200,17340,
20550,20605,23420,25810,35656,
39000,43204,43245,45310,45355,
47600,59025,69200,69210,
90000-99999
Line: 150   Category: 5

Diagnosis: ASTHMA
Treatment: MEDICAL THERAPY
ICD-9: 493
CPT: 90000-99999
Line: 151   Category: 5

Diagnosis: ULCERS, GASTRITIS AND
DUODENITIS
Treatment: MEDICAL THERAPY
ICD-9: 531-535
CPT: 90000-99999
Line: 152   Category: 5

Diagnosis: NON-INSULIN DEPENDENT
DIABETES
Treatment: MEDICAL THERAPY
ICD-9: 250.00
CPT: 10060,10100,11000,11042,
11050-1,11400-2,11420,11700-1,
11710-1,11730,11740,12001,
17000-2,17100,17110,17200,
17340,20550,20600-5,23420,
25810,35656,39000,43204,43245,
45310,45355,47600,59025,69200,
69210,90000-99999
Line: 153   Category: 5

Diagnosis: ACQUIRED HYPOTHYROID-
ISM, DYSHORMONOGENIC
GOITER
Treatment: MEDICAL THERAPY
ICD-9: 244,246.1
CPT: 90000-99999
Line: 154   Category: 5

Diagnosis: CALCULUS OF BILE DUCT
WITH OTHER CHOLECYSTI-
TIS
Treatment: MEDICAL THERAPY
ICD-9: 574.4
CPT: 90000-99999
Line: 155   Category: 5

Diagnosis: PHYSICAL AND SEXUAL
ABUSE INCLUDING RAPE
Treatment: MEDICAL TREATMENT
ICD-9: 992.91,994.2-.3,995.5,995.81,
V61.21
CPT: 90000-99999
Line: 156   Category: 1

Diagnosis: GONOCOCCAL INFECTION
OF EYE
Treatment: MEDICAL THERAPY
ICD-9: 098.4
CPT: 90000-99999
Line: 157   Category: 10

Diagnosis: HIV DISEASE INCLUDING
ACQUIRED IMMUNODE-
FICIENCY SYNDROME
Treatment: MEDICAL THERAPY
ICD-9: 042.9,043.9,044.9
CPT: 90000-99999
Line: 158   Category: 5

Diagnosis: EPILEPSY
Treatment: MEDICAL THERAPY
ICD-9: 345.1,345.9
CPT: 90000-99999
Line: 159   Category: 5

Diagnosis: HEREDITARY HEMOLYTIC
ANEMIAS (EG. SICKLE CELL)
Treatment: MEDICAL THERAPY
ICD-9: 282
CPT: 90000-99999
Line: 160   Category: 5

Diagnosis: STERILIZATION
Treatment: VASECTOMY
ICD-9: V25.2
CPT: 55250
Line: 161   Category: 6

Diagnosis: STERILIZATION
Treatment: TUBAL LIGATION
ICD-9: V25.2
CPT: 58600-11
Line: 162   Category: 6

Diagnosis: BIRTH CONTROL
Treatment: CONTRACEPTION MANAGE-
MENT
ICD-9: V25.0-.1,V25.4-.9

CPT: 90000-99999
Line: 163   Category: 6

Diagnosis: IMMINENT DEATH REGARD-
LESS OF DIAGNOSIS
Treatment: COMFORT CARE
ICD-9: 0
CPT: 90000-99999
Line: 164   Category: 7

Diagnosis: DENTAL SERVICES (EG. IN-
FECTIONS)
Treatment: RESTORATIVE DENTAL SER-
VICE
ICD-9: 0
CPT: 00415,00501,01550,02910,02920,
02940,03110,03120,03220,03310,
03320,03340,03350,05410-1,
05420,05510,05951,06930,07110,
07210,07440-1,07510,07520,
07910-12,07990,09110
Line: 165   Category: 10

Diagnosis: PREVENTIVE DENTAL SER-
VICES
Treatment: CLEANING AND FLUORIDE
ICD-9: V72.2
CPT: 00502,00999,01201,01203,01330,
01351,05931-5,05952-3,05956-7,
05982,05986,07260,07490,
07940-9,07955,09610
Line: 166   Category: 8

Diagnosis: PREVENTIVE SERVICES FOR
ADULTS WITH PROVEN
EFFECTIVENESS
Treatment: MEDICAL THERAPY
ICD-9: V01-V07,V10-V19,V41,V60-V65,
V70.0,V70.9,V71,V72.0-.3,
V72.8-.9,V73-V82
CPT: 90000-99999
Line: 167   Category: 9

Diagnosis: SOMATIC MEDICINE
Treatment: MEDICAL THERAPY
ICD-9: V70.4
CPT: 90000-99999
Line: 168   Category: 5

Diagnosis: CANCER OF CERVIX, TREAT-
ABLE
Treatment: MEDICAL AND SURGICAL

TREATMENT
ICD-9: 180
CPT: 37799,38770,44320,51040,
57452-54,57500,57505,57513,
57820,58150,58200,58210,
90000-99999
Line: 169   Category: 5

Diagnosis: GONOCOCCAL INFECTIONS
AND OTHER VENEREAL DIS-
EASES
Treatment: MEDICAL THERAPY
ICD-9: 098,099.0-099.2,099.4-099.0
CPT: 90000-99999
Line: 170   Category: 10

Diagnosis: DYSPLASIA OF CERVIX AND
CERVICAL CARCINOMA IN
SITU
Treatment: MEDICAL AND SURGICAL
TREATMENT
ICD-9: 078.1,233.1,622.0-.2,623.0-.1,
623.4,623.7,795.0
CPT: 11623,11960-70,15720,19120,
38745,45355,52240,56515,
58200-10,58960,56501,57061-
105, 57150,57180,57400,57454,
57510-20,90000-99999
Line: 171   Category: 5

Diagnosis: CANCER OF BREAST, TREAT-
ABLE
Treatment: MEDICAL AND SURGICAL
TREATMENT
ICD-9: 174-175,198.2,233.0,238.3,239.2
CPT: 11200,11401-02,11623,11950-70,
13132,13300,15720,17100,17200,
17999,19120,19160-240,19316-8,
19350,19499,20605,32000,37799,
38525-30,38745,45355,49000,
49080,49999,52240,56515,57510,
62192,57260,58200-10,58960,
62256,90000-99999
Line: 172   Category: 5

Diagnosis: UNDESCENDED TESTICLE
Treatment: ORCHIECTOMY, REPAIR
ICD-9: 752.5
CPT: 54520-54565,54300-440
Line: 173   Category: 5

Diagnosis: CANCER OF TESTIS, TREAT-
ABLE
Treatment: MEDICAL AND SURGICAL
TREATMENT
ICD-9: 186,236.4
CPT: 49200,54521-35,54660,55530,
38564,38780,64450,90000-99999
Line: 174   Category: 5

Diagnosis: COARCTATION OF THE
AORTA
Treatment: SURGICAL/EXCISION
ICD-9: 747.10
CPT: 33840-33851
Line: 175   Category: 5

Diagnosis: PYODERMA
Treatment: MEDICAL THERAPY
ICD-9: 686.0-.1
CPT: 90000-99999
Line: 176   Category: 3

Diagnosis: ANGINA PECTORIS; OTHER
FORMS OF CHRONIC
ISCHEMIC HEART DISEASE
Treatment: MEDICAL AND SURGICAL
TREATMENT
ICD-9: 412-414,996.03
CPT: 33210,33405,33510-33516,
92950-93799,33525,33570,
35001,35226,35286,35518,35661,
90000-99999
Line: 177   Category: 5

Diagnosis: CANCER OF ENDOCRINE
SYSTEM, TREATABLE
Treatment: MEDICAL AND SURGICAL
TREATMENT
ICD-9: 164.0,193-194,198.7,234.8,237.0-
.4,239.7
CPT: 11050-51,11600-46,12042,13132,
14060,17000-1,17100,17340,
31505,49081,21632,32095-100,
32480-90,32480-525,38510,
60200,60220-5,60240-5,60540,
63277,90000-99999
Line: 178   Category: 5

Diagnosis: CANCER OF OVARY, TREAT-
ABLE
Treatment: MEDICAL AND SURGICAL

TREATMENT
ICD-9: 183.0,198.6,236.2
CPT: 32000,32020,38760,44005,44320,
44625,49000,49085,49999,51010,
58180,58210,58720-40,58940-3,
58943,58951,58960-85,90000-
99999
Line: 179   Category: 5

Diagnosis: ADDISON'S DISEASE
Treatment: MEDICAL THERAPY
ICD-9: 255.4,255.5
CPT: 90000-99999
Line: 180   Category: 5

Diagnosis: CONSTITUTIONAL APLASTIC
ANEMIA
Treatment: MEDICAL THERAPY
ICD-9: 284.0
CPT: 90000-99999
Line: 181   Category: 5

Diagnosis: CORONARY ARTERY ANOM-
ALY
Treatment: ANOMALOUS CORONARY
ARTERY LIGATION
ICD-9: 746.85
CPT: 33502
Line: 182   Category: 2

Diagnosis: CONGENITAL ANOMALIES
OF URINARY SYSTEM
Treatment: RECONSTRUCTION
ICD-9: 753.0-.1,753.3-.9
CPT: 55899
Line: 183   Category: 5

Diagnosis: TOTAL ANOMALOUS
PULMONARY VENOUS CON-
NECTION
Treatment: COMPLETE REPAIR
ICD-9: 747.41
CPT: 33730
Line: 184   Category: 2

Diagnosis: ULCERS, GI HEMORRHAGE
Treatment: HEMIGASTRECTOMY
ICD-9: 531-534,578
CPT: 43204,43610-41,43825-40
Line: 185   Category: 5

Diagnosis: CANCER OF UTERUS, TREAT-
ABLE
Treatment: MEDICAL AND SURGICAL
TREATMENT
ICD-9: 179,182,236.0
CPT: 29811,38780,49201,56515,57065,
57452-54,57500,57513,58210,
58120,58150-285,58950-51,
90000-99999
Line: 186   Category: 5

Diagnosis: COAGULATION DEFECTS
Treatment: MEDICAL THERAPY
ICD-9: 286.0-.5,.7-.9
CPT: 90000-99999
Line: 187   Category: 5

Diagnosis: COMMON TRUNCUS
Treatment: TOTAL REPAIR/REPLANT
ARTERY
ICD-9: 745.0
CPT: 33786,33788
Line: 188   Category: 5

Diagnosis: HODGKIN'S DISEASE
Treatment: CHEMOTHERAPY, RADIA-
TION THERAPY
ICD-9: 201
CPT: 38100,49000,49200,49220,90000-
99999
Line: 189   Category: 5

Diagnosis: CONGENITAL STENOSIS AND
INSUFFICIENCY OF AORTIC
VALVE
Treatment: SURGICAL VALVE REPLACE-
MENT
ICD-9: 746.3-.4
CPT: 33405-33417
Line: 190   Category: 5

Diagnosis: ACQUIRED HEMOLYTIC
ANEMIAS
Treatment: MEDICAL THERAPY
ICD-9: 283
CPT: 90000-99999
Line: 191   Category: 5

Diagnosis: BULBUS CORDIS ANOM-
ALIES & ANOMALIES OF
CARDIAC SEPTAL CLOSURE:
DOUBLE OUTLET RIGHT

VENTRICLE
Treatment: SHUNT
ICD-9: 745.11
CPT: 33750-33766
Line: 192   Category: 2

Diagnosis: CONGENITAL PULMONARY
VALVE ATRESIA
Treatment: SHUNT
ICD-9: 746.01
CPT: 33750-33766
Line: 193   Category: 5

Diagnosis: NON-DISSECTING ANEUR-
YSM WITHOUT RUPTURE
Treatment: SURGICAL TREATMENT
ICD-9: 441.2,441.4,441.9,442
CPT: 33860-77,35081-103,35188,
35301-11,35331-51,35450-515,
35526-31,35536-52,35560-63,
35601-16,35626-46,35651,35663,
37618,61532,61700,61712
Line: 194   Category: 5

Diagnosis: PITUITARY DISORDERS:
PANHYPOPITUITARISM,
IATROGENIC AND OTHER
Treatment: MEDICAL THERAPY
ICD-9: 253.2,253.4,253.7,253.8
CPT: 90000-99999
Line: 195   Category: 5

Diagnosis: OTHER AND UNSPECIFIED
TYPE ENDOCARDIAL CUSH-
ION DEFECTS
Treatment: REPAIR ATRIOVENTRICU-

LAR
ICD-9: 745.60,745.69,745.8,745.9
CPT: 33670
Line: 196   Category: 5

Diagnosis: INTERRUPTED AORTIC
ARCH
Treatment: TRANSVERSE ARCH GRAFT
ICD-9: 747.11
CPT: 33870
Line: 197   Category: 2

Diagnosis: HEREDITARY FRUCTOSE IN-
TOLERANCE, INTESTINAL
DISACCHARIDASE AND
OTHER DEFICIENCIES
Treatment: MEDICAL THERAPY
ICD-9: 271.2-.9
CPT: 90000-99999
Line: 198   Category: 5

Diagnosis: CONGENITAL TRICUSPID
ATRESIA AND STENOSIS
Treatment: REPAIR
ICD-9: 746.1
CPT: 33649
Line: 199   Category: 5

Diagnosis: DISEASES AND DISORDERS
OF AORTIC VALVE
Treatment: AV REPLACEMENT, VAL-
VULOPLASTY, MEDICAL
THERAPY
ICD-9: 395,424.1,996.02
CPT: 33400,33411,90000-99999
Line: 200   Category: 5

————$87.12 Per Capita Cost Per Month————

Diagnosis: CONGENITAL MITRAL
VALVE STENOSIS
Treatment: MITRAL VALUE REPLACE-
MENT
ICD-9: 746.5
CPT: 33420-33430
Line: 201   Category: 2

Diagnosis: DISEASES OF MITRAL
VALVE
Treatment: VALVULOPLASTY, MV RE-
PLACE, MEDICAL THERAPY

ICD-9: 394,424.0,996.02
CPT: 33430,33425,90000-99999
Line: 202   Category: 5

Diagnosis: ADRENOGENITAL DIS-
ORDERS
Treatment: MEDICAL THERAPY
ICD-9: 255.2
CPT: 90000-99999
Line: 203   Category: 5

Diagnosis: CANCER OF VAGINA, VUL-

VA AND OTHER FEMALE
GENITAL ORGANS, TREAT-
ABLE
Treatment: MEDICAL AND SURGICAL
TREATMENT
ICD-9: 181,183.2-.9,184,236.1,236.3
CPT: 11400-22,17000-2,32000,44005,
46917,49000,49085,51010,56515,
56620,57065,57150,57513,58180,
58150,58200,58210,58240,58260,
58720,58960,90000-99999
Line: 204   Category: 5

Diagnosis: CANCER OF URINARY SYS-
TEM, TREATABLE
Treatment: MEDICAL AND SURGICAL
TREATMENT
ICD-9: 188-189,198.0-.1,233.7,236.7,
236.9,239.4
CPT: 11400,11440,11623, 11960-70,
15720,17000,19120,38745,45355,
56515,57510,58200-10,58960,
20550,50220-90,50650-60,51530,
51550-97,51700,51720,52234-40,
52281,52500,53670,53220,63277,
90000-99999
Line: 205   Category: 5

Diagnosis: CANCER OF EYE & ORBIT,
TREATABLE
Treatment: MEDICAL AND SURGICAL
TREATMENT
ICD-9: 190,234.0,238.8
CPT: 11050-51,11600-46,12042,13132,
14060,17000-1,17100,17340,
31505,49081,11401-02,11440,
65101-05,90000-99999
Line: 206   Category: 5

Diagnosis: CANCER OF SOFT TISSUE,
TREATABLE
Treatment: MEDICAL AND SURGICAL
TREATMENT
ICD-9: 164.1,171,238.1
CPT: 14040,21555-57,21925-35,
23075-77,24075-77,25075-77,
26115-17,27047-49,27075-79,
27327-29,27615-19,27899,
28043-46,32522,90000-99999
Line: 207   Category: 5

Diagnosis: ARTERIAL ANEURYSM OF

NECK
Treatment: REPAIR
ICD-9: 442.81-82
CPT: 35321,35355-81,35516-21,35533,
35556-58,35565-87,35621,
35650-61,35665-71
Line: 208   Category: 5

Diagnosis: HODGKIN'S DISEASE
Treatment: BONE MARROW TRANS-
PLANT (5-6 LOCI MATCH)
ICD-9: 201
CPT: 38230-41
Line: 209   Category: 5

Diagnosis: TETRALOGY OF FALLOT
(TOF)
Treatment: TOTAL REPAIR TETRALOGY
ICD-9: 745.2
CPT: 33692-33696
Line: 210   Category: 5

Diagnosis: COMPLETE, CORRECTED
AND OTHER TGA
Treatment: TRANSPOSITION OF VESSELS
ICD-9: 745.10,745.12,745.19
CPT: 33782-33784
Line: 211   Category: 2

Diagnosis: CONGENITAL CYSTIC LUNG
- MILD AND MODERATE
Treatment: LUNG RESECTION
ICD-9: 748.4
CPT: 32500
Line: 212   Category: 5

Diagnosis: CHRONIC HEPATITIS
Treatment: MEDICAL THERAPY
ICD-9: 571.4,571.8-.9
CPT: 90000-99999
Line: 213   Category: 5

Diagnosis: OTHER SPECIFIED APLASTIC
ANEMIAS
Treatment: BONE MARROW TRANS-
PLANT (5-6 LOCI MATCH)
ICD-9: 284.8
CPT: 38240
Line: 214   Category: 5

Diagnosis: CANCER OF PENIS AND OTH-
ER MALE GENITAL ORGAN,

TREATABLE
Treatment: MEDICAL AND SURGICAL
TREATMENT
ICD-9: 187,233.5
CPT: 11623,11960-70,15720,19120,
38745,45355,52240,56515,57510,
58200-10,58960,54120-35,90000-
99999
Line: 215   Category: 5

Diagnosis: BENIGN NEOPLASM OF THE
BRAIN
Treatment: CRANIOTOMY/
CRANIECTOMY
ICD-9: 225.0
CPT: 61304-61576,61712,62223,63276
Line: 216   Category: 5

Diagnosis: INFECTIOUS SKIN CONDI-
TIONS
Treatment: MEDICAL THERAPY
ICD-9: 526.4,706.2,757.32,757.39,757.9
CPT: 10000-61,10141,11000,
11100-446,17000-105,20000-05,
21030,21044,21501,23030,23040,
23930-31,25028-31,26010-30,
26990-91,27301,27603-04,28001,
40800-05,41800,90000-99999
Line: 217   Category: 5

Diagnosis: HEARING LOSS - AGE 3 OR
UNDER
Treatment: MEDICAL THERAPY
ICD-9: 388-389
CPT: 90000-99999
Line: 218   Category: 4

Diagnosis: URETERAL CALCULUS
Treatment: CYSTOURETHROSCOPY
W/FRAGMENTATION OF
CALCULUS, MEDICAL THER-
APY
ICD-9: 592.1
CPT: 50392,50561,50951-80,52320,
52325,52332,52335-36,53020,
90000-99999
Line: 219   Category: 5

Diagnosis: BENIGN CEREBRAL CYSTS
Treatment: DRAINAGE
ICD-9: 348.0,349.2
CPT: 61120-61152,61314-61315,

61522-61524,61680-61712
Line: 220   Category: 5

Diagnosis: CANCER OF BONES, TREAT-
ABLE
Treatment: MEDICAL AND SURGICAL
TREATMENT
ICD-9: 170,198.5,238.0,239.2
CPT: 14001,17002,21620,23140,23900,
24900-31,25900-31,26200,
26910-52,27290,27365,27590-98,
27880-89,28800-25,32500,
60252-54,60500-605,63276,
90000-99999
Line: 221   Category: 5

Diagnosis: AMEBIASIS
Treatment: MEDICAL THERAPY
ICD-9: 006.0-.1,006.9
CPT: 90000-99999
Line: 222   Category: 10

Diagnosis: LIVER ABSCESS AND
SEQUELAE OF CHRONIC
LIVER DISEASE
Treatment: MEDICAL THERAPY
ICD-9: 572.0-.2
CPT: 90000-99999
Line: 223   Category: 5

Diagnosis: PEMPHIGUS, PEMPHIGOID;
BENIGN MUCOUS MEM-
BRANE PEMPHIGOID, OTHER
AND UNSPECIFIED BULLOUS
DERMATOSES
Treatment: MEDICAL THERAPY
ICD-9: 694.4-.9
CPT: 90000-99999
Line: 224   Category: 5

Diagnosis: INTESTINAL MALABSORP-
TION
Treatment: MEDICAL THERAPY
ICD-9: 579
CPT: 90000-99999
Line: 225   Category: 5

Diagnosis: ACROMEGALY & GIGAN-
TISM, OTHER & UN-
SPECIFIED ANTERIOR PITU-
ITARY HYPERFUNCTION,
BENIGN NEOPLASM OF THY-

ROID GLANDS & OTHER EN-
DOCRINE GLANDS
Treatment: MEDICAL AND SURGICAL
TREATMENT
ICD-9: 253.0,253.1,253.6,253.9,226,
227.0-.1,227.4-.9
CPT: 11401,14000,17000,17102,17200,
52281,53670,60200-45,61712,
90000-99999
Line: 226   Category: 5

Diagnosis: MALIGNANT MELANOMA OF
SKIN, TREATABLE
Treatment: MEDICAL AND SURGICAL
TREATMENT
ICD-9: 172,238.2,239.2
CPT: 11400-46,11600-46,12032,13120,
14040-61,17000-110,17340,
17999,19200-29,19272,21555-7,
21632,21925-35,23075-7,24075-7,
25075-7,26115-7,27047-9,
27075-9,27327-9,27615-9,
28043-6,28315,32480,38500-780,
51575-95,54135,55842-45,
90000-99999
Line: 227   Category: 5

Diagnosis: PARALYTIC ILEUS
Treatment: MEDICAL THERAPY
ICD-9: 560.1
CPT: 90000-99999
Line: 228   Category: 5

Diagnosis: URETERAL STRICTURE OR
OBSTRUCTION
Treatment: OPEN RESECTION, PERCUTA-
NEOUS NEPHROSTO-
LITHOTOMY, NEPHRO-
LITHOTOMY, LITHOTRIPSY
ICD-9: 593.3-.4
CPT: 50060-81,50700-16,50590,52276
Line: 229   Category: 5

Diagnosis: TREATABLE DEMENTIA
Treatment: MEDICAL THERAPY
ICD-9: 291.2,290,40,292.82,293.9,294.8
CPT: 90000-99999
Line: 230   Category: 5

Diagnosis: CHRONIC OSTEOMYELITIS
Treatment: INCISION & DRAINAGE

ICD-9: 730.1-.2
CPT: 23035,23170-82,23189,23935,
24134-24147,25035,25145-25151,
26034,26230-36,26992,27303,
27075-79,27070-1,27607,28005,
27360,27640-1,28120-4
Line: 231   Category: 5

Diagnosis: CHRONIC PYELONEPHRITIS
Treatment: MEDICAL THERAPY
ICD-9: 590.0
CPT: 90000-99999
Line: 232   Category: 5

Diagnosis: TORSION OF TESTIS
Treatment: ORCHIECTOMY, REPAIR
ICD-9: 608.2
CPT: 54520-54560,54600,54640
Line: 233   Category: 10

Diagnosis: LEUKOPLAKIA OF CERVIX,
DYSTROPHY OF VULVA
Treatment: MEDICAL THERAPY
ICD-9: 622.2,624.0
CPT: 90000-99999
Line: 234   Category: 5

Diagnosis: CANCER OF LUNG, BRON-
CHUS, PLEURA, TRACHEA,
MEDIASTINUM & OTHER RE-
SPIRATORY ORGANS,
TREATABLE
Treatment: MEDICAL AND SURGICAL
TREATMENT
ICD-9: 162-163,164.2-.9,165,195.1,197.0,
197.2-.3,231.1-.2,235.7-.8
CPT: 11601,13151,17001-2,20605-10,
22900,31300,31540-1,31640-45,
31785-86,31899,32000,32020,
32095-100,32480-90,32440-50,
32500,32900,37799,38542,39010,
39200,39400,42415,45333,46917,
49421,63030,6471-21,66984,
69433,90000-99999
Line: 235   Category: 5

Diagnosis: ACUTE LYMPHOCYTIC LEU-
KEMIA (CHILD)
Treatment: CHEMOTHERAPY, RADIA-
TION THERAPY
ICD-9: 204.0

CPT: 90000-99999
Line: 236 Category: 5

Diagnosis: DISORDERS OF AMINO-ACID
TRANSPORT AND METAB-
OLISM (NON PKU)
Treatment: MEDICAL THERAPY
ICD-9: 270.0,270.2-270.9
CPT: 90000-99999
Line: 237 Category: 5

Diagnosis: PNEUMOCYSTIS CARINII
PNEUMONIA
Treatment: MEDICAL THERAPY
ICD-9: 136.3
CPT: 90000-99999
Line: 238 Category: 5

Diagnosis: NON-HODGKIN'S LYM-
PHOMAS
Treatment: CHEMOTHERAPY, RADIA-
TION THERAPY
ICD-9: 200,202.0-.2,202.8-.9
CPT: 11402,19340,20550,27125,38510,
49080,38100,38510-25,38720,
90000-99999
Line: 239 Category: 5

Diagnosis: CANCER OF STOMACH,
TREATABLE
Treatment: MEDICAL AND SURGICAL
TREATMENT
ICD-9: 151,230.2,235.2
CPT: 31300,31540-1,32100,38541,
39200,42415,45170,45333,45385,
46917,43120,43620-38,44100-30,
44140-47,44625,45111,45550,
46938,49000,60540, 90000-
99999
Line: 240 Category: 5

Diagnosis: DISORDERS OF THYRO-
CALCITONIN SECRETION
Treatment: THYROIDECTOMY
ICD-9: 246.0
CPT: 60240
Line: 241 Category: 5

Diagnosis: AORTIC PULMONARY FIS-
TULA
Treatment: REPAIR SINUS OF VALSALVA
ICD-9: 417.0

CPT: 33702-33710
Line: 242 Category: 5

Diagnosis: POLYARTERITIS NODOSA
AND ALLIED CONDITIONS
Treatment: MEDICAL THERAPY
ICD-9: 446.0,446.4,446.6-.7
CPT: 90000-99999
Line: 243 Category: 5

Diagnosis: MYELOID, MONOCYTIC,
ACUTE LYMPHOCYTIC AND
OTHER SPECIFIED LEU-
KEMIAS
Treatment: BONE MARROW TRANS-
PLANT (5-6 LOCI MATCH)
ICD-9: 204.0,205.1-.9,206.1-.9,207.1-.8
CPT: 38230-41
Line: 244 Category: 5

Diagnosis: CANCER OF COLON, REC-
TUM, SMALL INTESTINE
AND ANUS, TREATABLE
Treatment: MEDICAL AND SURGICAL
TREATMENT
ICD-9: 152-154,197.5,230.3-.4,235.5
CPT: 31300,31540-1,32100,39200,
42415,45333,46917,11042,32020,
32420,32900,37799,43630,
44140-50,44345,44620-25,
45110-12,45180,45360,45385,
45550,49000,49999,50230,50810,
60540,68760,90000-99999
Line: 245 Category: 5

Diagnosis: CARDIOMYOPATHY, HYPER-
TROPHIC MUSCLE
Treatment: MEDICAL AND SURGICAL
TREATMENT
ICD-9: 425
CPT: 21633,32100,33010,33245,33516,
33999,43030,43130-36,90000-
99999
Line: 246 Category: 5

Diagnosis: PERNICIOUS ANEMIA
Treatment: MEDICAL THERAPY
ICD-9: 281
CPT: 90000-99999
Line: 247 Category: 5

Diagnosis: CYSTIC FIBROSIS

Treatment: MEDICAL THERAPY
ICD-9: 277.0
CPT: 90000-99999
Line: 248   Category: 5

Diagnosis: AGRANULOCYTOSIS
Treatment: BONE MARROW TRANS-
PLANTATION (5-6 LOCI
MATCH)
ICD-9: 288.0
CPT: 38240
Line: 249   Category: 5

Diagnosis: ATRIAL SEPTAL DEFECT,
SECUNDUM
Treatment: REPAIR SEPTAL DEFECT
ICD-9: 745.5
CPT: 33640-33643
Line: 250   Category: 5

Diagnosis: ATRIAL SEPTAL DEFECT,
PRIMUM
Treatment: REPAIR SEPTAL DEFECT
ICD-9: 745.61
CPT: 33640
Line: 251   Category: 5

Diagnosis: STROKE
Treatment: MEDICAL THERAPY
ICD-9: 434,436
CPT: 90000-99999
Line: 252   Category: 3

Diagnosis: GANGRENE; ATHEROSCLER-
OSIS OF ARTERIES OF EX-
TREMITIES, DIABETES MEL-
LITUS W/PERIPHERAL

CIRCULATORY DISORDER,
CHRONIC ULCER OF SKIN,
GAS GANGRENE, OTHER
PERIPHERAL VASCULAR DIS-
EASE
Treatment: AMPUTATION
ICD-9: 785L4,440.2,
250.7,707.0,040.0,443.0
CPT: 11050-1,28800-25,27880-89,
27590-98,27290-95,26910-52,
25900-31,24900-40,23900-21,
23930,25020-28,26025-30,
26990-91,27301,27305,27600-03,
28001-03
Line: 253   Category: 5

Diagnosis: BUDD-CHIARI SYNDROME,
AND OTHER VENOUS
EMBOLISM AND THROM-
BOSIS
Treatment: THROMBECTOMY/LIGATION
ICD-9: 453
CPT: 34101,37140,37160,37500,34401
Line: 254   Category: 5

Diagnosis: OPPORTUNISTIC INFECTIONS
IN IMMUNOCOMPROMISED
HOSTS
Treatment: MEDICAL THERAPY
ICD-9: 003.9,007.2,
007.7,031.9,039,042.0-.2,042.9,
043.0-.2,043.9,047.9,053-054,
078.5,110,111.1,112.0,115,117.5,
118,130,136.3,173,295.9,287.5,
298.9,323.9,336.9,357
CPT: 90000-99999
Line: 255   Category: 5

————$92.10 Per Capital Cost Per Month————

Diagnosis: VENTRICULAR SEPTAL DE-
FECT
Treatment: CLOSURE
ICD-9: 745.4,745.7
CPT: 33681-33688
Line: 256   Category: 5

Diagnosis: CANCER OF SKIN, EXCLUD-
ING MALIGNANT MEL-
ANOMA, TREATABLE

Treatment: MEDICAL AND SURGICAL
TREATMENT
ICD-9: 173,198.2
CPT: 10040-61,11000-51,11400-46,
11600-46,12011,12031-2,13100-
52,14000-60,14300,15240-60,
15700,1700-999,19200-29,19272,
21555-7,21632,21925-35,23075-7,
24075-7,24075-7,25075-7,
26115-7,27047-9,27075-9,

27327-9,27615-9,28043-6,
38500-780,51575-95,54135,
55842-45,90000-99999
Line: 257   Category: 5

Diagnosis: CANCER OF PROSTATE
             GLAND, TREATABLE
Treatment: MEDICAL AND SURGICAL
             TREATMENT
ICD-9:   185,233.4,236.5
CPT: 11442-4,11623,11960-70,15720,
             17000-1,19120,38745,45355,
             52240,56515,57510,58200-10,
             58960,38564,38780,51700,52234,
             52281,52340,52601,52640,
             53600-1,54530,55000,55810-45,
             55899,90000-99999
Line: 258   Category: 5

Diagnosis: HEART FAILURE
Treatment: MEDICAL THERAPY
ICD-9:   428
CPT: 90000-99999
Line: 259   Category: 5

Diagnosis: APLASTIC ANEMIAS DUE TO
             DISEASE OR TREATMENT
Treatment: MEDICAL THERAPY
ICD-9:   284.8
CPT: 90000-99999
Line: 260   Category: 5

Diagnosis: ULCERATION OF INTESTINE
Treatment: COLECTOMY, EN-
             TEROSTOMY
ICD-9:   569.82
CPT: 44150-60,44300-16,45385
Line: 261   Category: 5

Diagnosis: CANCER OF RETRO-
             PERITONEUM, PERITONEUM,
             OMENTUM & MESENTERY,
             TREATABLE
Treatment: MEDICAL AND SURGICAL
             TREATMENT
ICD-9:   158,197.6,197.8,235.5
CPT: 31300,31540-1,32100,39200,
             42415,45333,46917,21044-45,
             30117-18,30500,32900,39010,
             40810-16,41116,41135,41150-55,
             42104-20,42842-45,42880,49081,
             90000-99999

Line: 262   Category: 5

Diagnosis: EBSTEIN'S ANOMALY
Treatment: REPAIR SEPTAL DEFECT
ICD-9:   746.2
CPT: 33640-33647
Line: 263   Category: 5

Diagnosis: DISEASES OF WHITE BLOOD
             CELLS
Treatment: MEDICAL THERAPY
ICD-9:   288.1-.9
CPT: 90000-99999
Line: 264   Category: 5

Diagnosis: CANCER OF ORAL CAVITY,
             PHARNYX, NOSE AND
             LARYNX, TREATABLE
Treatment: MEDICAL AND SURGICAL
             TREATMENT
ICD-9:   140-149,160-161,231.0,235.0-
             .1,235.6
CPT: 11050,11420,11440-2,11601,
             13132,13151,17000-2,17100,
             17201,27090,31300,31540-1,
             32100,32480,39200,40525-30,
             40899,41130,41110-16,41155,
             42415,42826,43200,45333,46917,
             67961,90000-99999
Line: 265   Category: 5

Diagnosis: BENIGN NEOPLASM OF IS-
             LETS OF LANGERHANS
Treatment: EXCISION OF TUMOR
ICD-9:   211.7
CPT: 60699
Line: 266   Category: 5

Diagnosis: PREMALIGNANT LESIONS
             AND CARCINOMA IN SITU
             OF SKIN
Treatment: DESTRUCT/EXCISION/MEDI-
             CAL THERAPY
ICD-9:   232,702
CPT: 10000,10040,11000,11400-46,
             13121,13131-2,14040-060,14300,
             17000-17200,17304,17340,11600-
             11646,19350,26116,30117,38745,
             58120,67405-13,67405-13,67450,
             69100,69110-20,69300,90000-
             99999

Line: 267   Category: 5

Diagnosis: ADRENAL OR CUTANEOUS
            HEMORRHAGE OF FETUS OR
            NEONATE
Treatment: MEDICAL THERAPY
ICD-9:   772.5-.9
CPT: 90000-99999
Line: 268   Category: 2

Diagnosis: SIALOADENITIS, ABSCESS,
            FISTULA OF SALIVARY
            GLANDS
Treatment: SURGERY
ICD-9:   527.2-.4
CPT: 42305,42325,42330,42340,42408,
            42410,42440-42507,42509,42600,
            42665,40810-40816,42650,42655
Line: 269   Category: 5

Diagnosis: LIPIDOSES AND OTHER DIS-
            ORDERS OF METABOLISM
Treatment: MEDICAL THERAPY
ICD-9:   272,277.1,277.5,277.9,330.1
CPT: 90000-99999
Line: 270   Category: 5

Diagnosis: LEUKOPLAKIA OF ORAL MU-
            COSA, INCLUDING TONGUE
Treatment: INCISION/EXCISION TONGUE,
            BIOPSY
ICD-9:   528.6
CPT: 41000-41599
Line: 271   Category: 5

Diagnosis: MALARIA AND RELAPSING
            FEVER
Treatment: MEDICAL THERAPY
ICD-9:   084,087
CPT: 90000-99999
Line: 272   Category: 1

Diagnosis: REGIONAL ENTERITIS, IDIO-
            PATHIC PROCTOCOLITIS
Treatment: MEDICAL AND SURGICAL
            TREATMENT
ICD-9:   555,556
CPT: 90000-99999,49000,44110,
            44140-60,44345,45112,44625,
            44650
Line: 273   Category: 5
Diagnosis: CONGENITAL PULMONARY

VALVE STENOSIS
Treatment: PULMONARY VALVE REPAIR
ICD-9:   746.02
CPT: 33470-33471
Line: 274   Category: 2

Diagnosis: URETERAL FISTULA
            (INTESTINAL)
Treatment: NEPHROSTOMY
ICD-9:   593.82
CPT: 50951-50980,50040-50045,
            50395-50398,50686-50688,50930
Line: 275   Category: 5

Diagnosis: DISORDERS OF ARTERIES,
            VISCERAL
Treatment: BYPASS GRAFT
ICD-9:   447.0,447.2-.9
CPT: 35501-15,35526-31,35536-51,
            35560-63,35601-16,35626-46,
            35663
Line: 276   Category: 5

Diagnosis: DISEASES OF EN-
            DOCARDIUM
Treatment: MEDICAL THERAPY
ICD-9:   424
CPT: 90000-99999
Line: 277   Category: 5

Diagnosis: CHRONIC LEUKEMIAS
Treatment: CHEMOTHERAPY, RADIA-
            TION THERAPY
ICD-9:   202.4,203.1,204.1-.9,205.1-.9,
            206.1-.9,207.1-.8,208.1-.9
CPT: 11402,11646,22899,36825,37799,
            38100,38308,38520-25,38760,
            38999,43832,45360,58150,58720,
            58805,59840,60500,90000-99999
Line: 278   Category: 5

Diagnosis: CYSTICERCOSIS, OTHER
            CESTODE INFECTION,
            TRICHINOSIS
Treatment: MEDICAL THERAPY
ICD-9:   123.1-.9,124
CPT: 90000-99999
Line: 279   Category: 5

Diagnosis: LEPTOSPIROSIS
Treatment: MEDICAL THERAPY

ICD-9: 100
CPT: 90000-99999
Line: 280   Category: 1

Diagnosis: ENCEPHALOCELE;
CONGENITAL HYDRO-
CEPHALUS
Treatment: SHUNT
ICD-9: 742.0,742.3
CPT: 62180-62258
Line: 281   Category: 2

Diagnosis: ANAL AND RECTAL POLYP
Treatment: EXCISION OF POLYP
ICD-9: 569.0
CPT: 45310,45333,45170
Line: 282   Category: 5

Diagnosis: BENIGN NEOPLASMS OF DI-
GESTIVE SYSTEM
Treatment: SURGICAL TREATMENT
ICD-9: 211.0-.6,211.8-.9
CPT: 11400-3,17000-2,43202,43251,
43450,43600,44100-20,44140-45,
44152,44369,44392,45310,45333,
45355-85,45383-5,46500,46610
Line: 283   Category: 11

Diagnosis: DIABETES INSIPIDUS
Treatment: MEDICAL THERAPY
ICD-9: 253.5
CPT: 90000-99999
Line: 284   Category: 5

Diagnosis: DISORDERS OF PLASMA
PROTEIN METABOLISM
Treatment: MEDICAL THERAPY
ICD-9: 273
CPT: 90000-99999
Line: 285   Category: 5

Diagnosis: CUSHING'S SYNDROME; HY-
PERALDOSTERONISM, OTH-
ER CORTICOADRENAL OVER-
ACTIVITY, MEDULLO-
ADRENAL HYPERFUNCTION
Treatment: MEDICAL THER-
APY/ADRENALECTOMY
ICD-9: 255.0,255.1,255.3,255.6
CPT: 90000-99999,60540,61546
Line: 286   Category: 5

Diagnosis: DISORDERS OF PANCREATIC
ENDOCRINE SECRETION
Treatment: MEDICAL THERAPY
ICD-9: 251.4-.9
CPT: 90000-99999
Line: 287   Category: 13

Diagnosis: GUILLAIN-BARRE SYN-
DROME
Treatment: MEDICAL THERAPY
ICD-9: 357.0
CPT: 90000-99999
Line: 288   Category: 3

Diagnosis: LEUKOPLAKIA OF ORAL MU-
COSA, INCLUDING TONGUE
Treatment: MEDICAL THERAPY
ICD-9: 528.6
CPT: 90000-99999
Line: 289   Category: 5

Diagnosis: HEREDITARY ANGIONEU-
ROTIC EDEMA
Treatment: MEDICAL THERAPY
ICD-9: 277.6
CPT: 90000-99999
Line: 290   Category: 5

Diagnosis: METASTATIC INFECTIONS
WITH LOCALIZED SITES
Treatment: MEDICAL THERAPY
ICD-9: 003.2,006.3-.9,014-018,022.1
CPT: 90000-99999
Line: 291   Category: 5

Diagnosis: CHRONIC RESPIRATORY DIS-
EASE ARISING IN THE NEO-
NATAL PERIOD
Treatment: MEDICAL THERAPY
ICD-9: 770.7
CPT: 90000-99999
Line: 292   Category: 5

Diagnosis: NON LIFE-THREATENING
ARRHYTHMIAS
Treatment: MEDICAL THERAPY, PACE-
MAKER
ICD-9: 426,427.3,427.6,996.01
CPT: 33201,33210,33212,33999,
90000-99999
Line: 293   Category: 5

Diagnosis: LYMPHOID LEUKEMIA
Treatment: BONE MARROW TRANS-
PLANT (5-6 LOCI MATCH)
ICD-9: 204.1-.9
CPT: 38240
Line: 294   Category: 5

Diagnosis: SYSTEMIC LUPUS ERYTHE-
MATOSUS, OTHER DIFFUSE
DISEASES OF CONNECTIVE
TISSUE
Treatment: MEDICAL THERAPY
ICD-9: 710.0,710.8,710.9
CPT: 90000-99999
Line: 295   Category: 5

Diagnosis: HYPOPLASIA AND DYSPLA-
SIA OF LUNG
Treatment: MEDICAL THERAPY
ICD-9: 748.5
CPT: 90000-99999
Line: 296   Category: 2

Diagnosis: PORTAL VEIN THROMBOSIS
Treatment: SHUNT
ICD-9: 452
CPT: 37140,49425
Line: 297   Category: 5

Diagnosis: TETANUS
Treatment: MEDICAL THERAPY
ICD-9: 037
CPT: 90000-99999
Line: 298   Category: 1

Diagnosis: VESICOURETERAL REFLUX
Treatment: MEDICAL THERAPY, RE-
PLANTATION
ICD-9: 593.7
CPT: 90000-99999
Line: 299   Category: 5

Diagnosis: CONGENITAL HYDRO-
NEPHROSIS
Treatment: NEPHRECTOMY/REPAIR
ICD-9: 753.2
CPT: 50230,50400-504
Line: 300   Category: 5

Diagnosis: DISORDERS OF PARA-

THYROID GLAND; BENIGN
NEOPLASM OF PARA-
THYROID GLAND
Treatment: MEDICAL AND SURGICAL
TREATMENT
ICD-9: 227.1,252
CPT: 60500-05,90000-99999
Line: 301   Category: 5

Diagnosis: PULMONARY FIBROSIS
Treatment: MEDICAL THERAPY
ICD-9: 515-517
CPT: 90000-99999
Line: 302   Category: 5

Diagnosis: INTRACEREBRAL HEMOR-
RHAGE
Treatment: MEDICAL THERAPY
ICD-9: 431
CPT: 90000-99999
Line: 303   Category: 3

Diagnosis: COARCTATION OF THE
AORTA
Treatment: BALLOON DILATION -
VALVE REPLACEMENT
ICD-9: 747.10
CPT: 33405-33417
Line: 304   Category: 5

Diagnosis: LEPROSY
Treatment: MEDICAL THERAPY
ICD-9: 030
CPT: 90000-99999
Line: 305   Category: 5

Diagnosis: CHRONIC OBSTRUCTIVE
PULMONARY DISEASE
Treatment: MEDICAL THERAPY
ICD-9: 492,496
CPT: 90000-99999
Line: 306   Category: 5

Diagnosis: CONSTITUTIONAL APLASTIC
ANEMIAS
Treatment: BONE MARROW TRANS-
PLANT (5-6 LOCI MATCH)
ICD-9: 284.0
CPT: 38240
Line: 307   Category: 5

Diagnosis: ACUTE LYMPHOCYTIC LEU-
KEMIAS (ADULT) AND MUL-
TIPLE MYELOMA
Treatment: CHEMOTHERAPY, RADIA-
TION THERAPY
ICD-9: 204.0,203.0,203.8
CPT: 45360,90000-99999
Line: 308   Category: 5

Diagnosis: DISORDERS RELATING TO
LONG GESTATION AND HIGH
BIRTHWEIGHT
Treatment: MEDICAL THERAPY

ICD-9: 766
CPT: 90000-99999
Line: 309   Category: 2

Diagnosis: NEPHROTIC SYNDROME
AND OTHER CHRONIC RE-
NAL FAILURE
Treatment: MEDICAL THERAPY INCLUD-
ING DIALYSIS
ICD-9: 581.0-581.2,581.8-.9,582,585,
587-589
CPT: 90000-99999
Line: 310   Category: 5

———$98.51 Per Capita Cost Per Month———

Diagnosis: ACUTE NON-LYMPHOCYTIC
LEUKEMIAS
Treatment: BONE MARROW TRANS-
PLANT (5-6 LOCI MATCH)
ICD-9: 205.0,206.0,207.0,208.0
CPT: 38230-41
Line: 311   Category: 5

Diagnosis: END STAGE RENAL DISEASE
Treatment: RENAL TRANSPLANT
ICD-9: 583.8-.9
CPT: 50360
Line: 312   Category: 5

Diagnosis: OTHER ANEURYSM OF AR-
TERY, PERIPHERAL
Treatment: SURGICAL TREATMENT
ICD-9: 442.0,442.3,442.9
CPT: 24900-31,25900-31,26910-52,
27080,27590-98,277880-89,
28800-25,37609,64510-20,
64802-18,35001-03,35011,
35013-21,35141-62
Line: 313   Category: 5

Diagnosis: DISORDERS MINERAL ME-
TABOLISM
Treatment: MEDICAL THERAPY
ICD-9: 275
CPT: 90000-99999
Line: 314   Category: 5

Diagnosis: NEONATAL CONJUNCTIV-
ITIS, DACRYOCYSTITIS AND

CANDIDA INFECTION
Treatment: MEDICAL THERAPY
ICD-9: 771.6-.7
CPT: 90000-99999
Line: 315   Category: 2

Diagnosis: ESOPHAGEAL VARICES
Treatment: MEDICAL THERAPY/SHUNT/
SCLEROTHERAPY
ICD-9: 456.0-.2
CPT: 90000-99999,37145,37160,37181,
38100,43400
Line: 316   Category: 5

Diagnosis: CHRONIC PANCREATITIS
Treatment: MEDICAL THERAPY
ICD-9: 577.1
CPT: 90000-99999
Line: 317   Category: 5

Diagnosis: HYPERPLASIA OF PROSTATE
Treatment: TRANSURETHRAL RESEC-
TION, MEDICAL THERAPY
ICD-9: 600
CPT: 52601,55040,55821,90000-99999
Line: 318   Category: 1

Diagnosis: END STAGE RENAL DISEASE
Treatment: MEDICAL THERAPY INCLUD-
ING DIALYSIS
ICD-9: 250.4,583.8-.9
CPT: 11060,90000-99999
Line: 319   Category: 5

Diagnosis: GIANT CELL ARTERITIS, KAWASAKI DISEASE, HYPERSENSITIVITY ANGITIS
Treatment: MEDICAL THERAPY
ICD-9: 446.1-.2,446.5
CPT: 90000-99999
Line: 320   Category: 3

Diagnosis: DERMATOMYOSITIS, POLYMYOSITIS
Treatment: MEDICAL THERAPY
ICD-9: 710.3,710.4
CPT: 90000-99999
Line: 321   Category: 5

Diagnosis: SYSTEMIC SCLEROSIS
Treatment: MEDICAL THERAPY
ICD-9: 710.1
CPT: 90000-99999
Line: 322   Category: 5

Diagnosis: UNWANTED PREGNANCY
(Note: This line item is not priced as part of the list.)
Treatment: ABORTION
ICD-9: 635-639,779.6
CPT: 59105-06,59840-52
Line: 323   Category: 6

Diagnosis: COMMON VENTRICLE
Treatment: TOTAL REPAIR TETRALOGY
ICD-9: 745.3
CPT: 33692-33696
Line: 324   Category: 5

Diagnosis: HERPES ZOSTER & HERPES SIMPLEX W/OPHTHALMIC COMPLICATIONS
Treatment: MEDICAL THERAPY
ICD-9: 053.2,054.4
CPT: 90000-99999
Line: 325   Category: 10

HYPHEMA
Diagnosis:
Treatment: REMOVAL OF BLOOD CLOT
ICD-9: 364.41
CPT: 65815,65930
Line: 326   Category: 10

Diagnosis: PENETRATING WOUND OF ORBIT
Treatment: SURGICAL TREATMENT
ICD-9: 870.3,870,8,870.9
CPT: 12011-3,12051-2,13132,13150-2, 67400-50
Line: 327   Category: 12

Diagnosis: PURULENT ENDOPHTHALMITIS
Treatment: VITRECTOMY
ICD-9: 360.0
CPT: 67005-67036
Line: 328   Category: 12

Diagnosis: PRIMARY AND OTHER ANGLE-CLOSURE GLAUCOMA
Treatment: IRIDECTOMY, LASER SURGERY
ICD-9: 365.20,365.22
CPT: 66761,66505,66625-66630
Line: 329   Category: 10

Diagnosis: GLAUCOMA ASSOCIATED WITH DISORDERS OF THE LENS
Treatment: EXTRACTION OF CATARACT
ICD-9: 365.5,360.19
CPT: 66920-66984
Line: 330   Category: 11

Diagnosis: PRIMARY AND OPEN ANGLE GLAUCOMA
Treatment: TRABECULECTOMY
ICD-9: 365.10-365.11
CPT: 66170
Line: 331   Category: 11

Diagnosis: GLAUCOMA: BORDERLINE, OPEN-ANGLE, CORTICO-STEROID-INDUCED, ASSOC. W/CONGENITAL ANOMALIES, DYSTROPHIES & SYSTEMIC SYNDROMES, ASSOC. W/DISORDER OF THE LENS, ASSOC. W/OTHER OCULAR DISORDERS, OTHER & UNSPECIFIED
Treatment: MEDICAL THERAPY
ICD-9: 365.0-365.1,365.3-365.9
CPT: 90000-99999

Line: 332   Category: 13

Diagnosis: DEGENERATION OF MACU-
LA AND POSTERIOR POLE
Treatment: VITRECTOMY, LASER SUR-
GERY
ICD-9: 362.5
CPT: 67038,67210
Line: 333   Category: 11

Diagnosis: VITREOUS HEMORRHAGE
Treatment: VITRECTOMY
ICD-9: 379.23
CPT: 67036
Line: 334   Category: 12

Diagnosis: PRIMARY AND OTHER OPEN-
ANGLE GLAUCOMA
Treatment: LASER TRABECULOPLASTY
ICD-9: 365.10-365.11
CPT: 65855
Line: 335   Category: 11

Diagnosis: PRIMARY AND OTHER OPEN-
ANGLE GLAUCOMA
Treatment: CYCLOCRYOTHERAPY
ICD-9: 365.10-365.11
CPT: 66720-66721
Line: 336   Category: 11

Diagnosis: CATARACT
Treatment: EXTRACTION OF CATARACT
ICD-9: 366.0-.3
CPT: 66920-84
Line: 337   Category: 11

Diagnosis: RETINAL DETACHMENT
WITH RETINAL DEFECT
Treatment: VITRECTOMY
ICD-9: 361.0
CPT: 67036-67112
Line: 338   Category: 12

Diagnosis: OPEN WOUND OF EYEBALL
Treatment: CORNEAL LACERATION RE-
PAIR
ICD-9: 871
CPT: 65280-65285
Line: 339   Category: 12

Diagnosis: CHRONIC INFLAMMATORY

DISORDER OF ORBIT
Treatment: MEDICAL THERAPY
ICD-9: 376.1
CPT: 90000-99999
Line: 340   Category: 13

Diagnosis: AFTER CATARACT
Treatment: DISCUSSION, LENS CAPSULE
ICD-9: 366.5
CPT: 66800-66821
Line: 341   Category: 11

Diagnosis: ACUTE, SUBACUTE,
CHRONIC AND OTHER
CERTAIN TYPES OF
IRIDOCYCLITIS
Treatment: MEDICAL THERAPY
ICD-9: 364.0-.3
CPT: 90000-99999
Line: 342   Category: 13

Diagnosis: DIABETIC AND OTHER
RETINOPATHY
Treatment: LASER SURGERY
ICD-9: 250.5,362.0-362.2
CPT: 67210,67227-8
Line: 343   Category: 11

Diagnosis: RETROLENTAL FIBROPLASIA
Treatment: CRYOSURGERY
ICD-9: 362.21
CPT: 67101-67122
Line: 344   Category: 11

Diagnosis: APHAKIA AND OTHER DIS-
ORDERS OF LENS
Treatment: INTRAOCULAR LENS
ICD-9: 379.3
CPT: 66985
Line: 345   Category: 11

Diagnosis: EXOTROPIA
Treatment: MEDICAL AND SURGICAL
TREATMENT
ICD-9: 378
CPT: 67311-67335,90000-99999
Line: 346   Category: 11

Diagnosis: FOREIGN BODY IN CON-
JUNCTIVAL SAC
Treatment: REMOVAL CONJUNCTIVAL

FOREIGN BODY
ICD-9: 930.1
CPT: 65205-22
Line: 347   Category: 10

Diagnosis: BENIGN NEOPLASM OF
PITUITARY GLAND
Treatment: MEDICAL AND SURGICAL
TREATMENT
ICD-9: 227.3
CPT: 11401,14000,17000,17102,17200,
52281,53670,60225,61070,61305,
61548,61546-48,61712,
90000-99999
Line: 348   Category: 5

Diagnosis: TRAUMATIC AMPUTATION
OF THUMB OR OTHER FIN-
GER (COMPLETE)(PARTIAL)
W/ & W/O COMPLICATION
Treatment: REPLANTATION/AMPUTATE
ICD-9: 885-886
CPT: 11000-1,11042,20812-28,26350-6,
26410-8,26910-52,64450,64830-2
Line: 349   Category: 12

Diagnosis: OPEN WOUNDS
Treatment: REPAIR
ICD-9: 872.0-.1,872.62-.69,872.7-.9,
878.4-.9,880.00,880.10,880.13,
880.20,880.23,881.00,001.02,
881.10,881.12,881.20,881.22,
883,884.2,890-891,892.2,893,
894.2
CPT: 11043,12001-13300,15000-15510,
15540-15550,15580-15625,
15650-15720,15710-15770,24999,
25260-72,56800,64856-7,69440,
69666,69667
Line: 350   Category: 10

Diagnosis: ABSCESSES AND CYSTS OF
BARTHOLIN'S GLAND AND
VULVA
Treatment: INCISION AND DRAINAGE,
MEDICAL THERAPY
ICD-9: 616.2-.9
CPT: 90000-99999,56400,56420,56440,
56501,56600
Line: 351   Category: 10

Diagnosis: PILONIDAL CYST WITH
ABSCESS
Treatment: MEDICAL AND SURGICAL
TREATMENT
ICD-9: 685.0
CPT: 10080-81,11770-72,90000-99999
Line: 352   Category: 14

Diagnosis: ACUTE THYROIDITIS
Treatment: MEDICAL THERAPY
ICD-9: 245.0
CPT: 90000-99999
Line: 353   Category: 10

Diagnosis: ACUTE OTITIS MEDIA
Treatment: MEDICAL THERAPY
ICD-9: 381.0-.4,381.8-.9,382.0,382.4,
382.9
CPT: 90000-99999
Line: 354   Category: 10

Diagnosis: CHRONIC OTITIS MEDIA
Treatment: PE TUBES/T & A/TYMPANO-
PLASTY
ICD-9: 381.5-.7,382.1-.3
CPT: 69400-69410,42820,69631-69633
Line: 355   Category: 11

Diagnosis: CHOLESTEATOMA
Treatment: SURGICAL TREATMENT
ICD-9: 385.30
CPT: 39501-5,69511,69601-5,69610,
69620,60131-7,69641-6,69670
Line: 356   Category: 13

Diagnosis: ACUTE SINUSITIS
Treatment: MEDICAL THERAPY
ICD-9: 461
CPT: 90000-99999
Line: 357   Category: 1

Diagnosis: ACUTE CONJUNCTIVITIS
Treatment: MEDICAL THERAPY
ICD-9: 372.0,077
CPT: 90000-99999
Line: 358   Category: 14

Diagnosis: SPINA BIFIDA WITHOUT HY-
DROCEPHALUS
Treatment: MEDICAL THERAPY
ICD-9: 741.9

CPT: 90000-99999
Line: 359   Category: 2

Diagnosis: EDEMA AND OTHER CONDI-
TIONS INVOLVING THE IN-
TEGUMENT OF THE FETUS
AND NEWBORN
Treatment: MEDICAL THERAPY
ICD-9: 778.5-.9
CPT: 90000-99999
Line: 360   Category: 2

Diagnosis: CONGENITAL RUBELLA AND
OTHER CONGENITAL IN-
FECTIOUS DISEASES
Treatment: MEDICAL THERAPY
ICD-9: 771.0-.2
CPT: 90000-99999
Line: 361   Category: 2

Diagnosis: FEEDING PROBLEMS IN
NEWBORN
Treatment: MEDICAL THERAPY
ICD-9: 779.3

CPT: 90000-99999
Line: 362   Category: 2

Diagnosis: DYSTONIA (UNCON-
TROLLABLE)
Treatment: MEDICAL THERAPY
ICD-9: 333
CPT: 90000-99999
Line: 363   Category: 5

Diagnosis: MULTIPLE VALVULAR DIS-
EASE
Treatment: SURGICAL TREATMENT
ICD-9: 396-397
CPT: 33450-74,33480-92
Line: 364   Category: 5

Diagnosis: BILIARY ATRESIA
Treatment: LIVER TRANSPLANT
ICD-9: 751.61
CPT: 47135
Line: 365   Category: 5

————$102.26 Per Capita Cost Per Month————

Diagnosis: CIRRHOSIS OF LIVER OR
BILIARY TRACT WITHOUT
MENTION OF ALCOHOL
Treatment: LIVER TRANSPLANT
ICD-9: 571.5-.6
CPT: 47135
Line: 366   Category: 5

Diagnosis: CHRONIC PULMONARY
HEART DISEASE, OTHER
DISEASES OF PULMONARY
CIRCULATION, ACUTE &
SUBACUTE ENDOCARDITIS,
ACUTE MYOCARDITIS,
CARDIOMYOPATHY,
OTHER CONG. ANOMALIES
OF HEART AND CIRC.
SYSTEM
Treatment: CARDIAC TRANSPLANT
ICD-9: 416-417,421-422,425,746-747
CPT: 33945
Line: 367   Category: 5

Diagnosis: ACUTE AND SUBACUTE
NECROSIS OF LIVER
Treatment: LIVER TRANSPLANT
ICD-9: 570
CPT: 47135
Line: 368   Category: 3

Diagnosis: DIVERTICULITIS OF COLON
Treatment: COLON RESECTION
ICD-9: 562.1
CPT: 44005,44140,44141,44143,44144,
44145,44147,44320,44620-25,
49000
Line: 369   Category: 3

Diagnosis: CYST AND PSEUDOCYST OF
PANCREAS
Treatment: DRAINAGE AND PAN-
CREATIC CYST
ICD-9: 577.2
CPT: 47480,47610,48100-45,48151,
48180,48500-40
Line: 370   Category: 5

Diagnosis: CANCER OF BRAIN AND NERVOUS SYSTEM, TREAT-ABLE
Treatment: MEDICAL AND SURGICAL TREATMENT
ICD-9: 191-192,198.3-.4,237.5-.9,239.6
CPT: 10060,61310,61516,61712,62141, 62223,61516,61712,61751,61770, 62223,63241,63275-90, 64774-818,90000-99999
Line: 371   Category: 5

Diagnosis: ATHEROSCLEROSIS, VIS-CERAL
Treatment: SURGICAL TREATMENT
ICD-9: 440.0-.1
CPT: 35501-15,35526-31,35536-51, 35560-63,35601-16,35626-46, 35663
Line: 372   Category: 5

Diagnosis: HYPERSOMNIA W/SLEEP APNEA
Treatment: MEDICAL THERAPY, TRACHEOTOMY
ICD-9: 780.53,347
CPT: 90000-99999,31600-10
Line: 373   Category: 5

Diagnosis: DISLOCATION KNEE & HIP, CLOSED
Treatment: RELOCATION
ICD-9: 835.0,836.3,836.5,718.35-.36
CPT: 27250-55,27550-27557
Line: 374   Category: 12

Diagnosis: DISLOCATION OF ELBOW, HAND, ANKLE, FOOT, CLAV-ICLE AND SHOULDER, CLOSED
Treatment: RELOCATION
ICD-9: 831.0,832.0,833.0,834.0,837.0, 838.0,718.30-.34,718.36-.39
CPT: 23520-52,23650-80,24600-24635, 25660-95,26641-715,27840-48
Line: 375   Category: 12

Diagnosis: TRACHOMA
Treatment: MEDICAL THERAPY
ICD-9: 076
CPT: 90000-99999

Line: 376   Category: 10

Diagnosis: CLEFT LIP, CONGENITAL FISTULA OF LIP
Treatment: LIP EXCISION AND REPAIR
ICD-9: 749.1,750.25
CPT: 40650-720
Line: 377   Category: 11

Diagnosis: CLEFT PALATE
Treatment: REPAIR & PALATOPLASTY
ICD-9: 749.0
CPT: 42200-26,42235-81
Line: 378   Category: 11

Diagnosis: CLEFT PALATE WITH CLEFT LIP
Treatment: EXCISION & REPAIR VESTIBULE OF MOUTH
ICD-9: 749.2
CPT: 40800-40899
Line: 379   Category: 11

Diagnosis: CLOSED FRACTURE OF EPIPHYSIS OF LOWER EX-TREMITIES
Treatment: REDUCTION
ICD-9: 820.01,821.22
CPT: 27516-27519
Line: 380   Category: 12

Diagnosis: FRACTURE OF SHAFT OF BONE, CLOSED
Treatment: REDUCTION
ICD-9: 812.2,813.2,813.8,818.0,821.0, 823.2,823.8
CPT: 24500-15,25500-25575, 25610-25620,27409,27500-06, 27664,27750-58,27800-06
Line: 381   Category: 10

Diagnosis: PARALEGIA, QUADRIPLEGIA
Treatment: MEDICAL THERAPY AND RE-HABILITATION
ICD-9: 343,344.0-.1
CPT: 90000-99999
Line: 382   Category: 13

Diagnosis: PARKINSON'S DISEASE
Treatment: MEDICAL THERAPY
ICD-9: 332

CPT: 90000-99999
Line: 383   Category: 13

Diagnosis: MULTIPLE SCLEROSIS AND
OTHER DEMYELINATING
DISEASES OF CENTRAL NER-
VOUS SYSTEM
Treatment: MEDICAL THERAPY AND RE-
HABILITATION
ICD-9: 340-341,334
CPT: 90000-99999
Line: 384   Category: 5

Diagnosis: CEREBRAL PALSY
Treatment: MEDICAL THERAPY
ICD-9: 343.0-.3,.9,344.1,741.9,335.21,
335.11,335.0
CPT: 90000-99999
Line: 385   Category: 13

Diagnosis: SUPERFICIAL INJURIES WITH
INFECTION
Treatment: MEDICAL THERAPY
ICD-9: 910.1,.3,.5,.7,.9,911.1,.3,.5,.7,.9,
912.1,.3,.5,.7,.9,913.1,.3,.5,.7,.9,
914.1,.3,.5,.7,.9,915.1,.3,.5,.7,.9,
916.1,.3,.5,.7,.9,917.1,.3,.5,.7,.9,
919.1,.3,.5,.7,.9
CPT: 12001-14,90000-99999
Line: 386   Category: 10

Diagnosis: LYME DISEASE
Treatment: MEDICAL THERAPY
ICD-9: 088
CPT: 90000-99999
Line: 387   Category: 13

Diagnosis: CHRONIC ULCER OF SKIN
Treatment: MEDICAL THERAPY
ICD-9: 707
CPT: 90000-99999,11000-44,15920-99
Line: 388   Category: 13

Diagnosis: CELLULITIS, NON-ORBITAL
Treatment: MEDICAL THERAPY
ICD-9: 527.3,566,597.0,607.2,608.4,
611.0,616.0,681-682,686.8
CPT: 90000-99999
Line: 389   Category: 10

Diagnosis: ATOPIC DERMATITIS

Treatment: MEDICAL THERAPY
ICD-9: 691.8
CPT: 90000-99999,11100
Line: 390   Category: 13

Diagnosis: CONTACT DERMATITIS AND
OTHER ECZEMA
Treatment: MEDICAL THERAPY
ICD-9: 692
CPT: 90000-99999,11900-11901
Line: 391   Category: 13

Diagnosis: ACNE
Treatment: MEDICAL AND SURGICAL
TREATMENT
ICD-9: 695.3
CPT: 90000-99999,10040-61,11450-71,
11900-11901,17100-05,17340
Line: 392   Category: 13

Diagnosis: PSORIASIS AND SIMILAR
DISORDERS
Treatment: MEDICAL THERAPY
ICD-9: 696
CPT: 90000-99999,11900-11901
Line: 393   Category: 13

Diagnosis: ABSCESS OF BURSA OR TEN-
DON
Treatment: INCISION AND DRAINAGE
ICD-9: 727.89
CPT: 27301,26990,26034,23930,23030,
28001,27603
Line: 394   Category: 10

Diagnosis: ABSCESS OF PROSTATE
Treatment: TURP, DRAIN ABSCESS
ICD-9: 601.2
CPT: 52601
Line: 395   Category: 10

Diagnosis: INFECTIVE OTITIS EXTERNA
Treatment: MEDICAL THERAPY
ICD-9: 380.1-.2,054.73,112.82
CPT: 90000-99999
Line: 396   Category: 14

Diagnosis: CHRONIC OTITIS MEDIA
Treatment: MEDICAL THERAPY
ICD-9: 381.5-.7,382.1-.3
CPT: 90000-99999

Line: 397   Category: 13

Diagnosis: DENTAL SERVICES (EG. DEN-
TAL CARIES, FRACTURED
TOOTH)
Treatment: RESTORATIVE DENTAL SER-
VICE
ICD-9: 0
CPT: 01110-20,02110-61,02210,
02330-35,02930-2,02951,
02970-80,03410-50,04910,
05983-5,07120-30,07220-50,
07285-6,07430-1,07450-65,
07530-50,07981,09210-40,
09310,09410-40
Line: 398   Category: 10

Diagnosis: RHEUMATOID ARTHRITIS,
OSTEOARTHRITIS, AND
ASEPTIC NECROSIS OF
BONE
Treatment: ARTHROPLASTY
ICD-9: 714.0,714.3,715.1-.3,715.9,733.4
CPT: 27437-27454,27457,27580,
23470-23472,23800-23802,
27284-27286,27122-27132,
27700-27703,27870-27871,
24360-24366,24800-24802,
26516-26536
Line: 399   Category: 11

Diagnosis: RHEUMATOID ARTHRITIS
AND OTHER IN-
FLAMMATORY POLY-
ARTHROPATHIES
Treatment: MEDICAL THERAPY
ICD-9: 714
CPT: 90000-99999
Line: 400   Category: 13

Diagnosis: GOUT
Treatment: MEDICAL THERAPY
ICD-9: 274
CPT: 90000-99999
Line: 401   Category: 13

Diagnosis: CRYSTAL ARTHROPATHIES
Treatment: MEDICAL THERAPY
ICD-9: 712
CPT: 90000-99999

Line: 402   Category: 13

Diagnosis: SYMPATHETIC UVEITIS AND
DEGENERATIVE DISORDERS
AND CONDITIONS
Treatment: ENUCLEATION
ICD-9: 360.11,360.2,360.4
CPT: 65105
Line: 403   Category: 12

Diagnosis: DISLOCATIONS OF NON-
CERVICAL VERTEBRA,
CLOSED
Treatment: REPAIR/RECONSTRUCTION
ICD-9: 839.2,839.4,839.6
CPT: 22315,22325-22327,22505,
22590-22650,22840-22855
Line: 404   Category: 12

Diagnosis: LUMBAR SPINAL STENOSIS
Treatment: LAMINECTOMY/LAMI-
NOTOMY
ICD-9: 344.6
CPT: 63005,63017,63031,63042,63047
Line: 405   Category: 11

Diagnosis: FISTULA INVOLVING FE-
MALE GENITAL TRACT
Treatment: CLOSURE OF FISTULA
ICD-9: 619
CPT: 57300,57310,57320,51900-51920,
50930,46715,44660
Line: 406   Category: 11

Diagnosis: HYMEN AND VAGINAL SEP-
TUM
Treatment: HYMENECTOMY
ICD-9: 623.2-.3,752.40,752.42
CPT: 56700-20
Line: 407   Category: 11

Diagnosis: RECTAL PROLAPSE
Treatment: PARTIAL COLECTOMY
ICD-9: 569.1
CPT: 44140-44
Line: 408   Category: 11

Diagnosis: CONGENITAL ABSENCE OF
VAGINA
Treatment: ARTIFICIAL VAGINA

ICD-9: 752.49
CPT: 57291-57292
Line: 409   Category: 11

Diagnosis: PLEURISY
Treatment: MEDICAL THERAPY
ICD-9: 511
CPT: 90000-99999,32000
Line: 410   Category: 10

Diagnosis: HYPOSPADIAS AND EPI-
SPADIAS
Treatment: REPAIR
ICD-9: 752.6
CPT: 54300-440
Line: 411   Category: 411

Diagnosis: FRACTURE OF VERTEBRAL
COLUMN WITH SPINAL
CORD INJURY, SACRUM AND
COCCYX
Treatment: LAMINECTOMY
ICD-9: 806.6-806.9
CPT: 61720-61793
Line: 412   Category: 10

Diagnosis: LOWER EXTREMITY: COM-
PARTMENT SYNDROME
Treatment: DECOMPRESSION
ICD-9: 958.8
CPT: 27600-02
Line: 413   Category: 3

Diagnosis: OCCLUSION AND
STENOSIS OF PRECEREBRAL
ARTERIES
Treatment: THROMBOENDARTEREC-
TOMY
ICD-9: 433
CPT: 35301
Line: 414   Category: 11

Diagnosis: ATHEROSCLEROSIS, PER-
IPHERAL
Treatment: SURGICAL TREATMENT
ICD-9: 440.2-.9,444.2
CPT: 20605,27590,34101,34201,35081,
35361,35381,35516-21,35533,
35556-58,35565-87,35621,
35650-61,35665-71,35721,37609,

64510-20,64802-19
Line: 415   Category: 11

Diagnosis: DISPLACEMENT OF CER-
VICAL INTERVERTEBRAL
DISC WITHOUT MYELO-
PATHY
Treatment: CERVICAL LAMINECTOMY,
MEDICAL THERAPY
ICD-9: 722.0,722.2
CPT: 63250,63265,63270,63275,63280,
63285,63001,63015,63020,
63035-40,63045,63048,63075-76,
63081-82,63300,63304,63170-72,
63180-82,63194,63196,63198,
90000-99999
Line: 416   Category: 11

Diagnosis: FRACTURE OF JOINT,
CLOSED (EXCEPT HIP)
Treatment: REDUCTION
ICD-9: 810.0,811.0,812.0,.4,813.0,813.4,
814.0,815.0,816.0,817.0,819.
0,821.20-.21,821.23-.29,822.0,
823.0,824.0,.2,.4,.6,.8,825.0,.2,
826.0,828.0
CPT: 23500-23515,23570-23630,
24530-88,24650-52,25350,25440,
25600-50,26600-15,26720-85,
27330,27409,27424,27508-14,
27520-40,27610,27760-62,
27780-92,27808-23,27846-8,
28400-530,28730,29874-9
Line: 417   Category: 12

Diagnosis: CALCULUS OF BLADDER OR
KIDNEY
Treatment: OPEN RESECTION, PERCUTA-
NEOUS NEPHROSTOLITHO-
TOMY, NEPHROLITHOTOMY,
LITHOTRIPSY
ICD-9: 592.0,594.1
CPT: 50060-81,50130,50392-93,
50700-16,50590,52317
Line: 418   Category: 11

Diagnosis: ANAL FISTULA
Treatment: FISTULECTOMY
ICD-9: 565.1
CPT: 46211,46270-85,46000-30

Line: 419   Category: 10

Diagnosis: RESIDUAL FOREIGN BODY
            IN SOFT TISSUE
Treatment: REMOVAL

ICD-9:   729.6
CPT: 28190,28192
Line: 420   Category: 10

————110.59 Per Capital Cost Per Month————

Diagnosis: GLYCOGENOSIS
Treatment: MEDICAL THERAPY
ICD-9:   271.0
CPT: 90000-99999
Line: 421   Category: 5

Diagnosis: MALUNION & NONUNION OF
            FRACTURE
Treatment: SURGICAL TX
ICD-9:   733.8
CPT: 24410,24430-35,23840-85,
            25400-25440,27165-27170,
            27470-27472,27720-25,
            28320-22,24400
Line: 422   Category: 11

Diagnosis: OSTEOPOROSIS
Treatment: MEDICAL THERAPY
ICD-9:   733.0
CPT: 90000-99999
Line: 423   Category: 13

Diagnosis: OPHTHALMIC INJURY:
            LACRIMAL SYSTEM
            LACERATION
Treatment: CLOSURE
ICD-9:   870.2
CPT: 68760
Line: 424   Category: 17

Diagnosis: DISORDERS OF REFRACTION
            AND ACCOMMODATION
Treatment: MEDICAL THERAPY
ICD-9:   367
CPT: 90000-99999
Line: 425   Category: 13

Diagnosis: VINCENT'S DISEASE
Treatment: MEDICAL THERAPY
ICD-9:   101
CPT: 90000-99999
Line: 426   Category: 1

Diagnosis: URETHRITIS
Treatment: MEDICAL THERAPY
ICD-9:   597
CPT: 90000-99999
Line: 427   Category: 10

Diagnosis: TRICHOMONAL URETHRITIS,
            TRICHOMONAL PROSTATITIS
Treatment: MEDICAL THERAPY
ICD-9:   131.02,131.03,131.8,131.9
CPT: 90000-99999
Line: 428   Category: 10

Diagnosis: UTERINE LEIOMYOMA
Treatment: TOTAL HYSTERECTOMY OR
            MYOMECTOMY
ICD-9:   218-219
CPT: 11422,49581,51010,51840,57410,
            57511,57820,58120-80,58200,
            58260-5,58340,58400,58720,
            58740,58925,58940,58951,
            58980-95,59050,59820,64435
Line: 429   Category: 11

Diagnosis: REDUCTION DEFORMITY OF
            LOWER LIMB
Treatment: EPIPHYSEAL, OSTEOPLASTY
ICD-9:   755.3
CPT: 27475-27485,27466-27468,
            27730-27742,27715
Line: 430   Category: 11

Diagnosis: MIGRAINE
Treatment: MEDICAL THERAPY
ICD-9:   346
CPT: 90000-99999
Line: 431   Category: 13

Diagnosis: ANAL FISSURE
Treatment: FISSURECTOMY
ICD-9:   565.0
CPT: 46200,46700,46940

Line: 432   Category: 10

Diagnosis: STRESS INCONTINENCE, FE-
MALE
Treatment: URETHROPEXY/PESSARY
ICD-9: 625.6
CPT: 51840-41,57160
Line: 433   Category: 11

Diagnosis: BODY INFESTATIONS (EG.
LICE, SCABIES)
Treatment: MEDICAL THERAPY
ICD-9: 132-134
CPT: 90000-99999
Line: 434   Category: 14

Diagnosis: SIALOLITHIASIS, MUCOCELE,
DISTURBANCE OF SALIVARY
SECRETION, OTHER AND UN-
SPECIFIED DISEASES OF SAL-
IVARY GLANDS
Treatment: SURGERY
ICD-9: 527.5-527.9
CPT: 42305,42325,42330,42340,42408,
42410,42440-42507,42509,42600,
42665,40810-40816,42650,42655
Line: 435   Category: 11

Diagnosis: ANOMALIES OF EXTERNAL
EAR W/ IMPAIRMENT OF
HEARING
Treatment: RECONSTRUCT OF EAR
CANAL
ICD-9: 744.0
CPT: 69320
Line: 436   Category: 11

Diagnosis: CERVICITIS, ENDOCERVIC-
ITIS, HEMATOMA OF VULVA,
OVARIAN CYSTS AND NON-
INFLAMMATORY DIS-
ORDERS OF THE VAGINA
Treatment: MEDICAL THERAPY
ICD-9: 616.0,620.0-.2,620.9,622.3-.4,
622.6-.7,623.6,623.8-.9,624.5,
626.7
CPT: 90000-99999
Line: 437   Category: 10

Diagnosis: BENIGN NEOPLASM OF KID-
NEY
Treatment: MEDICAL THERAPY

ICD-9: 233.1
CPT: 90000-99999
Line: 438   Category: 11

Diagnosis: NONINFLAMMATORY DIS-
ORDERS OF CERVIX
Treatment: MEDICAL THERAPY
ICD-9: 622.4-.9,624.2,624.5-.9
CPT: 90000-99999
Line: 439   Category: 11

Diagnosis: CEREBRAL PALSY
Treatment: REPAIR/RECONSTRUCTION
ICD-9: 343.0-.3,343.9,344.1,741.9,335.21,
335.11,335.0
CPT: 27097-122,27140-85,27315,
27320,27390-400,27605-06,
27685-92,28010-11,28030,
28130,28220-36,28240,28705-60,
27306-07,28300-13
Line: 440   Category: 11

Diagnosis: HYPOPLASTIC LEFT HEART
SYNDROME
Treatment: NORWOOD PROCEDURE
ICD-9: 746.7
CPT: 33480-33485
Line: 441   Category: 2

Diagnosis: OTHER SPECIFIED ANOM-
ALIES OF HEART
Treatment: APICAL-AORTIC CONDUIT
ICD-9: 746.8
CPT: 33404
Line: 442   Category: 5

Diagnosis: UTERINE PROLAPSE
Treatment: SURGICAL REPAIR
ICD-9: 618
CPT: 57160,58150,58260-85
Line: 443   Category: 11

Diagnosis: SHIGELLOSIS, GIARDIASIS,
INTESTINAL HELMINTHIASIS
Treatment: MEDICAL THERAPY
ICD-9: 004,007.1,120-122,123.0,125-129
CPT: 90000-99999
Line: 444   Category: 10

Diagnosis: CORNEAL ULCER
Treatment: MEDICAL THERAPY

ICD-9: 370.0
CPT: 90000-99999,65286
Line: 445 Category: 10

Diagnosis: CARPAL TUNNEL SYN-
DROME, CONTRACTURE OF
PALMAR FACIA
Treatment: SURGICAL TREATMENT
ICD-9: 354.0,354.2,728.6
CPT: 26035-60,26120-80,26440-597,
26820-63,27095-7,27100-22,
27140-85,27306-7,27448-55,
27466-8,27475-85,27715,
27730-42, 64702-4,64718-27,
64774-83,64788-95,64850-7,
64872-999
Line: 446 Category: 11

Diagnosis: DEFORMITIES OF UPPER
BODY & LIMBS
Treatment: REPAIR/REVISION/ RECON-
STRUCTION/RELOCATION/
FASCIECTOMY
ICD-9: 354.0,354.2,718.25,718.35,
732.1-.3,736.06,736.21-.22,
736.3-.5,736.8
CPT: 26035-60,26120-80,26440-597,
26820-63,27095-7,27100-22,
27140-85,27306-7,27448-55,
27466-8,27475-85,27715,
27730-42,64702-4,64718-27,
64774-83,64788-95,64850-7,
64872-999
Line: 447 Category: 11

Diagnosis: MENSTRUAL BLEEDING DIS-
ORDERS
Treatment: MEDICAL THERAPY
ICD-9: 626.2-.6,626.8,627.0
CPT: 90000-99999
Line: 448 Category: 10

Diagnosis: RUPTURE OF SYNOVIUM
Treatment: REMOVAL OF BAKER'S
CYST
ICD-9: 727.51
CPT: 27435
Line: 449 Category: 11

Diagnosis: DEFORMITIES OF FOOT
Treatment: FASCIOTOMY/

INCISION/REPAIR/
ARTHRODESIS
ICD-9: 727.1,736.73,700,736.74,736.71,
754.71,754.69,755.67,735.0-.2,
735.4-.9,732.5,355.6,355.5
CPT: 28008,28010,28035,28050-28092,
28110-28119,28126-28160,
28220-28238,28240-28360,
28705-28760,29425
Line: 450 Category: 11

Diagnosis: FOREIGN BODY IN UTERUS,
VULVA AND VAGINA
Treatment: MEDICAL AND SURGICAL
TREATMENT
ICD-9: 939.1-.2
CPT: 57410,58120,90000-99999
Line: 451 Category: 10

Diagnosis: VAGINITIS
Treatment: MEDICAL THERAPY
ICD-9: 112.1,131.00-
.01,131.09,623.5,625.1
CPT: 57150,90000-99999
Line: 452 Category: 10

Diagnosis: PRIAPISM, ORCHITIS, EPIDI-
DYMITIS, SEMINAL VESICUL-
ITIS, FOREIGN BODY IN PEN-
IS, URETHRAL STRICUTRE
Treatment: MEDICAL THERAPY, RE-
MOVAL OF FOREIGN BODY,
DILATION
ICD-9: 595.0,598,604,607.3,608.0,939.9
CPT: 51700,52275-76,53600-01,
53620-21,53660-61,53670,54115,
54154,54640,54700-861,55401,
55450,90000-99999
Line: 453 Category: 10

Diagnosis: BENIGN NEOPLASM OF EX-
TERNAL FEMALE GENITAL
ORGANS
Treatment: BIOPSY/EXCISION
ICD-9: 221.1-221.9
CPT: 56440,56501,56600,57105,57135
Line: 454 Category: 11

Diagnosis: BALANOPOSTHITIS AND
OTHER DISORDERS OF PENIS
Treatment: MEDICAL THERAPY

ICD-9: 607.1,607.8
CPT: 90000-99999
Line: 455   Category: 10

Diagnosis: NONINFLAMMATORY DIS-
ORDERS AND BENIGN NEO-
PLASMS OF OVARY AND
FALLOPIAN TUBES
Treatment: SALPINGECTOMY, OO-
PHORECTOMY
ICD-9: 620.4,620.8,220,221.0
CPT: 58140-50,58700-58720,58925,
58940
Line: 456   Category: 11

Diagnosis: BONE SPUR
Treatment: OSTECTOMY
ICD-9: 726.91
CPT: 28119,28899
Line: 457   Category: 11

Diagnosis: BELL'S PALSY, EXPOSURE
KERATOCONJUNCTIVITIS
Treatment: TARSORRHAPHY
ICD-9: 351.0,370,34
CPT: 67880
Line: 458   Category: 10

Diagnosis: NASAL POLYP, BENIGN NEO-
PLASM OF NASAL CAVITIES,
MIDDLE EAR & ACCESSORY
SINUSES
Treatment: RECONSTRUCTION
ICD-9: 471.9,212.0
CPT: 17000,31032,31201,31020,30425,
30520,39010,39400
Line: 459   Category: 11

Diagnosis: CYST OF THYROID
Treatment: SURGERY - EXCISION
ICD-9: 246.2
CPT: 60200,60100
Line: 460   Category: 11

Diagnosis: ORBITAL CYST
Treatment: ORBITOTOMY
ICD-9: 376.81
CPT: 67400-67450
Line: 461   Category: 11

Diagnosis: OTOSCLEROSIS

Treatment: STAPEDECTOMY
ICD-9: 387
CPT: 69650-62
Line: 462   Category: 11

Diagnosis: FOREIGN BODY: ACCIDEN-
TALLY LEFT DURING A
PROCEDURE, GRANULOMA
OF MUSCLE, GRANULOMA
OF SKIN & SUBCUTANEOUS
TISSUE
Treatment: REMOVAL OF FOREIGN
BODY
ICD-9: 998.4,728.82,709.4
CPT: 22330,22331,24200,24201,25248,
20520,20525,27086,27087,27372,
28190,28192,28193
Line: 463   Category: 11

Diagnosis: HYPERTROPHY OF BREAST
Treatment: SUBCUTANEOUS TOTAL
MASTECTOMY, BREAST RE-
DUCTION
ICD-9: 611.1
CPT: 19140,19318
Line: 464   Category: 11

Diagnosis: OBSTRUCTION OF NASO-
LACRIMAL DUCT, NEONA-
TAL
Treatment: PROBING NASOLACRIMAL
DUCT
ICD-9: 375.55
CPT: 68825-68830
Line: 465   Category: 11

Diagnosis: THROMBOSED AND COM-
PLICATED HEMORRHOIDS
Treatment: HEMORRHOIDECTOMY, INCI-
SION
ICD-9: 455.1-.2,455.4-.5,455.7-.8
CPT: 10140,45336,46083,46220,
46250-62,46320,46934-36
Line: 466   Category: 11

Diagnosis: STENOSIS OF NASO-
LACRIMAL DUCT (AC-
QUIRED)
Treatment: DACRYOCYSTOR-
HINOSTOMY
ICD-9: 375.4,375.56

CPT: 68720-68750
Line: 467   Category: 11

Diagnosis: URETHRAL FISTULA
Treatment: EXCISION, MEDICAL THER-
APY
ICD-9: 599.1
CPT: 50650-50660,90000-99999
Line: 468   Category: 11

Diagnosis: ENDOMETRIOSIS
Treatment: MEDICAL AND SURGICAL
TREATMENT WITHOUT HYS-
TERECTOMY
ICD-9: 617
CPT: 58145-50,58984,90000-99999
Line: 469   Category: 13

Diagnosis: PTOSIS (ACQUIRED) WITH
VISION IMPAIRMENT
Treatment: PTOSIS REPAIR
ICD-9: 374.3
CPT: 15823,67904
Line: 470   Category: 11

Diagnosis: ENTROPION AND TRICHIASIS
OF EYELID; ECTROPION; BE-
NIGN NEOPLASM OF EYELID
Treatment: ECTROPION/ENTROPION REP.
ICD-9: 216.1,374.0-374.1
CPT: 17340,67700-67850,67880,67914-
67924
Line: 471   Category: 11

Diagnosis: BENIGN NEOPLASM BONE &
ARTICULAR CARTILAGE,
OTHER BENIGN NEOPLASM
OF CONNECTIVE AND OTH-

ER SOFT TISSUE
Treatment: BIOPSY-EXCISION
ICD-9: 213,215,225.3-.4
CPT: 10003,11050,11400-46,13131,
17100-200,20550,21556,
21600,21920-21935,22106,
23065-23077,23140-23156,
23100-23101,24065-24077,24110,
25120-25136,25170,25100-25117,
25200-15,26250-62,26449, 27040-
49,27065-7,27075-9, 27323-
9,27637,28108,28122-4,
28285,64774, 69140
Line: 472   Category: 11

Diagnosis: FOREIGN BODY IN EAR &
NOSE
Treatment: REMOVAL OF FOREIGN
BODY
ICD-9: 931-932
CPT: 69200-69205,30300-20
Line: 473   Category: 10

Diagnosis: PTERYGIUM
Treatment: EXCISION OF TRANSPOSI-
TION OF PTERYGIUM W/O
GRAFT
ICD-9: 372.4
CPT: 65420
Line: 474   Category: 11

Diagnosis: OPEN WOUND OF EAR
DRUM
Treatment: TYMPANOPLASTY
ICD-9: 872.61
CPT: 69610-43
Line: 475   Category: 10

——$117.21 Per Capita Cost Per Month——

Diagnosis: ENOPHTHALMOS
Treatment: ORBITAL IMPLANT
ICD-9: 376.50
CPT: 67550
Line: 476   Category: 11

Diagnosis: HEARING LOSS - OVER AGE
OF THREE
Treatment: MEDICAL THERAPY
ICD-9: 388-389

CPT: 90000-99999
Line: 477   Category: 11

Diagnosis: PARALYSIS OF VOCAL
CORDS OR LARYNX, OTHER
DISEASES OF LARYNX
Treatment: INCISION/EXCISION/ENDO-
SCOPY
ICD-9: 478.3,478.7
CPT: 31300-31579,31580-31605

Line: 478   Category: 11

Diagnosis: DENTAL CARIES (PERI-
             APICAL INFECTION)
Treatment: SURGERY
ICD-9:   521.0
CPT: 41899
Line: 479   Category: 11

Diagnosis: IMPACTED TEETH
Treatment: SURGERY
ICD-9:   520.6,524.3-.4
CPT: 21254,30520,41899
Line: 480   Category: 11

Diagnosis: RECURRENT EROSION OF
             THE CORNEA
Treatment: CORNEAL TATTOO, RE-
             MOVAL OF CORNEAL EPI-
             THELIUM; WITH OR WITH-
             OUT CHEMO-
             CAUTERIZATION
ICD-9:   371.42
CPT: 65600,65435
Line: 481   Category: 11

Diagnosis: CHRONIC SINUSITIS, NASAL
             POLYPS, OTHER DISORDERS
             OF NASAL CAVITY AND
             SINUSES
Treatment: SURGICAL
ICD-9:   471,473,478.1
CPT: 11426-41,30000-31299
Line: 482   Category: 11

Diagnosis: OSTEOARTHRITIS AND AL-
             LIED DISORDERS
Treatment: MEDICAL THERAPY
ICD-9:   715
CPT: 90000-99999
Line: 483   Category: 13

Diagnosis: DEVIATED NASAL SEPTUM,
             ACQUIRED DEFORMITY OF
             NOSE, OTHER DISEASES OF
             UPPER RESPIRATORY TRACT
Treatment: EXCISION OF CYST/RHI-
             NECTOMY/PROSTHESIS
ICD-9:   470,738.0,478.0,478.2-.9
CPT: 14060,15823,20912,21325-35,
             30115-17,30124-30320,30400-30,

30520,20580,30620,30999,
31021-90,31200
Line: 484   Category: 11

Diagnosis: ADHESIVE CAPSULITIS OF
             SHOULDER, ARTICULAR
             CARTILAGE DISORDER OF
             SHOULDER, PERIOSTITIS OF
             SHOULDER
Treatment: REPAIR/RECONSTRUCTION
ICD-9:   718.01,726.0,726.2,730.31
CPT: 29815-29825,23410-23420,
             23440-23466,23107-23125,23190,
             23000,23020
Line: 485   Category: 11

Diagnosis: MENOPAUSAL MANAGE-
             MENT
Treatment: MEDICAL THERAPY OTHER
             THAN HORMONE REPLACE-
             MENT
ICD-9:   627.2-.9
CPT: 90000-99999
Line: 486   Category: 13

Diagnosis: EQUINUS DEFORMITY OF
             FOOT, ACQUIRED
Treatment: ARTHROTOMY
ICD-9:   736.72
CPT: 27612
Line: 487   Category: 11

Diagnosis: CYSTS OF ORAL SOFT TIS-
             SUES
Treatment: MEDICAL THERAPY
ICD-9:   528.4
CPT: 90000-99999
Line: 488   Category: 11

Diagnosis: STOMATITIS, CELLULITIS
             AND ABSCESS OF ORAL
             SOFT TISSUE, AND DISEASES
             OF LIPS
Treatment: MEDICAL THERAPY
ICD-9:   528.0,528.3,528.5
CPT: 90000-99999
Line: 489   Category: 10

Diagnosis: OTHER SPECIFIED CONDI-
             TIONS OF THE TONGUE
Treatment: EXCISION, BIOPSY

ICD-9: 529.8
CPT: 41100,41105,41110,41112-41114,
41599
Line: 490   Category: 11

Diagnosis: SPECIFIC DISORDERS OF THE
TEETH AND SUPPORTING
STRUCTURES
Treatment: EXCISION OF DENTO-
ALVEOLAR STRUCTURE
ICD-9: 525.8
CPT: 41822,41823,41830,41874,
41825-41827,41828,42299,41899,
40899,17999
Line: 491   Category: 11

Diagnosis: PARAPLEGIA
Treatment: SURGICAL PREVENTION OF
CONTRACTURES
ICD-9: 344.1
CPT: 27003
Line: 492   Category: 11

Diagnosis: PERIPHERAL ENTHESO-
PATHIES
Treatment: SURGICAL TREATMENT
ICD-9: 726.30-.32,726.4-.6,726.70,
726.8,726.90
CPT: 29105,29125-29131,24105,
27060-27062,29240,29260,29270,
29280,29345,29355,29365,
29405-50,20550,20600-10,29345,
29355,29365
Line: 493   Category: 11

Diagnosis: CHRONIC DISEASE OF
TONSILS AND ADENOIDS
Treatment: TONSILLECTOMY AND
ADENOIDECTOMY
ICD-9: 474
CPT: 42820-36,42860,42870
Line: 494   Category: 11

Diagnosis: GANGLION OF TENDON OR
JOINT
Treatment: EXCISION
ICD-9: 727.4
CPT: 28090
Line: 495   Category: 11

Diagnosis: KERATOCONJUNCTIVITIS
SICCA, NOT SPECIFIED AS
SJOGREN'S
Treatment: PUNCTAL OCCLUSION, TAR-
SORRHAPHY
ICD-9: 370.33
CPT: 68760,67880
Line: 496   Category: 11

Diagnosis: PARAPLEGIA
Treatment: ARTHRODESIS
ICD-9: 344.1
CPT: 27870
Line: 497   Category: 11

Diagnosis: OVARIAN CYST
Treatment: OOPHORECTOMY
ICD-9: 256.1,256.4
CPT: 58940
Line: 498   Category: 12

Diagnosis: HISTIOCYTOSIS
Treatment: MEDICAL THERAPY
ICD-9: 277.8
CPT: 90000-99999
Line: 499   Category: 5

Diagnosis: CANCER OF ESOPHAGUS,
TREATABLE
Treatment: MEDICAL AND SURGICAL
THERAPY
ICD-9: 150,195.2,230.1
CPT: 17002,38542,43260,44305,
47600-20,47710,43100-43120,
43340-41,44140-47,45111,45550,
49000,60540,90000-99999
Line: 500   Category: 5

Diagnosis: OCCUPATIONAL LUNG DIS-
EASES
Treatment: MEDICAL THERAPY
ICD-9: 500-505
CPT: 90000-99999
Line: 501   Category: 5

Diagnosis: LESION OF PLANTAR NERVE
Treatment: MEDICAL THERAPY, EXCI-
SION
ICD-9: 355.6
CPT: 28080,90000-99999
Line: 502   Category: 11

Diagnosis: NONTOXIC NODULAR GOITER
Treatment: THYROIDECTOMY
ICD-9: 241
CPT: 60245,60220
Line: 503 Category: 11

Diagnosis: HERNIA WITHOUT OBSTRUC-TION OR GANGRENE
Treatment: REPAIR
ICD-9: 550.9,553
CPT: 39502-41,43330-31,43885,44050, 44346,49000,49500-611,51500, 55540
Line: 504 Category: 11

Diagnosis: BENIGN NEOPLASM OF RES-PIRATORY AND IN-TRATHORACIC ORGANS
Treatment: LOBECTOMY, MEDICAL THERAPY
ICD-9: 212
CPT: 17000,31512,31599,90000-99999, 60220-60225
Line: 505 Category: 11

Diagnosis: MUSCULAR DYSTROPHY
Treatment: MEDICAL THERAPY
ICD-9: 359
CPT: 90000-99999
Line: 506 Category: 5

Diagnosis: TRANSIENT CEREBRAL ISCHEMIA
Treatment: MEDICAL THERAPY
ICD-9: 435
CPT: 90000-99999
Line: 507 Category: 10

Diagnosis: PERITONEAL ADHESION
Treatment: SURGICAL TREATMENT
ICD-9: 568
CPT: 44005,44610,45110,49000
Line: 508 Category: 1

Diagnosis: ALCOHOLIC FATTY LIVER OR ALCOHOLIC HEPATITIS
Treatment: MEDICAL THERAPY
ICD-9: 571.0-.1
CPT: 90000-99999
Line: 509 Category: 5

Diagnosis: SPINA BIFIDA WITH HYDRO-CEPHALUS
Treatment: MEDICAL THERAPY
ICD-9: 741.0
CPT: 90000-99999,63706
Line: 510 Category: 5

Diagnosis: OTHER DEFICIENCIES OF CIRCULATING ENZYMES (ALPHA 1-ANTITRYPSIN DE-FICIENCY)
Treatment: MEDICAL THERAPY
ICD-9: 277.6
CPT: 90000-99999
Line: 511 Category: 5

Diagnosis: DIABETES MELLITUS WITH END STAGE RENAL DISEASE
Treatment: PANCREAS/KIDNEY TRANS-PLANT
ICD-9: 250.4
CPT: 50389
Line: 512 Category: 5

Diagnosis: CANCER OF GALLBLADDER AND OTHER BILIARY, TREATABLE
Treatment: MEDICAL AND SURGICAL TREATMENT
ICD-9: 156,197.8,230.8
CPT: 36845,47600-20,47710,49000, 60540,90000-99999
Line: 513 Category: 5

Diagnosis: ACUTE POLIOMYELITIS
Treatment: MEDICAL THERAPY
ICD-9: 045
CPT: 90000-99999
Line: 514 Category: 3

Diagnosis: PITUITARY DWARFISM
Treatment: MEDICAL THERAPY
ICD-9: 253.3
CPT: 90000-99999
Line: 515 Category: 13

Diagnosis: UNSPECIFIED POLYNEURO-PATHY
Treatment: MEDICAL THERAPY
ICD-9: 357.9
CPT: 90000-99999

Line: 516   Category: 3

Diagnosis: HEREDITARY HEMORRHAG-
IC TELANGIECTASIA
Treatment: EXCISION
ICD-9: 448.0
CPT: 11400-11426
Line: 517   Category: 5

Diagnosis: DISEASES OF THYMUS
GLAND
Treatment: MEDICAL THERAPY
ICD-9: 254
CPT: 90000-99999
Line: 518   Category: 5

Diagnosis: CEREBRAL DEGENERATIONS
USUALLY MANIFEST IN
CHILDHOOD
Treatment: MEDICAL THERAPY
ICD-9: 330
CPT: 90000-99999
Line: 519   Category: 5

Diagnosis: CHRONIC RHEUMATIC PERI-
CARDITIS, RHEUMATIC
MYOCARDITIS
Treatment: MEDICAL THERAPY
ICD-9: 393,398.0
CPT: 90000-99999
Line: 520   Category: 5

Diagnosis: CANCER OF LIVER, TREAT-
ABLE
Treatment: MEDICAL AND SURGICAL
TREATMENT
ICD-9: 155,197.7,235.3
CPT: 31300,31540-1,32100,39200,
42415,45333,46917,11042,32900,
37617,43260,43630-38,43860,
44005,44025,44305,47010,48150,
44131,47120-30,47600-20,47710,
49000,49080,90000-99999
Line: 521   Category: 5

Diagnosis: ACUTE NON-LYMPHOCYTIC
LEUKEMIAS
Treatment: CHEMOTHERAPY
ICD-9: 205.0,206.0,207.0,208.0
CPT: 11646,37799,38100,38308,38760,
38999,45360,58150,58720,58805,

59840,60500,90000-99999
Line: 522   Category: 5

Diagnosis: MULTIPLE MYELOMA AND
CHRONIC LEUKEMIAS
Treatment: BONE MARROW TRANS-
PLANT (5-6 LOCI MATCH)
ICD-9: 202.4,203,205.1-.9,206.1-.9,
207.1-.8,208.1-.9
CPT: 38230-41
Line: 523   Category: 5

Diagnosis: MALIGNANT NEOPLASM OF
OTHER ENDOCRINE GLANDS
AND RELATED STRUCTURES,
TREATABLE
Treatment: BONE MARROW RESCUE
AND TRANSPLANT
ICD-9: 194
CPT: 38240,38230
Line: 524   Category: 5

Diagnosis: ANOMALIES OF GALL-
BLADDER, BILE DUCTS, AND
LIVER
Treatment: MEDICAL AND SURGICAL
TREATMENT
ICD-9: 751.6
CPT: 90000-99999,47400-47999
Line: 525   Category: 5

Diagnosis: CANCER OF PANCREAS,
TREATABLE
Treatment: MEDICAL AND SURGICAL
TREATMENT
ICD-9: 157,230.9
CPT: 31370-82,37799,42410-26,47760,
47721,49000,60540,90000-99999
Line: 526   Category: 5

Diagnosis: PARASITIC INFESTATION OF
EYELID
Treatment: MEDICAL THERAPY
ICD-9: 373.6
CPT: 90000-99999
Line: 527   Category: 10

Diagnosis: ATELECTASIS (COLLAPSE OF
LUNG)
Treatment: MEDICAL THERAPY
ICD-9: 518.0-.1

CPT: 90000-99999,31645
Line: 528   Category: 10

Diagnosis: HEMORRHAGE AND INFARC-
          TION OF THYROID
Treatment: MEDICAL THERAPY
ICD-9: 246.3
CPT: 90000-99999

Line: 529   Category: 10

Diagnosis: RETINAL TEAR
Treatment: LASER PROPHYLAXIS
ICD-9: 361.30
CPT: 67141-67145
Line: 530   Category: 10

————$120.76 Per Capita Cost Per Month————

Diagnosis: SPONTANEOUS AND MISSED
          ABORTION
Treatment: MEDICAL AND SURGICAL
          TREATMENT
ICD-9: 631-632,634.2-.9
CPT: 59820-21,90000-99999
Line: 531   Category: 10

Diagnosis: INFLAMMATION OF
          LACRIMAL PASSAGES
Treatment: MEDICAL THERAPY
ICD-9: 375
CPT: 90000-99999
Line: 532   Category: 10

Diagnosis: MINOR BURNS
Treatment: MEDICAL THERAPY
ICD-9: 941.0-.1,942.0-.1,943.0-.1,
       944.0-.1, 945.0-.1,946.0-.1,
       948.00, .10,.20,.30,.40,.50,.60,.70,
       .80,.90,949.0-.1
CPT: 11000-1,11040-4,11960-70,14020,
     14040-1,14060,15200,15220,
     15240,15260,15350,15400,
     15500-10,15770,16000-16035,
     20550,20610,35206,64450,
     90000-99999
Line: 533   Category: 10

Diagnosis: ALLERGIC RHINITIS AND
          CONJUNCTIVITIS
Treatment: MEDICAL THERAPY
ICD-9: 477,471,472,372.00-.14
CPT: 90000-99999
Line: 534   Category: 13

Diagnosis: CORNEAL ULCER
Treatment: CONJUNCTIVAL FLAP
ICD-9: 370.0
CPT: 68360
Line: 535   Category: 10

Diagnosis: HYPERESTROGENISM
Treatment: HYSTERECTOMY, MEDICAL
          THERAPY
ICD-9: 256.0
CPT: 58120,58150,90000-99999
Line: 536   Category: 10

Diagnosis: PELVIC PAIN SYNDROME
Treatment: MEDICAL AND SURGICAL
          TREATMENT
ICD-9: 614.1-.2,614.4,614.6-.9,615.1-.9,
       625.0-.2,625.4-.5,625.8-.9
CPT: 11043,58150,58805,58925,58980,
     90000-99999
Line: 537   Category: 13

Diagnosis: RETAINED DENTAL ROOT
Treatment: EXCISION OF DENTO-
          ALVEOLAR STRUCTURE
ICD-9: 525.3
CPT: 41822,41823,41830,41874,
     41825-41827,41828,42299,41899,
     40899,17999
Line: 538   Category: 10

Diagnosis: KERATITIS: CORNEAL UL-
          CER, SUPERFICIAL W/O CON-
          JUNCTIVITIS, OTHER AND
          UNSPECIFIED KERATOCON-
          JUNCTIVITIS, INTERSTITIAL
          & DEEP, CORNEAL NEO-
          VASCULARIZATION
Treatment: KERATOPLASY
ICD-9: 370.0,371.0-371.1,371.23,
       371.4-371.6
CPT: 65730,65920,66985
Line: 539   Category: 10

Diagnosis: TRANSIENT NEPHROTIC
          SYNDROME WITH LESION OF
          MINIMAL CHANGE GLOMER-

ULONEPHRITIS
Treatment: MEDICAL THERAPY
ICD-9: 581.3
CPT: 90000-99999
Line: 540   Category: 10

Diagnosis: TONGUE TIE AND OTHER
ANOMALIES OF TONGUE
Treatment: FRENOTOMY, TONGUE TIE
ICD-9: 750.0-.1
CPT: 40806,40819,41010,41115
Line: 541   Category: 11

Diagnosis: BRANCHIAL CLEFT CYST
Treatment: EXCISION
ICD-9: 744.42
CPT: 42810,42815
Line: 542   Category: 11

Diagnosis: ATROPHY OF EDENTULOUS
ALVEOLAR RIDGE
Treatment: VESTIBULOPLASTY, GRAFTS,
IMPLANTS
ICD-9: 525.2
CPT: 48040,40842,40845,15999,20902,
15350,15510,21210,21215,
21244-50
Line: 543   Category: 11

Diagnosis: SPINE DEFORMITIES
Treatment: ARTHRODESIS/REPAIR/RE-
CONSTRUCTION
ICD-9: 754.2,268.1,756.14,737.0,756.19,
737.11-.12,356.1,731.0,252.0,
737.30-.31,737.33-.39, 724.3
CPT: 22800-22812,22820,22840-22899,
22210-22230,22590-22650,
22554-22585,29010-29035
Line: 544   Category: 11

Diagnosis: BENIGN NEOPLASM OF MALE
GENITAL ORGANS: TESTIS,
PROSTATE, EPIDIDYMIS
Treatment: MEDICAL THERAPY
ICD-9: 222.0,222.2,222.3,222.8,222.9
CPT: 90000-99999
Line: 545   Category: 11

Diagnosis: DISORDERS OF BLADDER
Treatment: MEDICAL AND SURGICAL
TREATMENT
ICD-9: 596.0-.5,596.7-.9

CPT: 90000-99999,51800-45,
51880-980,53660-61,53670
Line: 546   Category: 11

Diagnosis: HYPERTELORISM OF ORBIT
Treatment: ORBITOTOMY
ICD-9: 376.41
CPT: 67400
Line: 547   Category: 11

Diagnosis: DENTAL SERVICES (EG.
TOOTH LOSS)
Treatment: RESTORATIVE DENTAL SER-
VICE
ICD-9: 0
CPT: 01510-25,04240-60,04345,
05110-40,05213-4,05860,
05911-21,05954-5,05949,07270,
07310-20,07560,07610-80,
07710-80,07950,09630
Line: 548   Category: 12

Diagnosis: DENTAL SERVICES (EG.
MALPOSITIONED TOOTH)
Treatment: RESTORATIVE DENTAL SER-
VICE
ICD-9: 0
CPT: 02960,05211-2,05520,05610,
05630-60,05710-21,05750-61,
06212,06242,06792,06972-80,
07271,07280-1,07290,07340-50,
07470-80,07810-50,07860-80,
07920,07960-80,079823,079914
Line: 549   Category: 11

Diagnosis: DENTAL SERVICES (EG. IN-
SUFFICIENT ROOM TO RE-
STORE TOOTH)
Treatment: RESTORATIVE DENTAL SER-
VICE
ICD-9: 0
CPT: 03950,04210-1,04320-1,05620,
05730-41,05810-05850,06211,
06241,06520-40,06752,06780,
06970
Line: 550   Category: 11

Diagnosis: UNSPECIFIED DISEASE OF
HARD TISSUES OF TEETH
(ALVUSION)
Treatment: INTERDENTAL WIRING

ICD-9: 525.9
CPT: 21497
Line: 551   Category: 12

Diagnosis: RETAINED INTRAOCULAR
FOREIGN BODY, MAGNETIC
& NONMAGNETIC
Treatment: FOREIGN BODY REMOVAL
ICD-9: 360.5-360.6
CPT: 65230,65260-65265
Line: 552   Category: 12

Diagnosis: INTERNAL DERANGEMENT
OF KNEE
Treatment: ARTHROSCOPIC REPAIR
ICD-9: 717.1-.3,717.40,717.42-.49
CPT: 29870-89,27403-29
Line: 553   Category: 12

Diagnosis: CLOSED FRACTURE OF
EPIPHYSIS OF UPPER EX-
TREMITIES
Treatment: REDUCTION
ICD-9: 812.09,812.44,813.43
CPT: 25350,25600-20
Line: 554   Category: 12

Diagnosis: CONGENITAL DISLOCATION
OF HIP; COXA VARA & VAL-
GA, CONGENITAL
Treatment: REPAIR/RECONSTRUCTION
ICD-9: 754.3,755.62,755.61
CPT: 27179,27181,27185
Line: 555   Category: 12

Diagnosis: MECHANICAL AND OTHER
COMPLICATION OF INTERN-
AL ORTHOPEDIC AND PROS-
THETIC DEVICE, IMPLANT
AND GRAFT; IMPLANT OR
GRAFT; INFECTION & IN-
FLAMMATORY REACTION
DUE TO INTERNAL PROS-
THETIC DEVICE
Treatment: TREATMENT, ARTHRO-
PLASTY
ICD-9: 996.4,99677,996.66
CPT: 27485-27488,27265,27266,27134,
27137,27138
Line: 556   Category: 12

Diagnosis: DISORDERS OF SHOULDER
Treatment: REPAIR/RECONSTRUCTION
ICD-9: 727.61,726.10,840.4
CPT: 29815-29825,23410-23420,
23440-23466,23107-23125,23190,
23000,23020
Line: 557   Category: 12

Diagnosis: CONGENITAL DISLOCATION
OF KNEE, GENU VARUM &
VALGUM (ACQ'D), CON-
GENITAL BOWING OF FE-
MUR, TIBIA & FIBULA, GENU
RECURVATUM (ACQ'D),
CONGITAL GENU RECUR-
VATUM LONG BONES OF
LEGS, CONGENITAL DE-
FORMITIES OF KNEE
Treatment: OSTEOTOMY
ICD-9: 736.42,754.40-.43,755.64
CPT: 27455,27448-27450
Line: 558   Category: 12

Diagnosis: CONGENITAL DEFORMITIES
OF KNEE
Treatment: ARTHROSCOPIC REPAIR
ICD-9: 755.64
CPT: 29870-89,27403-29
Line: 559   Category: 13

Diagnosis: UNSPECIFIED RETINAL VAS-
CULAR OCCLUSION; CEN-
TRAL RETINAL VEIN OCCLU-
SION, VENOUS TRIBUTARY
(BRANCH) OCCLUSION
Treatment: LASER SURGERY
ICD-9: 362.30,362.35,362.36
CPT: 67228
Line: 560   Category: 12

Diagnosis: EXFOLIATION OF TEETH
DUE TO SYSTEMIC CAUSES
Treatment: EXCISION OF DENTO-
ALVEOLAR STRUCTURE
ICD-9: 525.0
CPT: 41822,41823,41830,41874,
41825-41827,41828,42299,41899,
40899,17999
Line: 561   Category: 12

Diagnosis: RUBEOSIS IRIDIS

Treatment: LASER SURGERY
ICD-9: 364.42
CPT: 67228,66720-66721
Line: 562   Category: 12

Diagnosis: TRAUMATIC AMPUTATION
OF TOE (COMPLETE) (PAR-
TIAL) W/ & W/O COMPLICA-
TION
Treatment: REPLANTATION/AMPUTATE
ICD-9: 895
CPT: 20838-40,28810-25
Line: 563   Category: 12

Diagnosis: PERIPHERAL NERVE DIS-
ORDERS (NON-INJURY)
Treatment: NEUROPLASTY
ICD-9: 353.0-.4,354.1,354.9,355.0,
350.2,355.6,355.8
CPT: 64702-64727,64413-64450,
64774-64792
Line: 564   Category: 12

Diagnosis: DISORDERS OF SWEAT
GLANDS
Treatment: MEDICAL THERAPY
ICD-9: 705.0,705.81,705.89,705.9,780.8
CPT: 90000-99999
Line: 565   Category: 13

Diagnosis: CHONDROMALACIA
Treatment: MEDICAL THERAPY
ICD-9: 733.92
CPT: 90000-99999
Line: 566   Category: 13

Diagnosis: EPIPHYSEAL ARREST
Treatment: MEDICAL THERAPY
ICD-9: 733.91
CPT: 90000-99999
Line: 567   Category: 13

Diagnosis: DIAPHYSITIS
Treatment: MEDICAL THERAPY
ICD-9: 733.99
CPT: 90000-99999
Line: 568   Category: 10

Diagnosis: FRACTURE OF RIBS AND
STERNUM, CLOSED
Treatment: MEDICAL THERAPY

ICD-9: 807.0,807.2
CPT: 90000-99999
Line: 569   Category: 10

Diagnosis: FRACTURE OF ONE OR
MORE PHALANGES OF
FOOT
Treatment: SET
ICD-9: 826
CPT: 29425,28470,28480,28505,28550
Line: 570   Category: 10

Diagnosis: BRACHIAL PLEXUS
LESIONS
Treatment: MEDICAL THERAPY
ICD-9: 353.0
CPT: 90000-99999
Line: 571   Category: 13

Diagnosis: CHRONIC SINUSITIS
Treatment: MEDICAL THERAPY
ICD-9: 473
CPT: 90000-99999
Line: 572   Category: 13

Diagnosis: LUMBAGO; THORACIC OR
LUMBOSACRAL NEURITIS
OR RADICULITIS, UN-
SPECIFIED; POST-
LAMINECTOMY SYNDROME
Treatment: MEDICAL THERAPY
ICD-9: 724.2,724.4,722.8
CPT: 90000-99999
Line: 573   Category: 13

Diagnosis: DYSMENORRHEA
Treatment: MEDICAL THERAPY
ICD-9: 625.3
CPT: 90000-99999
Line: 574   Category: 13

Diagnosis: TIBIAL BURSITIS, OSTEO-
CHONDROPATHIES AND
CONGENITAL DEFORMITIES
OF KNEE
Treatment: MEDICAL THERAPY
ICD-9: 726.62,726.69,732.4,732.7, 755.64
CPT: 90000-99999
Line: 575   Category: 13

Diagnosis: EPICONDYLITIS AND RADIAL

STYLOID TENOSYNOVITIS
Treatment: MEDICAL AND SURGICAL
TREATMENT
ICD-9: 726.31-.32,727.04
CPT: 26035-60,26120-80,26440-597,
26820-63,27095-7,27100-22,
27140-85,27306-7,27448-55,
27466-8,27475-85,27715,
27730-42,64702-4,64718-27,
64774-95,64850-7,64872-999,
90000-99999
Line: 576 Category: 13

Diagnosis: POLYMYALGIA RHEUMA-
TICA
Treatment: MEDICAL THERAPY
ICD-9: 725
CPT: 90000-99999
Line: 577 Category: 13

Diagnosis: RAYNAUD SYNDROME
Treatment: MEDICAL THERAPY
ICD-9: 443
CPT: 90000-99999
Line: 578 Category: 13

Diagnosis: REITER'S DISEASE
Treatment: MEDICAL THERAPY
ICD-9: 099.3
CPT: 90000-99999
Line: 579 Category: 13

Diagnosis: URTICARIA, CHRONIC
Treatment: MEDICAL THERAPY
ICD-9: 708,995.1
CPT: 90000-99999,11000-11101
Line: 580 Category: 13

Diagnosis: KERATODERMA, ACQUIRED;
ACQUIRED ACANTHOSIS
NIGRICANS, STRIAE
ATROPHICAE, OTHER
AND UNSPECIFIED HYPER-
TROPHIC AND ATROPHIC

CONDITIONS OF SKIN
Treatment: MEDICAL THERAPY
ICD-9: 690,698,700,701.1-.3,701.8,
701.9,706.7
CPT: 11000-101,11900,11950-54,
90000-99999
Line: 581 Category: 13

Diagnosis: VERTIGINOUS SYNDROMES
AND OTHER DISORDERS OF
VESTIBULAR SYSTEM
Treatment: MEDICAL THERAPY
ICD-9: 386.0-.2,386.4-.9
CPT: 90000-99999
Line: 582 Category: 13

Diagnosis: DISORDERS OF CERVICAL
REGION
Treatment: CERVICAL LAMINECTOMY,
MEDICAL THERAPY
ICD-9: 721.0,722.4,722.81,723
CPT: 63250,63265,63270,63275,63280,
63285,63001,63015,63020,
63035-40,63045,63045,63048,
63075-76,63081-82,63300,63304,
63170-72,63180-82,63194,63196,
63198,90000-99999
Line: 583 Category: 13

Diagnosis: ERYTHEMATOUS CONDI-
TIONS: TOXIC, NODOSUM,
ROSACEA, LUPUS
Treatment: MEDICAL THERAPY
ICD-9: 695.0,695.2-.9
CPT: 90000-99999,11100-11101
Line: 584 Category: 13

Diagnosis: PLANTAR FASCIAL FIBRO-
MATOSIS
Treatment: MEDICAL THERAPY
ICD-9: 728.71
CPT: 90000-99999
Line: 585 Category: 13

————$127.01 Per Capita Cost Per Month————

Diagnosis: SPONDYLOSIS AND OTHER
CHRONIC DISORDERS OF
BACK
Treatment: MEDICAL AND SURGICAL

TREATMENT
ICD-9: 720,721.2-.5,721.7.721.9,722.3-.5,
722.7-.9,723.0,724,738.4,756.11,
847

CPT: 22100,22105,22110,22140-230,
22548-54,22590-650,22820-99,
62284,62290-1,63001-48,63075-8,
63081-2,63085-8,63090-1,
63300-4,90000-99999
Line: 586   Category: 13

Diagnosis: ESOPHAGITIS
Treatment: MEDICAL THERAPY
ICD-9: 530.1
CPT: 90000-99999
Line: 587   Category: 13

Diagnosis: INTERVERTEBRAL DISC DIS-
ORDERS
Treatment: THORACIC-LUMBAR LAMI-
NECTOMY, MEDICAL THER-
APY
ICD-9: 722.0-.1,722.7,952.1-.9
CPT: 63003,63005,63016,63017,
63030-31,63035,63042,63046-48,
63056-57,63064,63066,63077-78,
63085-91,63170,63173,
90000-99999
Line: 588   Category: 13

Diagnosis: CHRONIC PROSTATITIS,
OTHER DISORDERS OF PROS-
TATE
Treatment: MEDICAL THERAPY
ICD-9: 601.1,602
CPT: 90000-99999
Line: 589   Category: 13

Diagnosis: CHRONIC CYSTITIS
Treatment: MEDICAL THERAPY
ICD-9: 595.1-595.3
CPT: 90000-99999
Line: 590   Category: 13

Diagnosis: IMPETIGO HERPETIFORMIS
AND SUBCORNEAL PUSTU-
LAR DERMATOSIS
Treatment: MEDICAL THERAPY
ICD-9: 694.0-.3
CPT: 90000-99999
Line: 591   Category: 13

Diagnosis: TRIGEMINAL NERVE DIS-
ORDERS
Treatment: MEDICAL & SURGICAL

TREATMENT
ICD-9: 350
CPT: 64400,64600-64610,61450,61458,
90000-99999
Line: 592   Category: 13

Diagnosis: MYASTHENIA GRAVIS
Treatment: MEDICAL THERAPY, THY-
MECTOMY
ICD-9: 358
CPT: 90000-99999,60520
Line: 593   Category: 13

Diagnosis: SPRAINS, STRAINS AND
NON-ALLOPATHIC SPINAL
LESIONS: THORACIC, LUM-
BAR AND SCARUM ACUTE
Treatment: MEDICAL THERAPY
ICD-9: 847.0-.3,739.0-.4
CPT: 90000-99999
Line: 594   Category: 14

Diagnosis: HORDEOLUM AND OTHER
DEEP INFLAMMATION OF
EYELID; CHALAZION
Treatment: INCISION AND DRAIN-
AGE/MEDICAL THERAPY
ICD-9: 373.1-.2
CPT: 90000-99999,67700
Line: 595   Category: 14

Diagnosis: LABYRINTHITIS
Treatment: MEDICAL THERAPY
ICD-9: 386.3
CPT: 90000-99999
Line: 596   Category: 14

Diagnosis: VIRAL HEPATITIS
Treatment: MEDICAL THERAPY
ICD-9: 070
CPT: 90000-99999
Line: 597   Category: 14

Diagnosis: ANOVULATION (IN-
FERTILITY)
Treatment: MEDICAL THERAPY
ICD-9: 621.3,626.0-.1,628.0
CPT: 58100,58920-25,58940,61548,
90000-99999
Line: 598   Category: 15

Diagnosis: HYDROCELE
Treatment: MEDICAL THERAPY, EXCI-
SION
ICD-9: 603
CPT: 54840,55000,55040-41,55060,
55500,90000-99999
Line: 599   Category: 11

Diagnosis: ABSENCE OF BREAST AFTER
MASTECTOMY AS TREAT-
MENT FOR NEOPLASM
Treatment: BREAST RECONSTRUCT
ICD-9: 174,217,233.0,238.3
CPT: 11400-46,17340,19120-60,
19324-42,19360-96,19499
Line: 600   Category: 11

Diagnosis: SPASTIC DYSPHONIA
Treatment: MEDICAL THERAPY
ICD-9: 478.79
CPT: 90000-99999
Line: 601   Category: 11

Diagnosis: FEMALE INFERTILITY OF
CERVICAL ORIGIN, MALE IN-
FERTILITY
Treatment: ARTIFICIAL INSEMINATION,
MEDICAL THERAPY
ICD-9: 628.8-.9,606
CPT: 90000-99999,58310-58311
Line: 602   Category: 15

Diagnosis: TUBAL DISEASE
Treatment: MICROSURGERY
ICD-9: 256,628.2-.4
CPT: 58700,58740-70
Line: 603   Category: 15

Diagnosis: KELOID SCAR; OTHER AB-
NORMAL GRANULATION
TISSUE
Treatment: INTRALESIONAL INJEC-
TIONS/DESTRUCTION/EXCI-
SION
ICD-9: 701.4-.5
CPT: 11900-11901,17000-17105,
11200-11446
Line: 604   Category: 17

Diagnosis: CONJUNCTIVAL CYST
Treatment: EXCISION OF CON-
JUNCTIVAL CYST
ICD-9: 372.75
CPT: 68110
Line: 605   Category: 17

Diagnosis: HEPATORENAL SYNDROME
Treatment: MEDICAL THERAPY
ICD-9: 572.4
CPT: 90000-99999
Line: 606   Category: 3

Diagnosis: OTHER DEFICIENCIES OF
CIRCULATING ENZYMES
(ALPHA 1-ANTITRYPSIN DE-
FICIENCY)
Treatment: LUNG TRANSPLANT
ICD-9: 277.6
CPT: 33935
Line: 607   Category: 5

Diagnosis: LETHAL MIDLINE GRAN-
ULOMA
Treatment: MEDICAL THERAPY
ICD-9: 446.3
CPT: MEDICAL THERAPY
Line: 608   Category: 5

Diagnosis: AMYOTROPHIC LATERAL
SCLEROSIS (ALS)
Treatment: MEDICAL THERAPY
ICD-9: 335.20,335.22-.29
CPT: 90000-99999
Line: 609   Category: 5

Diagnosis: CANCER OF LIVER AND IN-
TRAHEPATIC BILE DUCTS
Treatment: LIVER TRANSPLANT
ICD-9: 155
CPT: 47135
Line: 610   Category: 5

Diagnosis: HEMATOMA OF AURICLE OR
PINNA AND HEMATOMA OF
EXTERNAL EAR
Treatment: DRAINAGE
ICD-9: 216.2,380.0,380.31
CPT: 69000-20
Line: 611   Category: 10

Diagnosis: ENOPHTHALMOS
Treatment: REVISION
ICD-9: 376.5
CPT: 67400

Line: 612   Category: 10

Diagnosis: ACUTE LYMPHADENITIS
Treatment: INCISION AND DRAINAGE
ICD-9: 683
CPT: 10060

Line: 613   Category: 10

Diagnosis: CONGENITAL ANOMALIES
OF FEMAL GENITAL ORGANS
Treatment: SURGICAL TREATMENT
ICD-9: 752.0-.3,752.41
CPT: 57135,57500,57720,58540,58700,
58940,58987,58995

Line: 614   Category: 11

Diagnosis: GENERALIZED CONVULSIVE
OR PARTIAL EPILEPSY WITH-
OUT MENTION OF IMPAIR-
MENT OF CONSCIOUSNESS
Treatment: FOCAL SURGERY
ICD-9: 345.1,345.5
CPT: 61720,61533-61536

Line: 615   Category: 11

Diagnosis: VARICOSE VEINS OF LOWER
EXTREMITIES
Treatment: STRIPPING/SCLEROTHERAPY
ICD-9: 454
CPT: 36468-71,37700,37720-35,37760,
37785-99

Line: 616   Category: 11

Diagnosis: DISEASE OF CAPILLARIES
Treatment: EXCISION
ICD-9: 448.1-.9
CPT: 11400-11426

Line: 617   Category: 11

Diagnosis: ANOMALIES OF RELATION-
SHIP OF JAW TO CRANIAL
BASE, MAJOR ANOMALIES
OF JAW SIZE, OTHER SPEC-
IFIED AND UNSPECIFIED
DENTOFACIAL ANOMALIES
Treatment: OSTEOPLASTY, MAX-
ILLA/MANDIBLE
ICD-9: 524.0-.2,524.5,524.85,524.9
CPT: 21110,21200-21208,21250-54,
21209,30520

Line: 618   Category: 11

Diagnosis: CONGENITAL ANOMALIES
OF THE EAR WITHOUT IM-
PAIRMENT OF HEARING
Treatment: OTOPLASTY, REPAIR & AM-
PUTATION
ICD-9: 744.1-.3
CPT: 69300,69110

Line: 619   Category: 11

Diagnosis: TMJ DISORDER
Treatment: TMJ SPLINTS
ICD-9: 524.6
CPT: 90000-99999

Line: 620   Category: 13

Diagnosis: TMJ DISORDERS
Treatment: TMJ SURGERY
ICD-9: 524.6,524.5,718.08,718.18,
718.28,718.38,718.58
CPT: 21499,21010,20910,21050-70,
21116,21240-21243,21480,21485,
21490,21210,21215,29909,21230,
21235,21254,20926,30520

Line: 621   Category: 11

Diagnosis: DISEASE OF NAILS, HAIR
AND HAIR FOLLICLES
Treatment: MEDICAL THERAPY
ICD-9: 703.8-.9,704.0,704.2-.9,757.4-.5
CPT: 11900,11700-11765,11000-11001,
90000-99999

Line: 622   Category: 13

Diagnosis: CIRCUMSCRIBED SCLERO-
DERMA
Treatment: MEDICAL THERAPY
ICD-9: 701.0
CPT: 90000-99999,11900-11901

Line: 623   Category: 13

Diagnosis: CAVUS DEFORMITY OF
FOOT
Treatment: MEDICAL THERAPY, OR-
THOTIC
ICD-9: 736.73
CPT: 90000-99999

Line: 624   Category: 13

Diagnosis: CERVICAL RIB
Treatment: SURGICAL TREATMENT
ICD-9: 756.2

CPT: 21615-16,21705
Line: 625   Category: 11

Diagnosis: ERYTHROPLAKIA, LEU-
KOEDEMA OF MOUTH OR
TONGUE
Treatment: MEDICAL THERAPY
ICD-9: 528.7
CPT: 90000-99999
Line: 626   Category: 13

Diagnosis: CHRONIC CONJUNCTIVITIS,
BLEPHAROCONJUNCTIVITIS
Treatment: MEDICAL THERAPY
ICD-9: 372.1-372.3
CPT: 90000-99999
Line: 627   Category: 13

Diagnosis: DERMATOPHYTOSIS
Treatment: MEDICAL THERAPY
ICD-9: 110-111
CPT: 90000-99999,11100
Line: 628   Category: 13

Diagnosis: KERATITIS: SUPERFICIAL
W/O CONJUNCTIVITIS, CER-
TAIN TYPES, OTHER AND
UNSPECIFIED K-CONJUNC-
TIVITIS, INTERSTITIAL &
DEEP, CORNEAL NEOVASCU-
LARIZATION, OTHER AND
UNSPECIFIED FORMS
Treatment: MEDICAL THERAPY
ICD-9: 370.2-370.9
CPT: 90000-99999
Line: 629   Category: 13

Diagnosis: DISORDERS OF SYNOVIUM,
TENDON AND BURSA; DIS-
ORDERS OF SOFT TISSUE
AND JOINTS
Treatment: MEDICAL THERAPY
ICD-9: 727.2-.3,729
CPT: 90000-99999
Line: 630   Category: 13

Diagnosis: TENDINITIS AND BURSITIS
Treatment: MEDICAL AND SURGICAL
THERAPY
ICD-9: 726.33,726.71-.72
CPT: 29105,29125-29131,24105,

27060-27062,29240,29260,29270,
29280,29345,29355,29365,
29405-50,20550,20600-10,29345,
29355,29365,90000-99999
Line: 631   Category: 14

Diagnosis: BLEPHARITIS
Treatment: MEDICAL THERAPY
ICD-9: 373.0
CPT: 90000-99999
Line: 632   Category: 13

Diagnosis: XEROSIS
Treatment: MEDICAL THERAPY
ICD-9: 706.8
CPT: 90000-99999,11000-11101
Line: 633   Category: 13

Diagnosis: OBESITY
Treatment: NUTRITIONAL AND LIFE
STYLE COUNSELING
ICD-9: 278
CPT: 90000-99999
Line: 634   Category: 13

Diagnosis: DISORDERS OF FUNCTION
OF STOMACH AND OTHER
FUNCTIONAL DIGESTIVE
DISORDERS
Treatment: MEDICAL THERAPY
ICD-9: 536,564
CPT: 90000-99999
Line: 635   Category: 13

Diagnosis: LICHEN PLANUS
Treatment: MEDICAL THERAPY
ICD-9: 697
CPT: 90000-99999,11900-11901
Line: 636   Category: 13

Diagnosis: MONOMEUROPATHY
Treatment: MEDICAL THERAPY
ICD-9: 354.0,354.2-.9
CPT: 90000-99999
Line: 637   Category: 13

Diagnosis: POSTCONCUSSION SYN-
DROME
Treatment: MEDICAL THERAPY
ICD-9: 310.2
CPT: 90000-99999

Line: 638　　Category: 13

Diagnosis: HERPES SIMPLEX WITHOUT COMPLICATIONS
Treatment: MEDICAL THERAPY
ICD-9: 054.0,054.2,054.6,054.8-.9
CPT: 90000-99999
Line: 639　　Category: 13

Diagnosis: TESTICULAR AND POLY-GLANDULAR DYSFUNCTION
Treatment: MEDICAL THERAPY
ICD-9: 257-258
CPT: 90000-99999
Line: 640　　Category: 13

——$134.61 Per Capita Cost Per Month——

Diagnosis: OTOSCLEROSIS
Treatment: MEDICAL THERAPY
ICD-9: 387
CPT: 90000-99999
Line: 641　　Category: 13

Diagnosis: PERIPHERAL EN-THESOPATHIES
Treatment: MEDICAL THERAPY
ICD-9: 726.30-.32,726.4-.6,726.70, 726.8,726.90
CPT: 90000-99999
Line: 642　　Category: 13

Diagnosis: CHRONIC BRONCHITIS
Treatment: MEDICAL THERAPY
ICD-9: 490-491,493.9
CPT: 90000-99999
Line: 643　　Category: 13

Diagnosis: SARCOIDOSIS
Treatment: MEDICAL THERAPY
ICD-9: 135
CPT: 90000-99999
Line: 644　　Category: 13

Diagnosis: BENIGN INTRACRANIAL HY-PERTENSION
Treatment: MEDICAL THERAPY
ICD-9: 348.2
CPT: 90000-99999
Line: 645　　Category: 13

Diagnosis: LYMPHEDEMA
Treatment: MEDICAL THERAPY, OTHER OPERATION ON LYMPH CHANNEL
ICD-9: 457,140-144
CPT: 90000-99999,38300-38308, 38382-38555,38700-38761

Line: 646　　Category: 13

Diagnosis: PHLEBITIS AND THROM-BOPHLEBITIS, SUPERFICIAL
Treatment: MEDICAL THERAPY
ICD-9: 451
CPT: 90000-99999
Line: 647　　Category: 13

Diagnosis: SYNOVITIS AND TENOSYNO-VITIS
Treatment: MEDICAL THERAPY
ICD-9: 727.0
CPT: 90000-99999,20550
Line: 648　　Category: 14

Diagnosis: DIAPER OR NAPKIN RASH
Treatment: MEDICAL THERAPY
ICD-9: 691.0
CPT: 90000-99999,11100
Line: 649　　Category: 14

Diagnosis: ORAL APHTHAE
Treatment: MEDICAL THERAPY
ICD-9: 528.2
CPT: 90000-99999
Line: 650　　Category: 14

Diagnosis: DERMATITIS DUE TO SUB-STANCES TAKEN INTER-NALLY
Treatment: MEDICAL THERAPY
ICD-9: 693
CPT: 90000-99999,11100
Line: 651　　Category: 14

Diagnosis: FOOD ALLERGY
Treatment: MEDICAL THERAPY
ICD-9: 692.5
CPT: 90000-99999

Line: 652   Category: 13

Diagnosis: SPRAINS OF JOINTS AND AD-
JACENT MUSCLES
Treatment: MEDICAL THERAPY
ICD-9: 717.5,717.8,840.1-844.2, 844.8-
.9,845.00-.03,845.1, 848.5
CPT: 29049-29085,29105-29131,
29200-29280,29305-29580,
29700-29799,90000-99999
Line: 653   Category: 14

Diagnosis: SUBLINGUAL, SCROTAL,
AND PELVIC VARICES
Treatment: VENOUS INJECTION, VASCU-
LAR SURGERY
ICD-9: 456.3-.5
CPT: 36470,37798-9,55530-35
Line: 654   Category: 11

Diagnosis: SPRAIN/STRAIN OF ACHILL-
ES TENDON
Treatment: MEDICAL THERAPY
ICD-9: 845.09
CPT: 90000-99999
Line: 655   Category: 14

Diagnosis: FRACTURE OF VERTEBRAL
COLUMN WITHOUT SPINAL
CORD INJURY, SACRUM AND
COCCYX
Treatment: LAMINECTOMY
ICD-9: 805.6-805.9
CPT: 22845,61720-61793
Line: 656   Category: 14

Diagnosis: ACUTE URTICARIA
Treatment: MEDICAL THERAPY
ICD-9: 708,995.1
CPT: 90000-99999
Line: 657   Category: 14

Diagnosis: CANDIDIASIS
Treatment: MEDICAL THERAPY
ICD-9: 112.0,112.3
CPT: 90000-99999
Line: 658   Category: 14

Diagnosis: SCLERITIS & EPISCLERITIS
Treatment: MEDICAL THERAPY
ICD-9: 379.0

CPT: 90000-99999
Line: 659   Category: 14

Diagnosis: INTERNAL INFECTIONS AND
OTHER BACTERIAL FOOD
POISONING
Treatment: MEDICAL THERAPY
ICD-9: 003.0,003.8-.9,005.0,005.2-.9,
008-009,027.1-.9
CPT: 90000-99999
Line: 660   Category: 14

Diagnosis: OPEN WOUND OF INTERNAL
STRUCTURES OF MOUTH
W/O COMPLICATION
Treatment: REPAIR SOFT TISSUES
ICD-9: 873.6
CPT: 13300,41251,41282,12001-57,
13131,13132,13151-2,40831
Line: 661   Category: 14

Diagnosis: VIRAL, SELF-LIMITING EN-
CEPHALITIS, MYELITIS AND
ENCEPHALOMYELITIS
Treatment: MEDICAL THERAPY
ICD-9: 056.0,323
CPT: 90000-99999
Line: 662   Category: 14

Diagnosis: ACUTE TONSILLITIS
Treatment: MEDICAL THERAPY
ICD-9: 463
CPT: 90000-99999
Line: 663   Category: 14

Diagnosis: ERYTHEMA MULTIFORME
Treatment: MEDICAL THERAPY
ICD-9: 695.1
CPT: 90000-99999,11100-11101
Line: 664   Category: 14

Diagnosis: CENTRAL SEROUS RETINO-
PATHY
Treatment: LASER SURGERY
ICD-9: 362.41
CPT: 67210
Line: 665   Category: 14

Diagnosis: VULVAL VARICES
Treatment: VASCULAR SURGERY
ICD-9: 456.6

CPT: 37799
Line: 666   Category: 14

Diagnosis: ASEPTIC MENINGITIS
Treatment: MEDICAL THERAPY
ICD-9: 047-049
CPT: 90000-99999
Line: 667   Category: 14

Diagnosis: INFECTIOUS MONONUCLE-
OSIS
Treatment: MEDICAL THERAPY
ICD-9: 075
CPT: 90000-99999
Line: 668   Category: 14

Diagnosis: OTHER NONFATAL VIRAL
INFECTIONS
Treatment: MEDICAL THERAPY
ICD-9: 051-053,055,056.9,057,072,
074,078.0,078.2-.8,079,480,
487.2-.9
CPT: 90000-99999
Line: 669   Category: 14

Diagnosis: ACUTE PHARYNGITIS AND
LARYNGITIS AND OTHER
DISEASES OF VOCAL CORDS
Treatment: MEDICAL THERAPY
ICD-9: 462,478.5
CPT: 90000-99999
Line: 670   Category: 14

Diagnosis: PREVENTIVE SERVICES FOR
ADULTS WITH QUESTION-
ABLE OR NO PROVEN EF-
FECTIVENESS
Treatment: MEDICAL THERAPY
ICD-9: 0
CPT: 90000-99999
Line: 671   Category: 16

Diagnosis: OLD LACERATION OF CER-
VIX AND VAGINA
Treatment: MEDICAL THERAPY
ICD-9: 622.3,624.4
CPT: 90000-99999
Line: 672   Category: 17

Diagnosis: BENIGN NEOPLASMS OF
SKIN

Treatment: MEDICAL THERAPY
ICD-9: 210,214,216,221,222.1,222.4
CPT: 10000-61,10120-61,11000,
11050-446,11600-46,12031-2,
13100-51,14001,17000-306,
19120,20000-5,20550,21030,
21044,21499,21501,23030,23040,
23930-1,25028-31,26010-30,
26989-91,27301,27603-4,28001,
31540,40800-12,41116,41800,
41826,41899,42415,42440,42808,
90000-99999
Line: 673   Category: 17

Diagnosis: REDUNDANT PREPUCE AND
PHIMOSIS
Treatment: MEDICAL THERAPY, DILA-
TION
ICD-9: 605
CPT: 54150-61,90000-99999
Line: 674   Category: 17

Diagnosis: VITILIGO, CONGENITAL PIG-
MENTARY ANOMALIES OF
SKIN
Treatment: MEDICAL THERAPY
ICD-9: 709.0,757.3,757.9
CPT: 90000-99999
Line: 675   Category: 17

Diagnosis: DENTAL SERVICES (MARG-
INAL IMPROVEMENT)
Treatment: RESTORATIVE DENTAL SER-
VICE
ICD-9: 0
CPT: 01204-5,09910,09940,09952,
07291,07272,06940,04261-72,
03910-20
Line: 676   Category: 17

Diagnosis: SEBORRHEIC KERATOSIS,
DYSCHROMIA, AND VASCU-
LAR DISORDERS, SCAR CON-
DITIONS, AND FIBROSIS OF
SKIN
Treatment: MEDICAL THERAPY
ICD-9: 702,709.1-.3,709.8-.9
CPT: 11000,11050,17000,90000-99999
Line: 677   Category: 17

Diagnosis: VIRAL WARTS

Treatment: MEDICAL THERAPY, CRYO-
SURGERY
ICD-9: 078.1
CPT: 90000-99999,17100,17110,
17340,17000,11900,28043,
46900-46924,54050-54065,56486,
11050,11100-11101,11901
Line: 678   Category: 17

Diagnosis: UPPER EXTREMITY: FINGER-
TIP EVULSION W/O PEDICLE
GRAFT
Treatment: REPAIR
ICD-9: 883.1,883.2
CPT: 12401
Line: 679   Category: 17

Diagnosis: AGENESIS OF LUNG
Treatment: MEDICAL THERAPY
ICD-9: 748.5
CPT: 90000-99999
Line: 680   Category: 17

Diagnosis: GALLSTONES WITHOUT
CHOLECYSTITIS
Treatment: MEDICAL THERAPY, CHO-
LECYSTECTOMY
ICD-9: 574.2,575.6
CPT: 90000-99999,47490,47600-20,
49000
Line: 681   Category: 17

Diagnosis: SIMPLE AND UNSPECIFIED
GOITER, NONTOXIC NODU-
LAR GOITER
Treatment: MEDICAL THERAPY
ICD-9: 240-241
CPT: 90000-99999
Line: 682   Category: 17

Diagnosis: SICCA SYNDROME
Treatment: MEDICAL THERAPY
ICD-9: 710.2
CPT: 90000-99999
Line: 683   Category: 17

Diagnosis: TRAUMATIC BRAIN INJURY,
STATIC DEMENTIA, BRAIN
ANOXIA DUE TO INFECTION
OR TRAUMA
Treatment: MEDICAL THERAPY
ICD-9: 295.9,299.0,319,348.1,348.3-.4,

851.0,850.2-.5,854.0,905.0
CPT: 61107,90000-99999
Line: 684   Category: 17

Diagnosis: ICHTHYOSIS
Treatment: MEDICAL THERAPY
ICD-9: 757.1
CPT: 90000-99999
Line: 685   Category: 17

Diagnosis: PROGRESSIVE DEMENTIA,
ORGANIC BRAIN SYNDROME
Treatment: MEDICAL THERAPY
ICD-9: 046.1,090.40,094.1,290.294.1,
310,331
CPT: 90000-99999
Line: 686   Category: 17

Diagnosis: INTRAVENTRICULAR AND
SUBARACHNOID HEMOR-
RHAGE OF FETUS OR NEO-
NATE
Treatment: MEDICAL THERAPY
ICD-9: 772.1-.2
CPT: 90000-99999
Line: 687   Category: 2

Diagnosis: CANCER OF VARIOUS SITES
WITH DISTANT METASTASES
WHERE TREATMENT WILL
NOT RESULT IN A 10% 5
YEAR SURVIVAL
Treatment: MEDICAL AND SURGICAL
TREATMENT
ICD-9: 140-198
CPT: 11600-46,38720-24,41110-14,
41130,42120,42842-45,42880,
47610,44131,47420-40,58951,
61500,61510,61518-21, 61546-48,
90000-99999
Line: 688   Category: 17

Diagnosis: SENSORINEURAL HEARING
LOSS
Treatment: COCHLEAR IMPLANT
ICD-9: 389.1
CPT: 69930
Line: 689   Category: 11

Diagnosis: ALCOHOLIC CIRRHOSIS OF
LIVER

Treatment: LIVER TRANSPLANT
ICD-9: 571.2
CPT: 47135
Line: 690   Category: 5

Diagnosis: NON-HODGKIN'S LYM-
PHOMAS
Treatment: BONE MARROW TRANS-
PLANT (5-6 LOCI MATCH)
ICD-9: 200,202.0-.2,202.8-.9
CPT: 38230-41
Line: 691   Category: 5

Diagnosis: OBESITY
Treatment: GASTROPLASTY
ICD-9: 278
CPT: 43845
Line: 692   Category: 11

Diagnosis: CONGENITAL CYSTIC LUNG
- SEVERE
Treatment: LUNG RESECTION
ICD-9: 748.4
CPT: 32500
Line: 693   Category: 17

Diagnosis: BENIGN POLYPS OF VOCAL
CORDS
Treatment: MEDICAL THERAPY
ICD-9: 478.4
CPT: 90000-99999
Line: 694   Category: 10

Diagnosis: ACUTE UPPER RESPIRATORY
INFECTIONS AND COMMON
COLD
Treatment: MEDICAL THERAPY
ICD-9: 460,465
CPT: 90000-99999
Line: 695   Category: 14

——$142.44 Per Capita Cost Per Month——

Diagnosis: TUBAL DYSFUNCTION AND
OTHER CASES OF IN-
FERTILITY
Treatment: IN-VITRO FERTILIZATION,
GIFT
ICD-9: 256
CPT: 58970-76
Line: 696   Category: 15

Diagnosis: DENTAL SERVICES (EG. OB-
SOLETE TREATMENTS FOR
VARIOUS CONDITIONS)
Treatment: RESTORATIVE DENTAL SER-
VICE
ICD-9: 0
CPT: 01310,01380-7,02410-30,
02510-630,02710-810,02950,
02952-4,02961-2,03460,03960,
05215-81,05862,05976,06210,
06240,06250-2,06545,06720-51,
06790-1,06950,08110-999,09950
Line: 697   Category: 17

Diagnosis: UNCOMPLICATED HEM-
ORRHOIDS
Treatment: HEMORRHOIDECTOMY
ICD-9: 455.0,455.3,455.6,455.9

CPT: 10140,45336,46083,46220-62,
46320,46500,46934-36
Line: 698   Category: 17

Diagnosis: MINOR HEAD INJURY:
HEMATOMA/EDEMA W/
NO/BRIEF LOSS OF CON-
SCIOUSNESS
Treatment: MEDICAL THERAPY
ICD-9: 851.02,851.12,851.82,
851.92,851.42,851.52, 850.9
CPT: 90000-99999
Line: 699   Category: 17

Diagnosis: GYNECOMASTIA
Treatment: MASTOPEXY
ICD-9: 611.1
CPT: 19316
Line: 700   Category: 17

Diagnosis: CYST OF KIDNEY, ACQUIRED
Treatment: MEDICAL AND SURGICAL
TREATMENT
ICD-9: 593.2
CPT: 50010,50390,90000-99999
Line: 701   Category: 17

Diagnosis: END STAGE HIV DISEASE
Treatment: MEDICAL THERAPY
ICD-9: 042-043
CPT: 90000-99999
Line: 702   Category: 17

Diagnosis: CHRONIC PANCREATITIS
Treatment: SURGICAL TREATMENT
ICD-9: 577.1
CPT: 48000,48999,49000
Line: 703   Category: 17

Diagnosis: SUPERFICIAL WOUNDS
WITHOUT INFECTION AND
CONTUSIONS
Treatment: MEDICAL THERAPY
ICD-9: 910.0,.2,.4,.6,.8,911.0,.2,.4,.6,.8,
912.0,.2,.4,.6, .8,913.0,.2,.4,.6,.8,
914.0,.2,.4,.6,.8,915.0,.2,.4,.6,.8,
916.0,.2,.4,.6,.8,917.0,.2,.4,.6,.8,
919.0,.2,.4,.6,.8,920-924
CPT: 10140,11740,12001-14,
90000-99999
Line: 704   Category: 17

Diagnosis: CONSTITUTIONAL APLASTIC
ANEMIA
Treatment: MEDICAL THERAPY
ICD-9: 284.0
CPT: 90000-99999
Line: 705   Category: 17

Diagnosis: PROLAPSED URETHRAL MU-
COSA
Treatment: SURGICAL TREATMENT
ICD-9: 599.5
CPT: 51840-41
Line: 706   Category: 11

Diagnosis: CENTRAL RETINAL ARTERY
OCCLUSION
Treatment: PARACENTESIS OF AQUEOUS
ICD-9: 362.31
CPT: 67015,67505
Line: 707   Category: 17

Diagnosis: EXTREMELY LOW BIRTH
WEIGHT (UNDER 500 GM)
AND UNDER 23 WEEK GES-
TATION
Treatment: LIFE SUPPORT
ICD-9: 765.0,765.11
CPT: 0
Line: 708   Category: 17

Diagnosis: ANENCEPHALOUS AND SIMI-
LAR ANOMALIES AND RE-
DUCTION DEFORMITIES OF
THE BRAIN
Treatment: LIFE SUPPORT
ICD-9: 740,742.2
CPT: 0
Line: 709   Category: 17

——$145.15 Per Capita Cost Per Month——

References

"A Call for Action." (1990). A final report of the Pepper Commission. Washington, D.C.: U.S. Government Printing Office.

Aaron, H. A., & Schwartz, W. B. (1990). Rationing health care: The choice before us. *Science* **247**, 418–422.

AFL–CIO Health Security Action News. (1989). UAW President calls for renewed drive for national health insurance program. February/March 1989.

American Academy of Pediatrics (1971). Committee on Fetus and Newborn. *Hospital care of newborn infants* (5th ed.). Winston, IL: American Academy of Pediatrics.

American Cancer Society (1991). *Cancer Facts and Figures-1990.* Atlanta: American Cancer Society.

American Public Health Association (1991). *An assessment of selected national health program concept papers.* Washington, D.C.: American Public Health Association (unpublished).

Anderson, N. H. (1979). Algebraic rules in psychological measurement. *American Scientist,* **67,** 555–563.

Anderson, J. P., Bush, J. W., Chen, M. M., & Dolenc, D. C. (1986). Policy space areas and properties of benefit-cost/utility analysis. *Journal of the American Medical Association,* **255**(6), 794–795.

Anderson, J. P., Kaplan, R. M., Berry, C. C., Bush, J. W., & Rumbaut, R. G. (1989). Interday reliability of function assessment for a health status measure: The quality of well-being scale. *Medical Care,* **27**(11), 1076–1084.

Balaban, D. J., Fagi, P. C., Goldfarb, N. I., & Nettler, S. (1986). Weights for scoring the quality of well-being instrument among rheumatoid arthritics. *Medical Care,* **24**(11), 973–980.

Ballugooie, E., Hooymans, J. M., Timmerman, Z., Reitsma, W. D., Sluiter, W. S., Schweitzer, N., & Doorenbos, H. (1984). Rapid deterioration of diabetic retinopathy during treatment with continuous subcutaneous insulin infusion. *Diabetes Care,* **7,** 236–242.

Bergner, M. (1989). Quality of life, health status, and clinical research. *Medical Care,* **27**(3), S148–S156.

Bernstein, H. (1989). After 40 years, Truman is proved right on health care. *Los Angeles Times,* May 9, 1989.

Berwick, D. M., Cretin, S., & Keeler, E. B. (1980) *Cholesterol, children, and heart disease: An analysis of alternatives.* Oxford University Press.

Blendon, R. J., & Edwards, J. N. (1991). Caring for the uninsured. Choices for reform. *Journal of the American Medical Association,* **265,** 2563–2565.

Bloom, B. (1990). Health Insurance and Medical Care: *Health of our nation's children, United States, 1988* (Report no. 188). Hyattsville, MD: National Center for Health Statistics.

Blue Cross and Blue Shield Association (1990). *Environmental Analysis, 1990.* Chicago.

Bombardier, C., Tugwell, P., & Sinclair, A. (1982). Preference for endpoint measures in clinical trials: Results of structured workshops. *Journal of Rheumatology,* **9,** 798–801.

Bombardier, C., Ware, J., Russell, I. J., Larson, Chalmers, & Read. (1986). Auranofin therapy and quality of life for patients with rheumatoid arthritis: Results of a multi-center trial. *American Journal of Medicine,* **81,** 565–578.

Boyle, M. H., Torrance, G. W., Sinclair, J. C., Horwood, S. P. (1983). Economic evaluation of neonatal intensive care of very-low-birth-weight infants. *New England Journal of Medicine,* **308**(22), 1330–1337.

Braumwald, E. (1977). Coronary artery surgery at the crossroad. *New England Journal of Medicine,* **297,** 661–663.

Bronow, R. S., Beltran, R. A., Cohen, S. C., Elliott, P. T., Goldman, G. M., & Spotnitz, G. (1991). The Physicians Who Care plan. Preserving quality and equitability in American medicine. *Journal of the American Medical Association,* **265,** 2211–2215.

Brook, R. H., & Lohr, K. (1986). Will we need to ration effective health care? *Issues in Science and Technology,* **3,** 68–77.

Brook, R. H., Park, R. E., Chassin, M. R., Kosecoff, J., Keesey, J., & Solomon, D. H. (1990). Carotid endarterectomy for elderly patients: Predicting complications. *Annals of Internal Medicine,* **113**(10), 747–753.

Buckingham, J. (1991). *Los Angeles Times,* December 16, 1991, p. A38.

Bush, J. W., Fanshel, S., & Chen, M. (1972). Analysis of a tuberculin testing program using a health status index. *Socio-economic Planning Sciences,* **6,** 49–68.

Bush, J. W., Chen, M. M., & Patrick, D. L. (1973). Cost-effectiveness using a health status index: Analysis of the New York State PKU screening program. In R. Berg (Ed.), *Health status index* (pp. 172–208). Chicago: Hospital Research and Educational Trust.

Bush, J. W., Chen, M. M., & Patrick, D. L. (1983). Cost-effectiveness using a health status index: Analysis of the New York State PKU screening program. *In* R. Berg (Ed.), *Health Status Indexes* (pp.172–208). Chicago: Hospital Research and Education Trust.

Butler, S. M., (1991). A tax reform strategy to deal with the uninsured. *Journal of the American Medical Association,* **265,** 2541–2548.

Campeau, L., Lesteiance, J., & Hermann, J. (1979). Loss of the improvement of angina between one and seven years after aortocoronary bypass surgery. *Circulation,* **60**(1), 51–55.

Cantor, J. C., Barrand, N. L., Desonia, R. A., Cohen, A. B., & Merrill, J. C. (1991). Business leaders views on American health care. *Health Affairs,* **10**(1), 98–105.

CASS Principle Investigators and Their Associates. (1983). Coronary artery surgery study (CASS). A randomized trial of coronary artery bypass survival data. *Circulation.* **68,** 939.

Centers for Disease Control (1991). Mortality attributable to HIV infection/AIDS, United States, 1981–1990. *Morbidity and Mortality Weekly Report,* **40**(3), 41.

Chollet, D., Folley, J., & Mages, C. (1990). Uninsured in the United States: The non-elderly population without health insurance, 1988. Washington, D.C.: Employee Benefit Research Institute.

Christiansen, E. H., & Nielsen, R. L. (1990). *Fourth annual Gallop California health care poll.* Unpublished document, The Gallop Organization, Irvine, CA.

Churchill, D. N., Lemon, B. C., Torrance, G. W. (1984). A cost-effectiveness analysis of continuous abulatory peritoneal dialysis and hospital hemodialysis. *Medical Decision Making,* **4**(4), 489–500.

Daniels, N. (1991). Is the Oregon rationing plan fair? *Journal of the American Medical Association,* **265,** 2232–2235.

Detsky, A. S., & Naglie, I. G. (1990). A clinician's guide to cost-effectiveness analysis. *Annals of Internal Medicine,* **113**(2), 147–154.

DiMatteo, M. R., & DiNicola, D. E. (1982). *Achieving patient compliance.* Elmsford, NY: Pergamon Press.

Doll, R., & Peto, R. (1981). *The causes of cancer* New York: Oxford University Press.

Doubelet, P., Weinstein, M. C., & McNeil, B. J. (1986). Use and misuse of the term "cost effectiveness" in medicine. *New England Journal of Medicine,* **314,** 253–256.

Drummond, M. F., Stoddard, G. L., & Torrance, G. W. (1987). *Methods for the economic evaluation of health care programmes.* Oxford: Oxford University Press.

The Economist. (1991). A survey of health care surgery needed. *The Economist,* July 6, 1991.

Eddy, D. M. (1989). Screening for breast cancer. *Annals of Internal Medicine,* **111,** 389–399.

Eddy, D. M. (1991). Oregon's methods: Did cost-effectiveness analysis fail? *Journal of the American Medical Association,* **266,** 2135–2141.

Eisenberg, J. M. (1991). Economics. (1991). *Journal of the American Medical Association,* **265**(23), 3113–3115.

Enthoven, A. C. (1980). Health plan: *The only practical solution to the soaring cost of medical care.* Redding, MA: Addison-Wesley Publishing Company.

Enthoven, A. C. (1991). Market forces and health care costs. *Journal of the American Medical Association,* **266,** 2751–2752.

Enthoven, A. C., & Kronick, R. (1991). Universal health insurance through incentives reform. *Journal of the American Medical Association,* **265,** 2532–2536.

Epstein, K. A., Schneiderman, L. J., Bush, J. W., & Zettner, W. R. (1981). The "abnormal" screening of thyroxine (T4): Analysis of physician response, outcome, cost and health effectiveness. *Journal of Chronic Disease,* **34,** 175–190.

Erickson, P., Kendal, E. A., Anderson, J. P., & Kaplan, R. M. (1989). Using composite health status measures to assess the nation's health. *Medical Care,* **27**(3), S66–S76.

European Coronary Surgery Study Group. (1979). Coronary-artery bypass surgery in stable angina pectoris: Survival at two years. *Lancet,* **i,** 889–893.

European Coronary Surgery Study Group. (1980). Prospective randomized study of coronary artery bypass surgery in stable angina pectoris. *Lancet* **ii**, 491–495.

Fanshel, S., & Bush, J. W. (1970). A health-status index and its applications to health-services outcomes. *Operations Research,* **18**, 1021–1066.

Fedson, D. S., Wajda, A., Nicol, J. P., Roos, L. L. (1992). Disparity between influenza vaccination rates and risks for influenza-associated hospital discharge and death in Manitoba in 1982–1983. *Annals of Internal Medicine,* **116**(7), 550–555.

Fein, R. (1991). The health security partnership. A federal-state universal insurance and cost-containment program. *Journal of the American Medical Association,* **265,** 2555–2558.

Feinstein, A. R. (1988). Statistical significance. *Quality of Life and Cardiovascular Diseases,* **4,** 1–10.

Fetter, R., Youngshoo, S., & Freeman, J. L. (1980). Case-mixed definition by diagnosis-related groups. *Medical Care,* **18**(suppl), 1.

Fischl, M. A., Richman, D. D. & Grieco, M. H. *et al.* (1987). The efficiency of azidothymidine (AZT) in the treatment of patients with AIDS and AIDS-related complex: A double-blind, placebo-controlled trial. *New England Journal of Medicine,* **317,** 185–191.

Fisher, E. S., Welch, H. G., & Wennberg, J. E. (1992). Prioritizing Oregon's hospital resources: An example bases on variations in descretionary medical utilization. *Journal of the American Medical Association,* **267,** 1925–1931.

Fitzgerald, J. F., Moore, P. S., & Dittus, R. S. (1988). The care of elderly patients with hip fracture. *New England Journal of Medicine,* **319,** 1392–1397.

Fries, J. F., Green, L. W., & Levine, S. (1989). Health promotion and the compression of morbidity. *Lancet,* **1**(8636), 481–483.

Fuchs, V. R., & Hahn, J. S. (1990). How does Canada do it? A comparison of expenditures for physicians' services in the United States and Canada. *New England Journal of Medicine,* **323**(13), 884–890.

Ganiats, T. G., Humphrey, J. D. C., Tares, H. L., & Kaplan, R. M. (1991). Routine neonatal circumcision: A cost–utility analysis. *Medical Decision Making,* **11,** 282–293.

Gerber, A. (1992). *Under the knife: A surgeon dissects America's health care.* Manuscript in preparation, University of California, San Diego.

Gillette, R. D. (1991). Setting health care priorities in Oregon. *Journal of the American Medical Association,* **266,** 1080.

Greely, H. (1992). Implementing the model proposal: Three hard questions and one proposed answer. *In* D. Hadorn (Ed.) *Health care needs, basic benefits, and clinical guidelines.* New York: Waverly Press.

Grumbach, K., Bodenheimer, T., Hemmilstein, D. U., & Woolhandler, S. (1991). Liberal benefits, conservative spending, the physicians for a national health program proposal. *Journal of the American Medical Association,* **265,** 2549–2554.

Guyatt, G., Walter, S., & Norman, G. (1987). Measuring change over time: Assessing the usefulness of evaluative instruments. *Journal of Chronic Disease,* **40,** 171.

Hadorn, D. C. (1991a). Setting health care priorities in Oregon: Cost-effectiveness meets the rule of rescue. *Journal of the American Medical Association,* **265,** 2218–2225. Copyright 1991, American Medical Association.

Hadorn, D. C. (1991b). Reply to doctors Gillette & MacLean. *Journal of the American Medical Association,* **266,** 1081.

Hadorn, D. C., & Brook, R. H. (1991). The health care resource allocation debate. Defining our terms. *Journal of the American Medical Association, 266*(23), 3328–3331.

Hall, J., Gerard, K., Salkeld, G., & Richardson, J. (1992). A cost/utility analysis of mammography screening in Australia. *Social Science and Medicine,* in press.

Hasnain, R., & Garland, M. (1990). Report to the health services commission to identify public values for use in the health services prioritization process. Technical Report, Oregon Health Services Commission. April, 1990.

Haynes, R. B., Sackett, D. L., Gibson, E. S., Taylor, D. W., Hackett, B. C., Roberts, R. S., & Johnson, A. L. (1976). Improvement of medication compliance in uncontrolled hypertension. *Lancet,* **i,** 1265–1268.

Health Care Financing Administration (1988). Office of the Actuary. Expenditures and percent of gross national product for national health expenditures by private and public funds, hospital care, and physician services: Calendar years 1960–87. *Health Care Financing Review,* **10,** 2.

Healthy people 2000: National health promotion and disease prevention objectives (1991). [Washington, D.C.]: U.S. Dept. of Health and Human Services, Public Health Service: For sale by the Supt. of Docs., U.S. G.P.O.

Health Care Financing Administration (1990). Metropolitan Life Insurance Company, Statistical Bulletin, January–March 1990.

Hewitt, M., Recker, D., & Sa'adah, S. (1991). Method of prioritizing health services under Oregon's proposed Medicaid demonstration project. Washington, D.C.: U.S. Congress Office of Technology Assessment.

Hillman, A. L. (1990). Health maintenance organizations, financial incentives, and physicians' judgments. *Annals of Internal Medicine,* **112**(12), 891–893.

Hillman, A. L., Pauly, M. V., & Kerstein, J. J. (1989). How do financial incentives affect physician's clinical decisions and the financial performance of health maintenance organizations? *New England Journal of Medicine,* **321,** 86–92.

Hillman, B. J., Joseph, C. A., Mabry, M. R., Sunshine, J. H., Kennedy, S. D., & Noether, M. (1990). Frequency and costs of diagnostic imaging in office practice—a comparison of self-referring and radiologist-referring physicians. *New England Journal of Medicine,* **323**(23), 1604–1608.

Himmelstein, D. U., & Woolhandler, S. (1991a). Who care for the care givers? Lack of health insurance among health and insurance personnel. *Journal of the American Medical Association,* **266**(3), 399–401.

Hsaio, W. C., Braun, P., Dunn, D., & Becker, E. R. (1988a). Resource-based relative values. An overview. *Journal of the American Medical Association,* **260**(16), 2347–2353.

Hsaio, W. C., Yntema, D. B., Braun, P., Dunn, D., & Spencer, C. (1988b). Measurement and analysis of intraservice work. *Journal of the American Medical Association,* **260**(16), 2361–2370.

Hsaio, W. C., *et al.* (1990). A national study of resource-based relative value scales for physician services: Phase two final report. Boston: Harvard School of Public Health.

Hsaio, W., Braun, P., Becker, E. R., & Dunn, D. (1992). RBRVS: Objections to Maloney, I. *Journal of the American Medical Association,* **267,** 1822–1823.

Hu, T., Bai, J., Keeler, T. E., & Barnett, P. G. (1991). The impact of a large tax increase on cigarette consumption: The case of California. Unpublished manuscript, School of Public Health, University of California, Berkeley.

Hultgren, H. N., Shettigar, R., & Miller, D. C. (1982). Medical versus surgical treatment of unstable angina. *American Journal of Cardiology, 50,* 663–670.

Iacocca, L. (1989). We've had a ten-year war on rising costs of health care-and lost it. *Durham Morning Herald,* April 3, 1989.

Inglehart, J. F. (1991). Efforts to address the problems of physician self-referral. *New England Journal of Medicine, 325,* 1820–1824.

Inglehart, J. K. (1992). The American health care system. *New England Journal of Medicine. 396,* 962–967.

Jackson-Beck, B. M., & Kleinman, J. K. (1983). Evidence for self-selection among health maintenance organization enrollees. *Journal of the American Medical Association,* **250,** 2826.

Jajich-Toth, C., & Roper, B. W. (1990). Americans' views on health care: A study in contradictions. *Health Affairs, 9*(4), 149–157.

Job, D., Eschwege, B., Guyot-Argenton, C., Aubry, J. P., & Tchobroutsky, G. (1976). Effect of multiple daily injections on the course of diabetic retinopathy. *Diabetes, 25,* 463–469.

Jonsen, A. (1986). Bentham in a box: Technology assessment and health care allocation. *Law Medicine and Health Care, 14,* 172–174.

Kahneman, D., & Tversky, A. (1983). Choices, values, and frames. *American Psychologist,* **39,** 341–350.

Kansas Employer Coalition on Health (1991). A framework for reform of the US health care financing and provision system. *Journal of the American Medical Association,* **265,** 2529–2531.

Kaplan, R. M. (1982). Human preference measurement for health decisions and the evaluation of long-term care. In R. L. Kane & R. A. Kane (Eds.), *Values and long-term care* (pp. 157–188). Lexington, MA: Lexington Books.

Kaplan, R. M. (1984). The connection between clinical health promotion and health status: A critical review. *American Psychologist, 39,* 755–765.

Kaplan, R. M. (1985a). Behavioral epidemiology, health promotion, and health services. *Medical Care, 23,* 564–583.

Kaplan, R. M. (1985b). Quantification of health outcomes for policy studies in behavioral epidemiology. In R. M. Kaplan & M. H. Criqui (Eds.), *Behavioral epidemiology and disease prevention* (pp.31–54). New York: Plenum.

Kaplan, R. M. (1988). New health promotion indicators: The general health policy model. *Health Promotion 3*(1), 35–49.

Kaplan, R. M. (1990a). Models of health outcome for policy analysis. *Health Psychology,* **8,** 723–735.

Kaplan, R. M. (1990b). Behavior as a central outcome in health care. *American Psychologist, 45,* 1211–1220.

Kaplan, R. M. (1991a). Value for money in management of HIV: Health-related quality of life. In A. Maynard (Ed.), *Economic aspects of HIV management.* London: Colwood Press.

Kaplan, R. M. (1991b). Health-related quality of life in patient decision making. *Journal of Social Issues, 47*(4), 69–90.

Kaplan, R. M., & Anderson, J. P. (1988a). A general health policy model: Update and applications. *Health Services Research, 23,* 203–235.

Kaplan, R. M., & Anderson, J. P. (1988b). The quality of well-being scale: Rationale for a single quality of life index. *In* S. R. Walker & R. Rosser (Eds.), *Quality of life assessment and applications* (pp. 51–77). London: MTP Press.

Kaplan, R. M., & Anderson, J. P. (1990). The general health policy model: An integrated approach. *In* B. Spilker (Ed.), *Quality of life assessments in clinical trials* (pp. 131–149). New York: Raven.

Kaplan, R. M., & Bush, J. W. (1982). Health-related quality of life measurement for evaluation research and policy analysis. *Health Psychology,* **1,** 621–680.

Kaplan, R. M., & Davis, W. K. (1986). Evaluating the costs and benefits of outpatient diabetes education and nutritional counseling. *Diabetes Care,* **9,** 81–86.

Kaplan, R. M., & Ernest, J. A. (1983). Do category rating scales produce biased preference weights for a health index? *Medical Care* **21**(2), 193–207.

Kaplan, R. M., Bush, J. W., & Berry, C. C. (1976). Health status: Types of validity and the index of well-being. *Health Services Research,* **11**(4), 478–507.

Kaplan, R. M., Bush, J. W., & Berry, C. C. (1978). The reliability, stability, and generalizability of a health status index. *American Statistical Association, Proceedings of the Social Status Section,* 704–709.

Kaplan, R. M., Bush, J. W., & Berry, C. C. (1979). Health status index: Category rating versus magnitude estimation for measuring levels of well-being. *Medical Care,* **17**(5), 501–525.

Kaplan, R. M., Atkins, C. J., & Timms, R. (1984). Validity of a quality of well-being scale as an outcome measure in chronic obstructive pulmonary disease. *Journal of Chronic Diseases,* **37**(2), 85–95.

Kaplan, R. M., Hartwell, S. L., Wilson, D. K., & Wallace, J. P. (1987). Effects of diet and exercise interventions on control and quality of life in non-insulin-dependent diabetes mellitus. *Journal of General Internal Medicine,* **2,** 220–228. [Republished in *Diabetes Spectrum,* 1989, **2**(1), 20–25.]

Kaplan, R. M., Kozin, F., & Anderson, J. P. (1988). Measuring quality of life in arthritis patients. *Quality of Life in Cardiovascular Diseases,* **4,** 131–139.

Kaplan, R. M., DeBon, M., & Anderson, B. F. (1991). Effects of number of rating scale points upon utilities in a quality of well-being scale. *Medical Care,* **29,** 1061–1064.

Kinosian, B. P., and Eisenberg, J. M. (1988). Cutting into cholesterol: cost-effective alternatives for treating hypercholesterolemia. *Journal of the American Medical Association,* **259**(15), 2249–2254.

Kinzer, D. M. (1990). Universal entitlement to health care: Can we get there from here? *New England Journal of Medicine,* **322**(7), 467–470.

Kirkman-Liff, B. L. (1991). Health insurance values and implementation in the Netherlands and the Federal Republic of Germany. An alternative path to universal coverage. *Journal of the American Medical Association,* **265,** 2496–2506.

Kitzhabar, J. (1990). *The Oregon basic health services act.* Oregon State Senate. Salem, Oregon.

Klein, R., & Klein, B. (1985). Vision disorders in diabetes. In *National diabetes data group—Diabetes in America* (pp. 85–1468). NIH Publication.

Kopans, D. B. (1991). Breast screening in women under fifty. *Lancet,* **338,** 447.

Lasker, R. D., Marquis, M. S., & Morrow, M. N. (1991). *Physician payment Review* commission: *Survey of visits and consultations, 1991.* Washington, D.C.: Physician Payment Review Commission.

Ledy, L. L. (1991). Carotid endarterectomy. When and why. *Journal of American Medical Association,* **266,** 332–333.

Lee, P. R., & Estes, C. L. (1990). *The nation's health* (3rd ed.). Boston: Jones and Bartlett Publishers.

Lee, P. R., & Ginsburg, P. B. (1991). Trials of Medicare physician payment reform. *Journal of the American Medical Association,* **266,** 1562.

Levy, L. L. (1991). Carotid endarterectomy. When and why. *Journal of the American Medical Association,* **266**(23), 3332–3333.

Liang, M. H., Cullen, K. E., Larson, M. G., *et al.* (1986). Cost-effectiveness of total joint arthroplasty in osteoarthritis. *Arthritis Rheum.,* **29, 937–943.**

Liang, M. H. Fossell, A. H., & Larons, M. G. (1990). Comparisons of five health status instruments for orthopedic evaluation. *Medical Care,* **28,** 632–642.

Lipid Research Clinics Coronary Prevention Trial Results (1984). 1. Reduction in incidence in coronary heart disease. *Journal of the American Medical Association,* **251,** 351–364.

Localio, A. R., Lawthers, A. G., Brennan, T. A., Laird, N. M., Hebert, L. E., Peterson, L. M., Newhouse, J. P., Weiler, P. C., Hiatt, H. H. (1991). Relation between malpractice claims and adverse events due to negligence. Results of the Harvard Medical Practice Study III. *New England Journal of Medicine,* **325**(4), 245–251.

Los Angeles Times (1991). Study finds rise in ranks of state's medically uninsured. July 17, 1991, pp. A1, A14.

Los Angeles Times (1991). Health costs spiral. L.A. Employers pay the steepest rate in the U.S. for their group insurance survey shows. October 5, 1991, Section D, pg. 1.

Luft, H. S. (1985). Competition and regulation. *Medical Care,* **23,** 383–400.

MacLean, D. S. (1991). Setting health care priorities in Oregon. *Journal of the American Medical Association,* **266,** 1080–1081.

Marwick, C. (1991). Groups survey health care costs, charges. *Journal of the American Medical Association,* **265**(19), 2454–2458.

Mauldoon, M. F., Manuck, S. B., & Matthews, K. A. (1990). Effects of cholesterol lowering on mortality: A quantitative review of primary prevention trials. Presented at the annual meeting of the American Psychological Association, Boston.

Mayberg, M. R., Wilson, S. E., Yatsu, F., Weiss, D. G., Messina, L., Hershey, L. A., Colling, C., Eskridge, J., Deykin, D., Winn, H. R. (1991). Carotid endarterectomy and prevention of cerebral ischemia in symptomatic carotid stenosis. *Journal of the American Medical Association,* **266,** 3289–3294. Copyright 1991, American Medical Association.

Maloney, J. V., Jr. (1991). A critical analysis of the resource-based relative value scale. *Journal of the American Medical Association,* **266,** 3453–3458.

Maynard, A. (1991). Economic issues in HIV management. In A. Maynard (Eds.), *Economic aspects of HIV management* (pp. 6–12). London: Colwood House Medical Publications.

Mehlman, M. J. (1990). *The Oregon medicaid program: Is it just?* Unpublished manuscript, Case Western Reserve Universities, School of Law.

Mosteller, R. (1981). Innovation and evaluation. *Science,* **211,** 881–886.

Mulley, H. J. (1989). Assessing patient's utilities: Can the ends justify the means? *Medical Care,* **27,** S269–S281.

National Cancer Institute (1991). *Cancer Statistics Review 1973-1988.* Bethesda, Maryland, July 1991.

National Center for Health Statistics (1986). *Current estimates from the National Health Interview Survey.* Hyattsville, MD: National Center for Health Statistics.

Nations Health (1991). Medical care costs rising as twice as the economy's average. *The Nation's Health,* November 1991, p. 7.

Nelson, C., & Short, K. (1990). *Health Insurance Coverage, 1986–1988. Current population reports, household economic studies* (Series p-70, #17). Washington D.C.: U.S. Department of the Census.

Nerenz, D. R., Golob, K., & Trump, D. L. (1990). *Preference weights for the quality of well-being scale as obtained from oncology patients.* Unpublished paper, Henry Ford Hospital, Detroit, MI.

Nicod, P., Gilpin, E. A., Dittrich, H., Henning, H., Maisel, A., Blacky, A. R., Smith, S. C., Jr., Ricou, F., & Ross, J. J., (1991). Trends in use of coronary angiography in subacute phase of myocardial infarction. *Circulation* **84**(3), 1004–1015.

Office of Technology Assessment, United States Congress (1979). *a review of selected federal vaccine and immunization policies: Based on case studies of pneumococcal vaccine.* Washington D.C.: U.S. Government Printing Office.

Office of Technology Assessment, United States Congress (1992). *Evaluation of the Oregon Medicaid proposal.* Washington D.C.: U.S. Government Printing Office.

Oregon Health Services Commission (1991). Prioritization of Health Services: A Report to the Governor and the Legislature: State of Oregon.

Palmer, R. M., Saywell, R. M., Jr., Zollinger, T. W., Erner, B. K., LaBov, A. D., Freund, D. A., Garber, J. E., Misamore, G. W., Throop, F. B. (1989). The impact of the prospective payment system on the treatment of hipfractures in the elderly. *Archives of Internal Medicine,* **10,** 2237–2241.

Patrick, D. L., & Erickson, P. (1992). *Health status and health policy: Allocating resources to health care.* Manuscript in preparation.

Patrick, D. L., Bush, J. W., & Chen, M. M. (1973a). Toward an operational definition of health. *Journal of Health and Social Behavior,* **14**(1), 6–23.

Patrick, D. L., Bush, J. W., & Chen, M. M. (1973b). Methods for measuring levels of well-being for a health status index. *Health Services Research,* **8,** 228–245.

Patrick, D., Sittanpalam, Y., & Somerville, S. (1985). A cross-cultural comparison of health status values. *American Journal of Public Health,* **75**(12), 1402–1407.

Peto, R. (1990). Future world-wide effects of present smoking patterns. Presented at the 15th International Cancer Congress, Hamburg, Germany, August.

Pierce, J. P., Burns, D. M., Berry, C., Rosbrook, B., Goodman, J., Gilpin, E., Winn, D., Bal, D. (1991). Reducing tobacco consumption in California: Proposition 99 seems to work. *Journal of the American Medical Association,* **265**(10), 1257–1258.

Radecki, S. E., Ginsburg, P. B., & Lasker, R. D. (1992). RBRVS: Objection to Maloney, II. *Journal of the American Medical Association,* **267,** 1824–1825.

Reinhardt, U. E. (1990). Rationing the health care surplus: An American tragedy. In P. R. Lee & C. L. Estes (Eds.), *The nation's health* (3rd ed.). Boston: Jones & Bartlett.

Relman, A. (1989). Confronting the crisis in health care. *Technology Review,* July, 31–40.

Reynolds, W. J., Rushing, W. A., & Miles, D. L. (1974). The validation of a function status index. *Journal of Health and Social Behavior,* **15,** 271.

Richardson, J. (1991). *Economic assessment in health care: Theory and practice.* Monash University: National Centre for Health Program Evaluation.

Richman, D. D., Fischl, M. A., & Grieco, M. H. *et al.* (1987). The toxicity of azidothymidine (AZT) in the treatment of patients with AIDS and AIDS-related complex: A double-blind, placebo-controlled trial. *New England Journal of Medicine,* **317,** 192–197.

Ries, D. P. (1990). The medical care system: Past, trends and future projections. In P. R. Lee & C. L. Estes (Eds.), *The nation's health* (3rd ed.). Boston: Jones & Bartlett.

Rimm, A. A. (1985). Trends in cardiac surgery in the United States. *New England Journal of Medicine,* **312,** 119–120.

Robinson, J. C. (1991). HMO market penetration and hospital cost inflation in California. *Journal of the American Medical Association,* **266,** 2719–2723.

Rockefeller, J. D., IV (1990). The Pepper Commission report on comprehensive health care. *New England Journal of Medicine,* **323,** 1005–1007.

Rockefeller, J. D., IV (1991). A call for action: The Pepper Commission's blue print for health care reform. *Journal of the American Medical Association,* **265,** 2507–2510.

Rogers, W. H., Draper, D., Kahn, K. L., Keeler, E. B., Rubenstein, L. V., Kosecoff, J., Brook, R. H. (1990). Quality of care before and after implementation of the DRG-based prospective payment system. A summary of effects. *Journal of the American Medical Association,* **264**(15), 1989–1994.

Rokeach, M. (1973). *The nature of human values.* New York: The Free Press.

Roos, N. P. (1989). Using administrative data from Manitoba, Canada, to study treatment outcomes: Developing control groups and adjusting for case severity. *Social Science and Medicine,* **28**(2), 109–113.

Roos, L. L., Fisher, E. S., Sharp, S. M., Newhouse, J. P., Anderson, G., & Bubolz, T. A. (1990). Postsurgical mortality in Manitoba and New England. *Journal of the American Medical Association,* **263**(18), 2453–2458.

Rosenbaum, S. (1992). Poor Women, poor children, poor policy: The Oregon medicaid experiment. *In* M. A. Strosberg, J. M. Wiener, R. Baker, & I. A. Fein (Eds.), *Rationing America's Medical Care: The Oregon Plan and Beyond* (pp. 91–106). Washington: The Brookings Institution.

Rosser, R. M. (1992). The history of health related quality of life in ten and a half paragraphs. *Journal of the Royal Society of Medicine,* in press.

Roybal, E. R. (1991). The USHealth Act. Comprehensive reform for a caring America. *Journal of the American Medical Association,* **265,** 2545–2548.

Russell, L. (1986). *Is prevention better than cure?* Washington, D.C.: The Brookings Institution.

Russell, L. B. (1987). *Evaluating preventive care.* Washington: The Brookings Institution.

Sachs, H., Chalmers, T. C., & Smith, H. (1982). Randomized versus historic controls for clinical trials. *American Journal of Medicine,* **72,** 233–240.

Salive, M. E., Mayfield, J. A., & Weissman, N. W. (1990). Patient outcomes research teams in the Agency for Health Care Policy and Research. *Health Services Research,* **25,** 697–708.

Samuelson, P. A. (1970). *Economics* (8th ed.). New York: McGraw-Hill.

Schade, D., Santiago, J., Skyler, J., & Rizza, R. (1983). Effects of intensive treatment on long-term complications. In Intensive Insulin Therapy, Chapter 5. *Princeton Excerpta Medica.*

Schneiderman, L. J., Pearlmen, R. A., Kaplan, R. M., Anderson, J. P., & Rosenberg, E. M. (1992). Relationship of general advance directive instructions to specific life-sustaining treatment preferences in patients with serious illness. *Archives of Internal Medicine,* in press.

Schramm, C. J. (1991). Health care financing for all Americans. *Journal of the American Medical Association,* 265(24), 3296–3299.

Schroeder, S. A. (1987). Strategies for reducing medical costs by changing physician's behavior. *International Journal of Technology in Health Care,* 3, 39–50.

Schulman, K. A., Lynn, L. A., Glick, H. A., & Eisenberg, J. M. (1991). Cost-effectiveness of low-dose zidovudine therapy for asymptomatic patients with human immunodeficiency virus (HIV) infection. *Annals of Internal Medicine,* 114(7), 798–802.

Schwartz, W. B., & Mendelson, D. N. (1991). Hospital cost containment in the 1980s. Hard lessons learned and prospects for the 1990s. *New England Journal of Medicine,* 324(15), 1037–1042.

Sheets, L. (1991). Health care reform: Congress suddenly awash in new proposals. *Retirement Life,* September 1991, 4–8.

Short, P. F. (1990). *National medical expenditure survey: Estimates of the uninsured population, calendar year 1987: Data summary 2.* Rockville, MD: National Center for Health Services Research and Health Care Technology Assessment.

Short, P. F., Monheit, A., & Beauregard, K. (1989). *National medical expenditure survey: A profile of uninsured Americans: Research findings 1.* Rockville, MD: National Center for Health Services Research and Health Care Technology Assessment.

Sick Health Services (1988). *The Economist.* July 16, 1988, pp. 19–22.

Starfield, B. (1991). Primary care and health. A cross-national comparison. *Journal of the American Medical Association,* 266, 2268–2271.

Steering Committee of the Physicians' Health Study Research Group (1988). Preliminary report: Findings from the aspirin component of the ongoing Physicians' Health Study. *New England Journal of Medicine,* 318, 262–264.

Steering Committee of the Physicians' Health Study Research Group (1989). Final report on the aspirin component of the ongoing Physicians' Health Study. *New England Journal of Medicine,* 321, 129–135.

Stewart, A. L., Ware, J. E., Jr., Brook, R. H., & Davies-Avery, A. (1978). *Conceptualization and measurement of health for adults* (Vol. 2. *Physical health in terms of functioning*). Santa Monica, CA: Rand Corp.

Tchobroutsky, G. (1978). Relation of diabetic control to development of microvascular complications. *Diabetologia,* 15, 143–152.

Terris, M. (1990). Public health policy for the 1990s. *Annual Review of Public Health,* 11, 39–51.

Thompson, M. S., Read, J. L., Hutchins, H. C., Patterson, M., & Harris, E. D. (1988). The cost effectiveness of auranofin: Results of a randomized clinical trial. *Journal of Rheumatology,* 12, 35–42.

Thorpe, K. E., & Spencer, C. (1991). How do uncompensated care pools affect the level and type of care? Results from New York State. *Journal of Health Politics, Policy and Law,* 16(2), 363–381.

Todd, J. S., Seekins, S. V., Krichbaum, J. A., & Harvey, L. K. (1991). Health access America–Strengthening the US health care system. *Journal of the American Medical Association,* **265,** 2503–2506.

Toevs, C. D., Kaplan, R. M., & Atkins, C. J. (1984). The costs and effects of behavioral programs for chronic obstructive pulmonary disease. *Medical Care* **22,** 1088–1100.

Torrance, G. W. (1986). Measurement of health state utilities for economic appraisal: A review. *Journal of Health Economics,* **5,** 1.

Torrance, G. W. (1987). Utility approach to measuring health-related quality of life. *Journal of Chronic Diseases,* **40,** 593–600.

Torrance, G. W., & Zipursky, A. (1984). Cost-effectiveness of antepartum prevention of RH immunization. *Clinics in Perinatology,* **11**(2), 267–268.

U.S. Department of Commerce (1989). *Business Conditions Digest,* September, 1989.

U.S. Preventive Services Task Force. (1989). *Guide to clinical preventive services: An assessment of the effectiveness of 169 interventions.* Report of the U.S. Preventive Services Task Force. Baltimore: Williams & Wilkins.

U.S. Surgeon General (1989). *Reducing the health consequences of smoking: Twenty-five years of progress.* Rockville, MD: U.S. Department of Health and Human Services, Centers for Disease Control.

Vall-Spinosa, A. (1991). Lessons from London: British are reforming their national health service. *American Journal of Public Health,* **81,** 1566–1570.

Vital and Health Statistics (1989). *National hospital discharge survey, 1987* (Series 13, U.S. DHHS, Publication No (PHS) 89-1760). April 1989.

von Neuman, J., & Morganstern, O. (1944). *Theory of games and economic behavior.* Princeton, NJ: Princeton University Press.

Voulgaropolous, D., Schneiderman, L. J., & Kaplan, R. M. (1989). *Recommendations against the use of medical procedures: Evidence, judgment and ethical implications.* Submitted for publication.

Walker, S. R., & Rosser, R. (Eds.). (1988). *Quality of life: Assessment and application.* London: MTP Press.

Wallerstein, E. (1985). Circumcision—The unique American medical enigma. *Urological Clinics of North America,* **12,** 123–132.

Warner, K. E. (1986). Smoking and health implications of a change in federal cigarette excise tax. *Journal of the American Medical Association,* **255,** 1028–1032.

Washington Post (1991). Ad sponsored by Pharmaceutical Manufacturers Association, May 20, 1991, p. A8.

Weiler, P. C., & Brennan, T. A. (1990). Medical malpractice. In *A call for Comprehensive health care* (Vol. 2). Washington, D.C.: U.S. Government Printing Office.

Weiner, S. J. (1991). Bad debt and uncompensated care. *Journal of the American Medical Association,* **266**(18), 2563.

Weinstein, M. C., & Feinberg, H. V. (1980). *Clinical decision analysis.* Philadelphia: Saunders.

Weinschrott, D. J. (1991). Self-interest reigns in health care reform. *Wall Street Journal,* August 6, 1991, p. A14.

Weinstein, M. C. (1980). Estrogen use in postmenopausal women—costs, risks, benefits. *New England Journal of Medicine,* **303,** 308–316.

Weinstein, M. C., & Stason, W. B. (1976). *Hypertension: A policy perspective.* Cambridge, MA: Harvard University Press.

Weinstein, M. C., & Stason, W. B. (1977). Foundations of cost-effectiveness analysis for health and medical practice. *New England Journal of Medicine, 296,* 716–721.

Weinstein, M. C., & Stason, W. B. (1982). Cost-effectiveness of coronary artery bypass surgery. *Circulation,* Suppl. 3, 56–66.

Weinstein, M. C., & Stason, W. B. (1983). *Cost-effectiveness of coronary artery bypass surgery.* Cambridge, MA: Harvard University Center for Analysis of Health Practice.

Weinstein, M. C., & Stason, W. B. (1985). Cost-effectiveness of interventions to prevent or treat coronary heart disease. *American Review of Public Health, 6,* 41–63.

Wenger, N., Mattson, M., Furberg, C., & Elinson, J. (1984). *Assessment of quality of life in clinical trials of cardiovascular therapies.* New York: Le Jacq Publishing, Inc.

Wennberg, J. E. (1990). Small area analysis and the medical care outcome problem. *In* L. Sechrest, E. Perrin, & J. Bunker (Eds.), *Research Methodology: Strengthening Causal Interpretations of Nonexperimental Data.* Agency for Health Care Policy and Research, USPHS/DHHS, Publication No. (PHS) 90-3454, pp. 177–206.

Wickizer, T. M. (1990). Effect of utilization review on hospital use and expenditures: A review of the literature and an update on recent findings. *Medical Care Review, 47*(3), 327–364.

Wiener, J. M. (1992). Oregon's plan for health care rationing. *Brookings Review.* Winter, 26–31.

Williams, A. (1988). The importance of quality of life in policy decisions. In S. Walker and R. Rosser (Eds.), *Quality of life: Assessment and Application* (pp. 279–290). London: MTP Press.

Wines, M. (1992). Bush unveils plan for health care. *New York Times.* February 7, 1992, pg. A1, A15.

Wiswell, T. E., & Roscelli, J. D. (1986). Corroborative evidence for the decreased evidence of urinary tract infections in circumcised male infants *Pediatrics, 78,* 96–99.

Woolhandler, S., & Himmelstein, D. U. (1991). The deteriorating administrative efficiency of the U.S. health care system. *New England Journal of Medicine, 324*(18), 1253–1258.

World Health Organization (1984). *Health promotion: A discussion document on the concept and principles.* Copenhagen: WHO Regional Office for Europe.

World Health Organization (1987). *Tobacco price and the smoking epidemic: Smoke-free Europe.* Copenhagen: World Health Organization.

Wu, A. W., Matthews, W. C., Brysk, L. T., Atkinson, J. H., Grant, I., Abramson, I., Kennedy, C. J., McCutchan, J. A., Spector, S. A., & Richman, D. D. (1990). Quality of life in a placebo-controlled trial of zidovudine in patients with AIDS and AIDS-related complex. *Journal of Acquired Immune Deficiency Syndromes, 3*(7), 683–690.

Yates, B. T., & DeMuth, N. M. (1981). Alternative funding and incentive mechanisms for health systems. In A. Broskowski, E. Marks, & S. H. Budman (Eds.), *Linking health and mental health* (pp. 77–99). Beverly Hills, CA: Sage.

Index